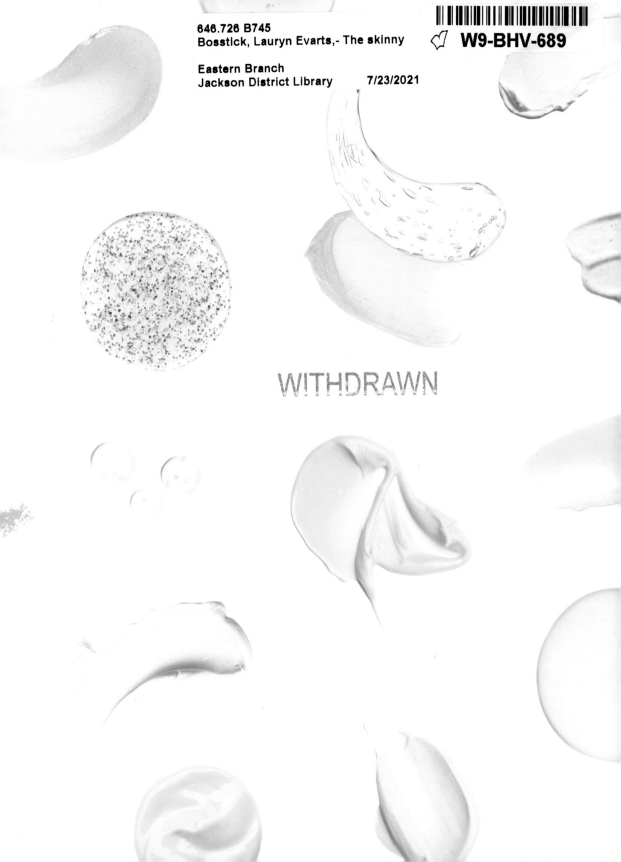

WITHDRAWN

THE SKINNY CONFIDENTIAL'S

GET
THE F♥CK
OUT OF
THE SUN

THE SKINNY CONFIDENTIAL'S

GET
THE F♥CK
OUT OF
THE SUN

LAURYN EVARTS BOSSTICK

FOREWORD BY DR. DENNIS GROSS

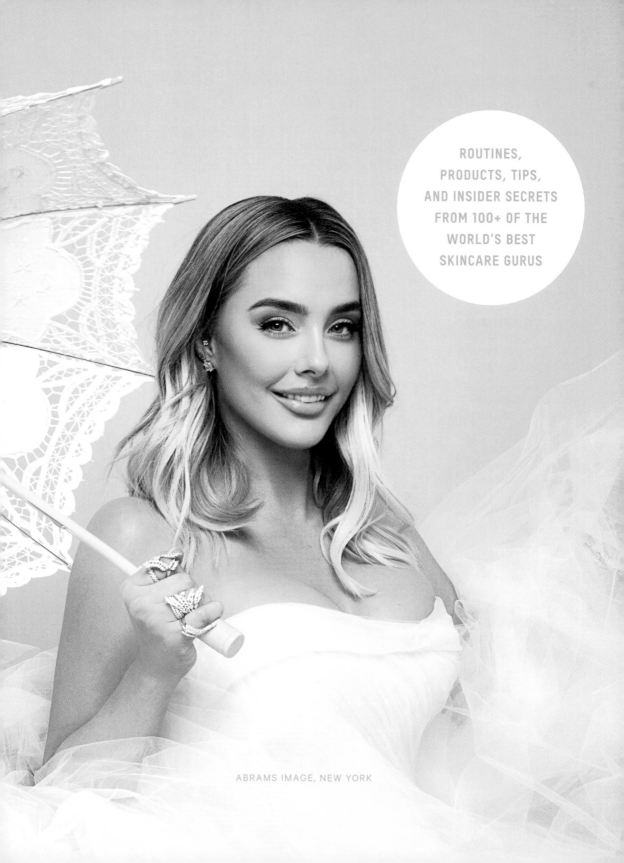

ROUTINES,
PRODUCTS, TIPS,
AND INSIDER SECRETS
FROM 100+ OF THE
WORLD'S BEST
SKINCARE GURUS

ABRAMS IMAGE, NEW YORK

Editor: Rebecca Kaplan
Designer: Danielle Deschenes
Production Manager: Kathleen Gaffney

Library of Congress Control Number: 2020944913

ISBN: 978-1-4197-4787-8
eISBN: 978-1-64700-041-7

Printed and bound in the United States
10 9 8 7 6 5 4 3 2 1

All of the material contained in this book, including text,
graphics, and images, is presented only for informational and
artistic purposes. Every effort has been made to ensure that the
information provided is accurate and up to date. The publisher
and author make no representation, assume no responsibility,
and accept no liability for any accidents, injuries, loss, legal
consequences, or incidental or consequential damage incurred
by any reader in reliance on the information or advice provided in
this book. The information provided in this book is not intended
or implied to be a substitute for professional medical advice,
diagnosis or treatment. Readers should review all skincare,
health or medical information regarding any medical condition or
treatment with a physician or other medical professional.

Abrams Image books are available at special discounts when
purchased in quantity for premiums and promotions as well
as fundraising or educational use. Special editions can also
be created to specification. For details, contact specialsales@
abramsbooks.com or the address below.

Abrams Image® is a registered trademark of Harry N. Abrams, Inc.

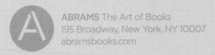

ABRAMS The Art of Books
195 Broadway, New York, NY 10007
abramsbooks.com

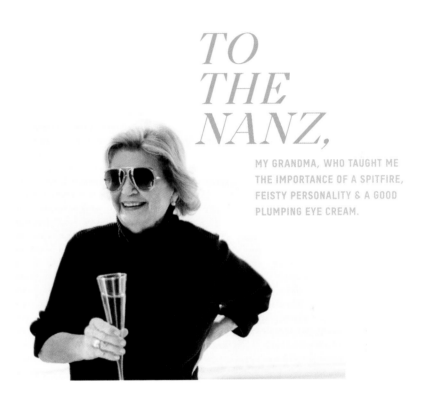

TO
THE
NANZ,

MY GRANDMA, WHO TAUGHT ME
THE IMPORTANCE OF A SPITFIRE,
FEISTY PERSONALITY & A GOOD
PLUMPING EYE CREAM.

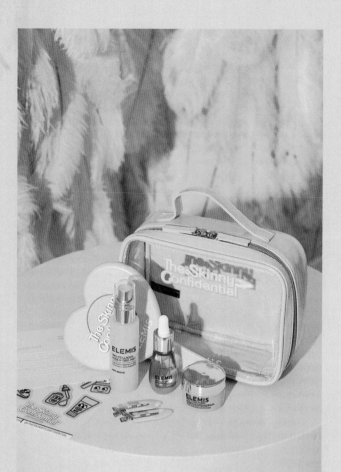

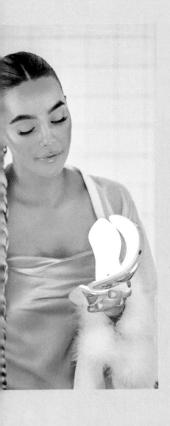

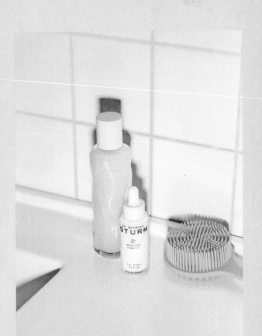

BY

Dr. Dennis Gross

TOP NYC
DERMATOGIST
AND CO-FOUNDER
OF DR. DENNIS
GROSS SKINCARE

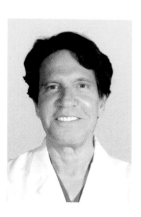

Lauryn's reputation preceded her—particularly among dermatologists. When I met her in person for the first time, I already knew about her militant skincare routine and her compulsive sun avoidance, specifically her driving gloves. I will never forget the first time that I saw those white gloves.

I would never have been able to convince my teenage daughters to wear them, but it was easy after Lauryn's endorsement.

I remember thinking, *How f***ing cool is that?!* She has just made sun protection trendy and stylish while also protecting her skin from UVA/UVB and the sun spots and wrinkles they cause.

After speaking more with Lauryn about her skincare routine, she checked all the boxes to earn the distinction of my best patient. She was the first to admit she's addicted to skincare and obsessed with beauty. Her passion is a good thing.

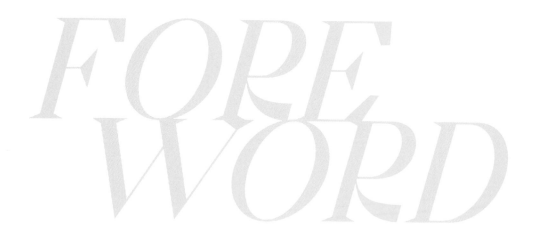

FORE WORD

Dermatologically speaking, Lauryn's alabaster skin is pristine. Her complexion is radiant, poreless, and clear, with no sun spots or signs of any sun damage whatsoever.

But as impressive as her complexion is, I have always been most impressed with Lauryn's ability to make skincare and science cool and relatable. That is not an easy task.

Trust me, I spend all day long at my practice groveling, *begging* patients to use sunscreen. After one blog post, Lauryn has people running to buy full-face sun shields and hot pink UVA/UVB protective ski masks. I remembered thinking, *What is her secret!?*

After spending more time with Lauryn, it became clear that her super power is her ability to connect with people. Lauryn bridges the gap between skincare guru and unapologetic content creator. If you know Lauryn, you know she keeps it REAL.

She loves everything having to do with skin and is an avid student, always wanting to learn more. She appreciates science, which to me is fantastic. I am a self-proclaimed science nerd, and we bonded right away when discussing skincare on her podcast. Seriously, we could have talked skin for hours.

From a very young age, I knew I wanted to be a doctor. I've always had an underlying desire to help people. I remember there was a moment when I saw a mole on the back of a bus driver's hand—it was a black growth that I feared might be skin cancer. I mentioned something to him as I got off the bus. That's when I realized dermatology was for me. I loved that you could make a visual diagnosis—I didn't need an X-ray machine.

When I met Lauryn, I recognized she had the same desire to help others. I immediately saw her hunger for knowledge and admired how she used that knowledge to help others. Whether she is tackling a taboo topic head-on, opening up a conversation that was previously nonexistent, or asking "if I am going to sweat today," she is always advocating for people to be the best, most curious version of themselves.

Regarding skincare specifically, Lauryn and I share a lot of the same philosophies. For at-home skincare, there is no magic formula. You need to create a regimen of different ingredients that are working to build collagen, protect against free radicals, and target your specific concerns. Modern clinical skincare can change your life if you do it right. For in-office procedures, treatments like Botox or fillers should be used to enhance your natural features—the goal is to achieve your best "undone look." You don't want to look like a completely new person when you leave the dermatologist's office.

Lauryn's dedication to being a lifelong student is just one of the many characteristics that sets her apart from her peers. Skincare and science go hand in hand—and there are constantly new innovations, new ingredients, and studies that require ongoing education and understanding of how skin works.

If you are just starting skincare now, don't freak out! It is never too late to start a skincare routine. This book is not only filled with Lauryn's knowledge, but also tips and advice from the best in the industry.

Oh, and by the way, with Lauryn's help, Michael (Lauryn's husband) lost his Botox virginity that day in my office.

Dennis Gross, MD

/ @drdennisgross

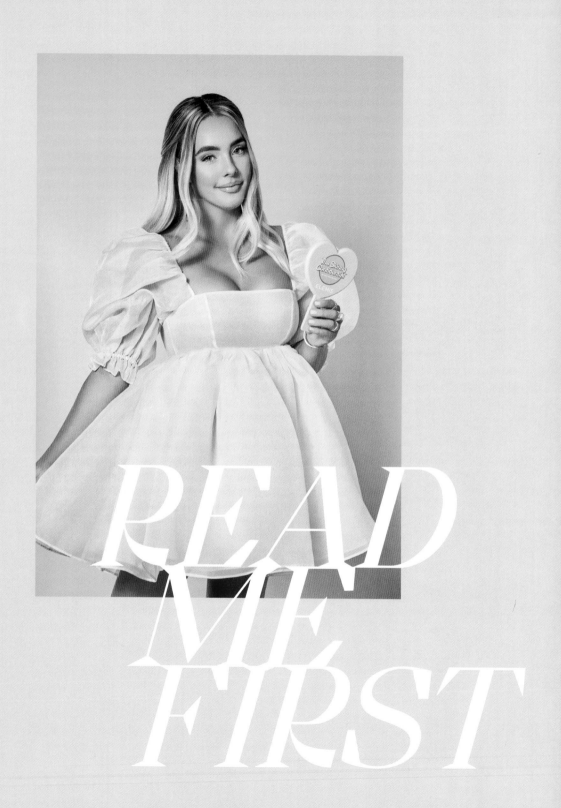

READ ME FIRST

How to Use This Book Like a Boss

This is one of those books that you have displayed on your coffee table for a casual Instagram... BUT you will actually—wait for it—USE IT. Sure, it's on your coffee table looking all pink and cute, but you're also going to dog-ear the fuck out of it. Whether you bend the pages or use little bookmarks, my hope is that you find SO MUCH value in this book that it becomes your one-stop shop for all things SKIN.

Think of it as an encyclopedia for your skin, but an easy-to-digest, cheeky encyclopedia. I hope you grab a glass of rosé, kick your feet up, and read through this book, laughing along like we're at happy hour together. Maybe you'll even ice roll your face as you learn tons of beauty secrets. You could read this from start to finish, OR you could also crack open any page and find some hot tips and on-the-pulse skin secrets.

But before we get into that, let me introduce myself. Why, hello, fancy seeing you here—I'm Lauryn Evarts Bosstick. I'm a wife to my husband, Michael, a mom to my daughter, Zaza, a dog mom to my two chihuahuas, and also the creator of *The Skinny Confidential*, a blog, podcast, book, and brand. *The Skinny Confidential* blog started 12 years ago as a platform to "get the skinny," get the juice, stalk the scoop. My first book, *The Skinny Confidential: A Babe's Sassy, Sexy Fitness & Lifestyle Guide*, included a big chapter on skin, but I felt like there was a need to write *much* more for this incredible community of women. So! Voilà! A full-blown resource completely dedicated to the subject. I mean, right? It only made sense to compile all things SKIN into one place for you guys. The hope is that you think of this book as your go-to collection of skincare advice.

If you're dealing with a specific problem like acne, there's a chapter for you. If you're looking to de-puff your face after too many spicy margaritas with your friends, there's a chapter for you. If you're looking to switch up your wellness routine so you glow from the inside out, yes, there's a chapter for you. And if you're looking for Hollywood skincare tips, I went straight to the influencers and celebs to get the 411 for you.

We'll go over sunscreen in specific detail, lymphatic drainage, how to get rid of brown spots, freezing-cold shower benefits, fatty acids, humidifier secrets, Botox, fillers, preventative measures, all the tools you have to have—think jade rollers, extra-chilled ice rollers, *gua sha*, facial steamers, etc.—we'll even get into facial exercises for tightening the turkey neck.

Expect buttery silk pillowcases, injectable realness, microneedling tips, everything to know about oil, hyperpigmentation, brow grooming, lasers, Korean skincare, and of course, making sure that you don't just focus on your face, but TAKE IT TO YOUR TITS. Even to your toes, really?

FEEL FREE TO MOVE AROUND. You can obtain tons of knowledge about everything, from how to use your baby's diaper cream for an irritated zit (YES INDEED) to substituting a vibrator for a facial massager to using soap (like SOAP soap) to brush up your brows for that youthful look. Honestly, you don't even have to read every section—read whatever speaks to you.

I've spent my entire career interviewing people from all different walks of life. The podcast I host with my husband Michael, *The Skinny Confidential HIM & HER,* has hundreds of interviews with dynamic, charismatic, talented people, so you should not be surprised that this book is also filled with tips and tricks from some of your favorite sparkly experts. I mean, let me pull out my scroll here: Dr. Harold Lancer, Dr. Barbara Sturm, Dr. Dennis Gross, Kate Somerville, Sonya Dakar, Dr. Kay Durairaj, Dr. Anjali Mahto, Dr. Daniel Barrett, and Dr. Andrew Jacono. While doctors' opinions are amazing, you'll also hear from people who themselves struggle with acne, hyperpigmentation, and lackluster skin. These people also happen to be top-tier influencers and celebrities like Aimee Song, *The LadyGang*, Katherine Schwarzenegger Pratt, Chriselle Lim, Patrick Starrr, Kristin Cavallari, *The Bachelor*'s Kaitlyn Bristowe, Molly Sims, Drunk Elephant's Tiffany Masterson, and even The Fat Jew (be prepared to laugh your fucking ass off for that one). I've also included many tips from the community—meaning YOU. Yes, you. Over the past 12 years, I've compiled so many tips from readers and listeners via DMs, tweets, Facebook, and Instagram comments. And geez—you guys have the juice, let me tell you.

I'm not an expert, a doctor, or a facialist—I'm a practitioner who has immersed herself in the skincare industry for the last decade. In addition to all the experts I get to interview, I have tried *everything*. I consider myself a human guinea pig, wanting to test everything so I can report back to my audience about what's worth their time and what isn't.

My other longtime love—besides reading, scrapbooking, taking Pilates, practicing photography, baking, and traveling—is *researching*. But I've always felt there's been a lack of research presented in a flamboyant, pretty way. Research is typically dull and boring . . . kinda like a limp dick, if you will. There was a need for someone to present skincare in a way that was EASY to digest and wrapped in a hot pink neon bow. There's one thing I don't do, and that's boring—I don't want you to read a boner-stiff medical study, I want you to ENJOY yourself. So grab a glass of rosé—and your visor, driving gloves and umbrella—and let's begin, shall we?

Cheers,

xx lauryn ♡

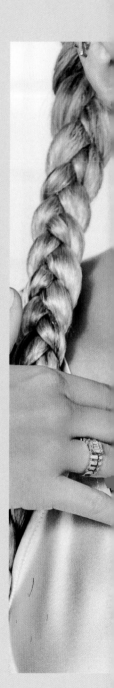

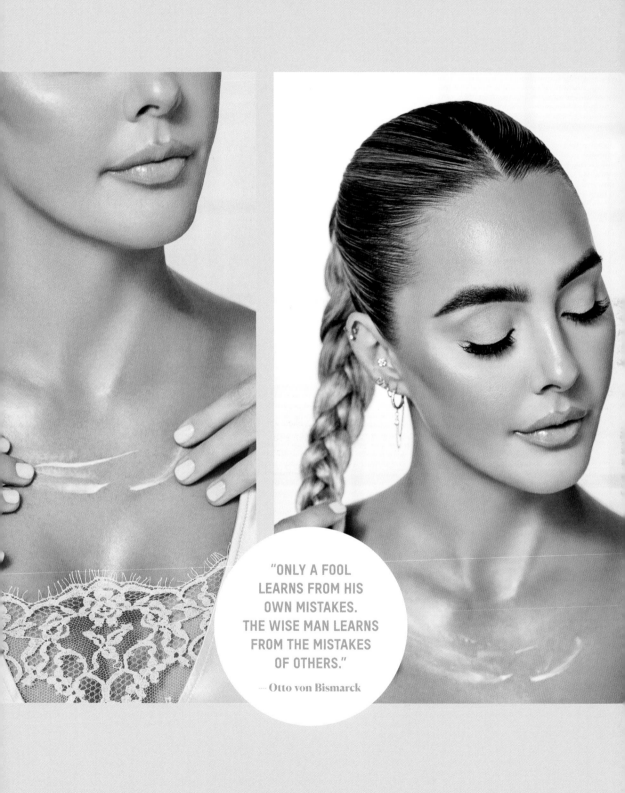

"ONLY A FOOL LEARNS FROM HIS OWN MISTAKES. THE WISE MAN LEARNS FROM THE MISTAKES OF OTHERS."

— Otto von Bismarck

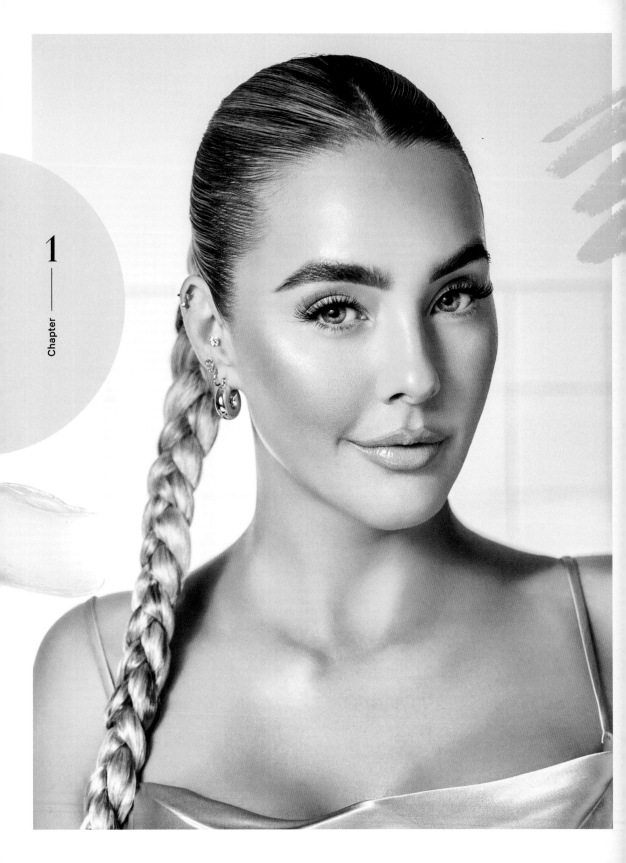

PREVENT-ATIVE BEAUTY IS IN:

Millennial Skincare

As a practitioner in the industry, I've observed something super interesting. For a while, I've been lucky enough to speak to women via DM. And these women from all over the world talk to me about their skincare routines. I've noticed that instead of covering up zits, acne, and hyperpigmentation, women are more interested in solving the problems that cause them. They want to look fresh-faced and dewy . . . but actually *be* fresh-faced and dewy—not just hiding skin issues with pounds of makeup. WHO CAN RELATE?!

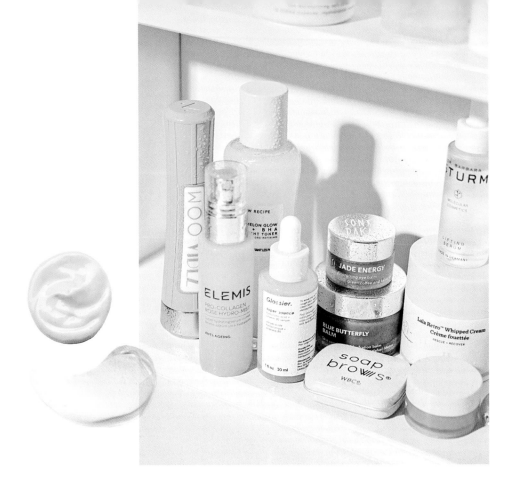

"Dewy" has been a buzzword since 2015. People seem to be moving away from the matte look—because a matte finish tends to showcase fine lines and wrinkles more, it's aging and not as youthful. So, as you can imagine, oils are in, glowy is all the rage, and you can see a bunch of dewy millennials rocking a bit of tinted moisturizer and pale pink rosé-colored lip gloss. And if you pay close attention, you'll notice brands are now marketing skincare to women, as opposed to cosmetics.

You see it on Instagram and TikTok: Selfies are now more about the skin and less about the cover-up. Sure, everyone is still very much into cosmetics, but people are more interested in being the best version of themselves. Millennials seem to agree that what's *under* the makeup is most important these days.

Instead of waiting for their skin to get wrinkled, millennials are taking ACTION. Women want to prevent problems from ever occurring, rather than fix them down the road. And that action is spreading like wildfire because of social media. We're using Instagram, Instagram Stories, and Snapchat to showcase our skincare. We've seen what happened to our mothers' skin and heard too many skin cancer horror stories to not realize the importance of covering up our face, hands, and neck with sunscreen. We're stocking up on cleansers, oils, masks, and Korean beauty products to keep our skin healthy. We're also paying more attention to how we can take care of our skin from the inside out, like drinking more water, getting in a good detoxifying sweat, and eating cleaner foods. Also, preventative Botox is mainstream now—no longer taboo. This generation will look younger for longer than any generation before it.

*SOME VERY
THE SKINNY
CONFIDENTIAL-
ESQUE
RESEARCH
FOR YA*

The global cosmetic products market was valued at $532.43 billion (USD) in 2017, and is expected to reach a market value of $805.61 billion by 2023. To get micro: Millennials aren't banking on saving face when they get older. They want great skin right now, and they want to preserve that youthful glow for as long as possible. As a result, they're spending serious cash on skincare, in addition to investing in preventative procedures, like Botox and fillers. We're talking spending more money on more products than *any other generation*. And instead of going the route of "anti-aging" products, they're shelling out for lotions, serums, spritzes, and tools that are perfectly suited for their skincare needs. Talk about from the mouths (or faces) of babes.

That doesn't mean that no one cares about wrinkles these days. It's just that now it's all about prevention rather than treatment—and besides stocking up on more sunscreen with higher SPF levels, prevention often means heading to the dermatologist for Botox, fillers, peels, and laser treatments. In fact, a recent survey by the West Coast aesthetics chain Skin by Lovely found this to be especially true of women aged 30 to 34: Nearly 47 percent had already tried injectables, compared to only 28 percent of women aged 35 to 39 and 11 percent of women aged 40 to 49. "This group understands that it's easier to prevent than reverse signs of aging," says the company's founder, Lovely Laban. In this case, the splurge seems worth it. "The long-lasting results fillers deliver make the cost manageable and something they can plan for."

BOTTOM LINE:

Easy to use, cute and cool Korean products have set the tone for affordable, preventative skincare accessible to millennials on a budget. The new approach to skincare is skin*care*. As in giving a shit about your skin and being an active participant in how healthy it is. This is something I had to learn the hard way, but it informed how I've been taking care of my skin ever since. So before we get into other shifts and trends I've been seeing, I'd like to share my skincare journey with you. Let's go back, shall we?

Ever since I can remember, I've always been interested in lotions and potions. When I was little, my Hollywood-lit vanity was filled with drugstore finds: Cetaphil, Tinkerbell Cosmetics, stick-on earrings, Dr Pepper Lip Smacker, hot pink tubes of Maybelline Great Lash mascara, Pink Sugar perfume, Aqua Net Professional Hairspray, Bath & Body Works "Sun-Ripened Raspberry," and St. Ives apricot scrub . . . all next to my glitter Caboodle. Anyone else? (continued on page 21)

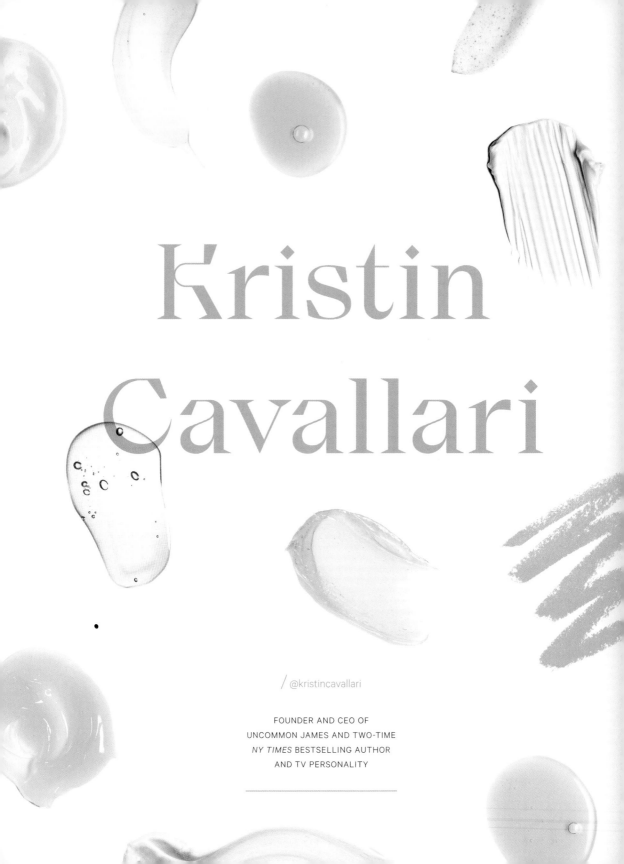

Kristin Cavallari

/ @kristincavallari

FOUNDER AND CEO OF
UNCOMMON JAMES AND TWO-TIME
NY TIMES BESTSELLING AUTHOR
AND TV PERSONALITY

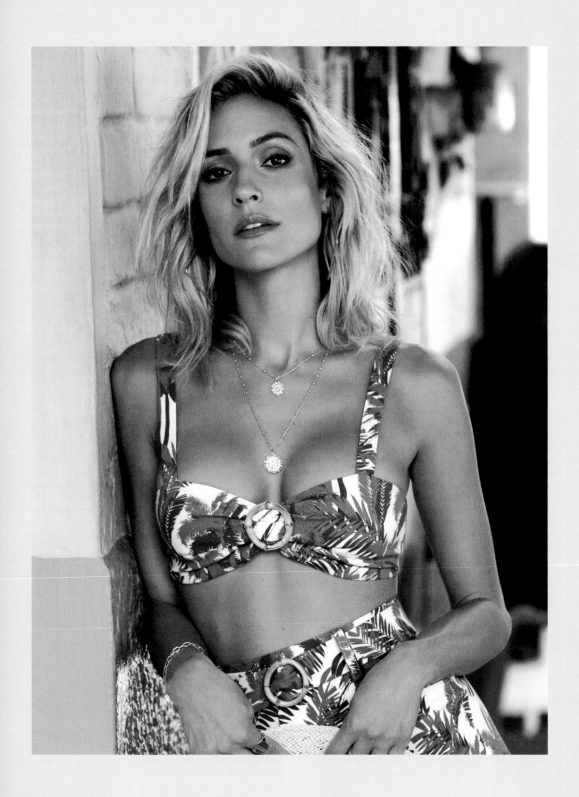

WHAT HAVE YOU FOUND TO BE THE MOST EFFECTIVE SKINCARE PRODUCT UNDER $50, AND WHAT'S YOUR BIGGEST SPLURGE?

I love the black mask by Revision for under $50. Biggest splurge is Koji pads from Karee Hays—the pads are customized to your skin's needs, focusing on pigmentation and texture.

WHAT IS THE MOST PRACTICAL, RELATABLE ADVICE YOU'VE RECEIVED FOR PREVENTATIVE SKINCARE?

That your face is a muscle, so you have to work it out the same way you would any other muscle in your body.

WHAT IS THE WORST ADVICE YOU'VE EVER HEARD WHEN IT COMES TO TAKING CARE OF YOUR SKIN?

To start getting Botox in your early 20s because it's preventative. Full disclaimer: I've never done Botox, but I imagine it's the type of thing that once you start, you can't stop. If you start in your early 20s, that's years and years of pumping those chemicals into your face when we don't know the long-term effects of that stuff. Plus, I think there's something to aging gracefully and showing expression on your face.

WHAT HABIT HAVE YOU DEVELOPED OVER THE YEARS THAT MAKES A DIFFERENCE IN YOUR SKIN?

Using at-home devices. You name it, I have it. I go through phases: red light therapy, electrocurrent, microneedling. I really do think they help, because again, it goes back to working your face out the same way you would your body.

> **"...your face is a muscle, so you have to work it out the same way you would any other muscle in your body."**

WHAT STEPS DO YOU TAKE DURING YOUR DAILY SKIN ROUTINE?

In the morning, I rinse with water, then do a peptide gel and vitamin C serum, followed by a moisturizer. At night, I wash my face, then do a retinol three times a week and the other nights I do a retexturize cream. I always do eye cream and put oil on my neck and chest. I exfoliate twice a week, and I also love masks.

WHAT WOULD YOU SAY TO YOUR YOUNGER SELF ABOUT SKINCARE IF YOU COULD?

It's going to be very important to you—and it should! Don't worry about the zits now, because it will all work out.

WHAT IS AN UNUSUAL OR SOMEWHAT WEIRD PRACTICE YOU DO TO KEEP YOUR SKIN YOUTHFUL?

Before a big event, I will shave my face. Yes, I will literally shave my face. The technical term is called dermaplane, but you can easily do it yourself with a razor. My facialist in Nashville told me to do it years ago, and it makes such a difference—your skin looks so smooth and glows.

WHAT ARE YOUR THOUGHTS ON PLASTIC SURGERY, BOTOX, FILLERS, LASERS, AND OTHER COSMETIC MEDICAL PROCEDURES?

Personally, I'm not a fan. I've seen firsthand how that stuff sucks you in, and then nothing is ever good enough. I think it starts with accepting ourselves for how we are. With that being said, if one little tweak here or there is going to make you that much happier, then by all means, go for it. It's when people chase an unrealistic outcome and are looking for happiness in a procedure that it scares me. ♥

GET THE F♥CK OUT OF THE SUN

(continued) My skincare journey and my wisdom on protecting myself from the tanning bed came from my mom. She was a REAL sunscreen psycho who very much believed in staying out of the sun because she was convinced that it was super aging. She would always encourage me to apply SPF, even before school—I was that girl on the beach with blue zinc all over her (remember those different colored zincs? Horrendous), covered by a hat and an umbrella. Never did I see my mom without a huge pink bottle of Coppertone—really, though . . . Little Miss Coppertone with her underwear being pulled down by a black cocker spaniel is forever ingrained in my brain. I can even smell it as I write this. Anyway, at the time I was annoyed with all that sunscreen . . . so much sunscreen!

Maggie MacDonald

/ @maggiemacdonald

LIFESTYLE INFLUENCER
AND YOUTUBER

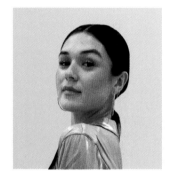

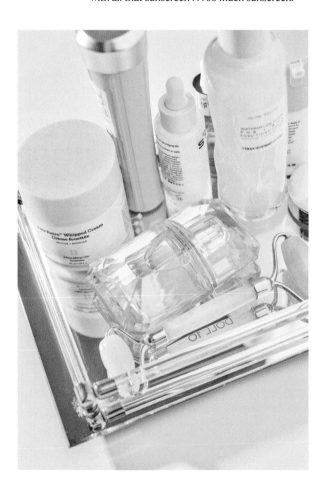

The worst advice I've ever heard when it comes to taking care of your skin is, "If it ain't broke, don't fix it," meaning if you don't have any "problems" with your skin, you don't need to put anything on it. I disagree. I definitely don't think your skincare routine has to consist of 50 different products and be super expensive—I know it's not for everyone, and some people like to keep it simple, which I totally get! A serum (vitamin C in the morning, retinol at night for me), moisturizer and sunscreen are SO important and crucial in my routine. Having a skincare routine is so much more than using products to make your skin "perfect." I always think about the long-term effects taking care of my skin will have. I am always looking to protect my skin and reduce anything that can cause premature aging. I want to glow from within and have a radiant complexion. Skincare is self-love, and I love creating rituals to make myself feel good and accomplished!

As the years went on and I got older, I didn't take my mom's recommendations too seriously and instead I focused on my tan. Hello, red Playboy Bunny sticker on my hip coming out of the tanning bed. There was always a spray bottle of Banana Boat tanning oil in my bag when I went to camp and I mean, the darker the better. Paris Hilton was all the rage at this time, and if you remember, her tan was a moment. My hair was bleached, my tan was orange, my Playboy Bunny was poppin'. I remember every Friday I would go lie in the tanning bed and just bake with no sun protection for 20 MINUTES!! FAKE AND BAKE time was the best time.

Cut to my later teenage years, when I started to get into facials. Facials were a luxury; they weren't as mainstream as they are now. Typically, you could only find them at bougie hotels. So picture me, 18 years old, going to get a facial, and insisting I needed a peel, too. (I didn't even know what a fucking peel was, but I needed one.) I instructed my facialist to give me a pumpkin glycolic peel (because I, with the Playboy Bunny on my hip, was the expert). This was around Thanksgiving, so I thought I was being festive and creative.

During my hour-long pampering facial, she applied glycolic acid to my face with a paintbrushlike tool, and I lay there waiting for it to take effect. The peel was tingly and smelled delicious— I really thought I had this skincare thing in the bag.

The facialist applied some light SPF—I'm thinking 15 probably—and I went on my merry way, making the 10-minute trek to my car with no hat. Over the next week, I did what I always did: went to school, ran errands, drove with the window down and the sunroof open. And on Friday, it was time for my weekly tanning session, so I applied my Playboy Bunny sticker to my left hip and hopped in.

The next morning, I looked in the mirror and noticed a shadow above my upper lip.

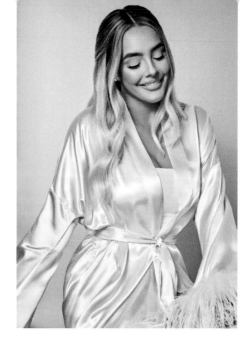

What the facialist didn't tell me was that after you get any kind of peel, you HAVE to stay out of the sun. And when I say stay out of the sun, I mean *stay out of the sun*. Even incidental sun exposure is not acceptable! This means SPF and covering up even if you're just getting out of your car at 7-Eleven to grab Flamin' Hot Cheetos or walking from your parking garage into your house or strolling across the street to get an iced cinnamon coffee. (While we're at it, I should also mention this same rule goes for microneedling, IPL, and lasers, too—but more on those later.)

Two more weeks went by, and out of nowhere I had this huge, brown hyperpigmentation mustache. Then tiny, little brown spots started to form on my face, my freckles became more noticeable, and the whole situation was bleak. At the time, I didn't know it was from sun exposure and tanning right after getting a peel, but I noticed that when I tanned or lay in the sun, the spots would get worse. I realized I was stuck with hyperpigmentation.

For anyone who isn't familiar with the term, "hyperpigmentation" is darkening of the skin. So, when you get brown spots from the sun, or a darker scar from going nuts on a zit, or a darker spot from eczema or something, that is hyperpigmentation. Melasma is a form of hyperpigmentation that's caused by the sun and hormones, and it can occur during pregnancy or as a result of taking birth control pills.

LITTLE DID I KNOW that this was such a blessing in disguise, because it really kick-started a whole new journey for me when it came to taking care of my skin. This is what really gave me momentum when it came to skincare. Through my own experiences I learned how powerful the sun can be, how aging it is and how it has the potential to create fine lines and wrinkles and cause hyper-pigmentation. Call it one big kick in the ass to get the fuck out of the tanning bed.

From that whole experience, I realized hats needed to be in my handbag; I had to wear sunscreen every day; I needed to use foundations, CC creams, and concealers that have SPF; I had to find a good facialist and no more tanning bed.

Hello, Mystic level 3 spray tan with violet tones!!

Then the transformation happened: I started to take my skin health into my own hands and committed myself to becoming a science experiment. This is all pre-*The Skinny Confidential*. I was 18, still in high school, and didn't know shit. At this point I had no money and was working at a boutique and hostess-ing at night. I kept trying to find ways to make skincare work for me, and I realized one of my favorite things to utilize was oils.

I remember I was on a Korean website and saw how a lot of girls were using olive oil on their skin. (Olive oil is high in a fatty acid called oleic acid, which is known to reduce inflammation.) So I ran to my nearest Rite Aid rocking a wide-brimmed hat (don't think I was screwing with that incidental sun exposure) and got an oversized bottle of organic cold-pressed olive oil for $5.99. And I just started using it all over. I'd take my makeup off with it (never been a wipe

fan, it pulls down on your skin). I used it in the morning before I applied makeup (and sunscreen, of course) and at night all over my body—neck, arms, tits, the works—and I noticed that every morning I'd wake up with pretty, dewy skin. This started my love affair with oils.

I also found a sunscreen I loved and ta-da!

During this time, I realized the importance of taking off my makeup at night, too. I mean, I was 18, partying and drinking, hanging off the bar with my tits hanging out (LOL), so I would fall asleep with my makeup and drugstore fake lashes on and wake up with dry, flaky skin. One day, I made a promise to myself that I'd remove my makeup with olive oil every night and then slather on some more to moisturize. Slowly, my hyper-pigmentation started to get better. That's the kind of party I wanted to attend: a "say goodbye to melasma" gala, HA!

Two years later, I was attending San Diego State University full-time, teaching Pure Barre and Pilates, broke as hell, and living at my godparents' house. I joined a sorority for LIKE A MINUTE, then immediately dropped out because they were charging an arm and a leg to be part of it. (I couldn't believe it—$800 a semester to be a part of a community? No thanks. I barely had money for creamy chicken-flavored Top Ramen) During my junior year, the idea came: I saw a blank space for creating a sorority . . . online. I wanted to have this hub where women from all over the world could go to learn tips, tricks, and hacks about anything and everything. I wanted to create a whole experience for women every-where, not just for sharing *my* tips and tricks but theirs, too. I wanted to know what was on their vanities, what they used to exfoliate, what they were eating for stronger hair and nails, and how much water they were drinking to notice a difference in their skin. Like an online sorority FOR FREE. A hot pink beauty and wellness resource.

And that just about brings us to how *The Skinny Confidential* came to be.

I didn't launch the blog until a year after I had this idea, though. I wanted everything to be perfect, so I had this pink Trapper Keeper that I would put all my ideas in.

Finally, I launched. It started as a health and fitness blog but quickly became very beauty/wellness/skin–focused and in no time I was sharing all the products I was testing on myself and the ones recommended by readers . . . and then I had double jaw surgery. That is what REALLY got me into skincare.

Part of why I love skincare so much is that it's turned into a creative, artistic, therapeutic experience. It's a way to start the day and end the night, and it's something millennials are truly committed to. Like, it's not a fad—it's here to stay. Ten years ago, most women were committed to one brand to take care of their skin. Take Proactiv, for example: It's a five-step (aka five-product) program and you stick to it. Although this is nice and efficient, in my opinion, it's working against the consumer because not everyone's skin is the same and not everyone likes using the same products in the same order. It's boring, too, right?

On my vanity, you can expect to find an all-natural, delicious, buttery serum that I found in Cabo San Lucas alongside a plastic surgeon–approved eye cream, a vibrating facial massager, and even coconut oil lube (but OMG have you tried it? *You have to*). It's a medley of different brands, and as the consumer, I have the power to handpick my own unique collection. It's not only empowering, but also works best for my own skin.

After stalking my community's Instagram accounts, I've found that their "shelfies" (that's selfie + shelf) are also covered in multiple different products. What millennials are doing now is finding their favorite products from various brands and forming their own unique skincare collections, rather than buying all their products from one line. It's not all about the Proactiv five-step collection anymore. It's about mixing things up from different brands and curating what works for YOU.

MEET YOUR CHEER SQUAD

Gone are the days of celebs hawking products online that they don't even use. Now it's all about the everyday girl and relatable people sharing what they do in real life. To help you figure out what works best for you, I've personally hand-picked some of my favorite influencers and experts who'll bring the goods, answer questions you're all wondering, and giving us their "Hot Tips," from their favorite products to their quirkiest hacks. Many of them have struggled with skin issues themselves and now have the whole self-care thing under control. And, most importantly, none of this is sponsored; it's just exactly what's plumping their skin and showcased on their vanity. You'll find these interviews and tasty tidbits scattered throughout the book. In this section you'll meet Chriselle Lim and Sivan Ayla on why they love cleansing balms, and their ride-or-die products.

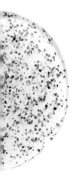

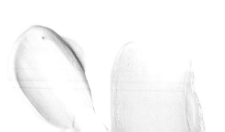

Chriselle

Lim

/ @chrisellelim

STYLIST, INFLUENCER, AND FOUNDER OF
THE CHRISELLE FACTOR AND BÜMO

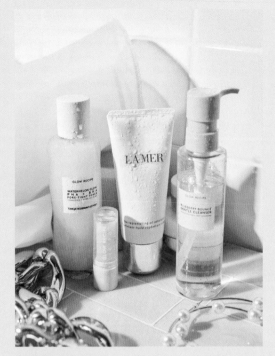

WHAT HAVE YOU FOUND TO BE THE MOST EFFECTIVE SKINCARE PRODUCT UNDER $50, AND WHAT'S YOUR BIGGEST SPLURGE?

iS Clinical Cleansing Complex, which is $42. Hands down the best cleanser I've used. I've been using this on and off for 3 years. It's a lightweight cleansing gel with mild resurfacing ingredients that gently cleanses the surface and pores of the skin without stripping away any natural oils. My biggest splurge is anything La Mer or Dior beauty. I love the cooling gel cream from La Mer (great for combination/oily skin like mine) and the Capture Youth revitalizing serum. The Capture Youth serum and toner always leaves my skin incredibly glowy and hydrated. It also sits under makeup really well. Sometimes I put a few drops of the Capture Youth serum in my foundation to add a glow to my makeup. My little secret.

WHAT STEPS DO YOU TAKE DURING YOUR DAILY SKIN ROUTINE?

Double cleanse (oil and cleanser), mask (usually a sheet mask but if I'm feeling oily I'll do a clay mask), essence/toner, serum, oil, moisturizer, eye cream.

WHAT WOULD YOU SAY TO YOUR YOUNGER SELF ABOUT SKINCARE IF YOU COULD?

Spend more money on skin vs. clothes. You live with your skin forever. Study ingredients and know what you are applying to your skin vs. buying into all the hype of trendy brands. Also: ALWAYS wash off your face at the end of the day.

WHAT IS THE MOST PRACTICAL, RELATABLE ADVICE YOU'VE RECEIVED FOR PREVENTATIVE SKINCARE?

Sunscreen, sunscreen, sunscreen, and stay out of the sun as much as you can. I grew up in Korea, and I would watch women (including my own mom) protect their skin by using an umbrella even on a sunny day to block the sun from hitting their face. Not only does it leave their skin like porcelain but also free from wrinkles. Anti-sun is the best antiaging defense, but living in California can be quite hard, so I'm always slathering on SPF before my makeup every day (even on cloudy and overcast days).

WHAT IS THE WORST ADVICE YOU'VE EVER HEARD WHEN IT COMES TO TAKING CARE OF YOUR SKIN?

The more the better. Just because you are applying more skincare products doesn't mean it'll serve you better. You need to know what ingredients work for your skin type and how to layer your skincare on properly. Also, just because it has an expensive price tag, it does NOT mean that it's better for your skin.

WHAT IS A HABIT YOU'VE DEVELOPED OVER THE YEARS THAT MAKES A DIFFERENCE IN YOUR SKIN?

Hydrating and sheet masking every day! If I don't have time for a sheet mask, I'll add an overnight mask onto my skin before bedtime. It keeps the skin hydrated all night long, supercharging your skin for the next day. In Korea, women use sheet masks every day as a part of their skin-care routine. ♥

Sivan

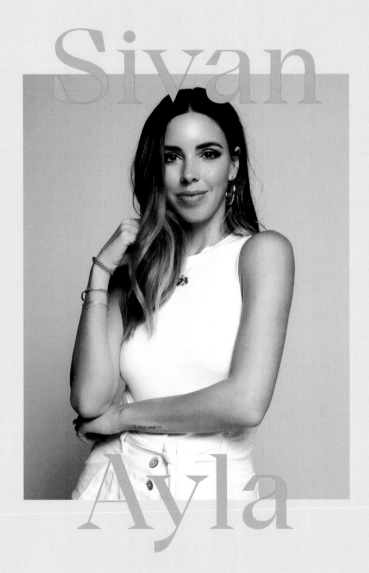

Ayla

/ @sivanayla

LIFESTYLE BLOGGER, DIGITAL
ENTREPRENEUR, AND FOUNDER OF
TAN + LINES AND + LUX UNFILTERED

WHAT HAVE YOU FOUND TO BE THE MOST EFFECTIVE SKINCARE PRODUCT UNDER $50, AND WHAT'S YOUR BIGGEST SPLURGE?

Best skincare product under $50 is KNC Beauty eye gel pads. I keep them in the fridge to help de-puff my whole eye area and leave them on for up to an hour. In fact, ANY eye patch is made more effective by storing in the fridge. The cooling sensation after taking it off not only feels great, but I always notice less puffiness and hollowness after doing this.

My favorite skincare splurge would have to be Augustinus Bader The Rich Cream. Holy shit, that stuff is amazing. BUT, because I love to try out so many different products, I'm not the ideal person to use it because you're not supposed to use other products with it. When I was trying out The Rich Cream, I was so impressed by the thickness of the formula. So many creams claim to be rich and emollient, but my skin drinks them right up. This one (without any additional products under or over it) was exactly as it claimed!

While I love to invest in skincare and test new products (that are some-times super pricey), I also know that you don't have to use the most expen-sive products on the market to have an effective skincare routine that works. There are so many great brands today that offer affordable skincare products that target specific needs, so as long as you are using the right products for you in the right order, I think that is truly all that matters.

WHAT IS THE MOST PRACTICAL, RELATABLE ADVICE YOU'VE RECEIVED FOR PREVENTATIVE SKINCARE?

Protect your face!!! I don't LOVE SPF on my face, but when I'm out in the sun I go all the way. Full-brim visor, zinc on the lips, face SPF, the works. When I was younger, I thought I was invincible in the sun, getting the most amazing tan and not giving a shit about sun damage. Fast-forward to today and it's a whole different story. The age spots alone are enough to make me change my habits, and that's just the surface!

Incorporating products with vitamin C has truly made a big difference in my complexion. I love SkinCeuticals C E Ferulic Serum to help block free radicals in the environment that we cannot control. It smells a little funky, but I find it incredibly effective. I also love Summer Fridays CC Me Serum—it's super hydrating, light, non-irritating, and gives a pretty glow to the face.

Today, when I want a tan on my face I just use + LUX UNFILTERED Nº12 Bronzing Drops and I instantly look more alive and tan. Problem solved!

WHAT IS THE WORST ADVICE YOU'VE EVER HEARD WHEN IT COMES TO TAKING CARE OF YOUR SKIN?

A celebrity dermatologist once told me to cure my dry skin I need to dry it out further with a product she developed for acne (FYI, I don't have acne). I was peeling and flaking like a lizard for weeks before I realized that it was complete bullshit! It seemed counterintuitive to me at the time, but I trusted her, as she services some of Hollywood's biggest names. To this day, I'm not sure if she was just trying to push her product on me or if my skin just had a bad reaction, but either way I learned in that situation to listen to your skin. If something is irritating or making your problem WORSE, it's probably not the answer.

WHAT IS A HABIT YOU'VE DEVELOPED OVER THE YEARS THAT MAKES A DIFFERENCE IN YOUR SKIN?

This might sound gross, but I stopped using face soaps, and I cannot believe the difference it has made in my skin. I switched to cleansing balms rather than using foaming, soapy cleansers, and my skin has never felt or looked better. Soaps tend to dry out my skin and leave it feeling tight and leathery. Balms deep clean without stripping all your hydration, and for someone with dry skin, that is exactly what I need.

My favorite balm is the Elemis Pro-Collagen Rose Cleansing Balm (a rec from Lauryn, actually!), and I don't think I'll ever go back to regular soap. It melts off my makeup, cleans my pores, smells fresh, and leaves my skin super dewy and hydrated.

On shoot days or days I feel like my skin needs an extra good cleaning, I either double cleanse, exfoliate, or just go get a facial to get rid of any buildup.

WHAT STEPS DO YOU TAKE DURING YOUR DAILY SKIN ROUTINE?

First thing I want to note is make sure to apply your skincare products in the correct order. Applying in the wrong order counteracts its effectiveness. Rule of thumb: Apply from thinnest to thickest.

/ A.M. /

1 Rinse face with cool water and pat dry. I prefer to not wash my face in the morning, as I feel it dries out my skin. Instead, I like to splash cool water on my face to help me wake up and just give my skin a nice, clean canvas for the rest of my products.

2 Apply a vitamin C serum for brightness. I like SkinCeuticals, Summer Fridays, and Ole Henriksen, to name a few. Vitamin C serums always immediately brighten up my complexion, which is a win first thing in the morning.

3 Apply a day cream with SPF. Since I don't love SPF on its own, I like to find a moisturizer with SPF in it. Currently loving RéVive Day Cream with SPF 30.

4 Every 3 days I finish my A.M. routine with a few + LUX UNFILTERED Nº12 Bronzing Drops on my face to keep it looking tan and healthy. I like to do this AFTER applying all of my skincare products to ensure my skin is getting the essentials first, and it also helps keep the color more subtle.

/ P.M. /

1 Remove eye makeup first using Bioderma micellar water in Sensitive. I got this years ago in a pharmacy in France, and I have not stopped using it since. It's super gentle but effective. If I don't use this product, I find mascara residue even days later!

2 Melt off face makeup and cleanse skin with Elemis Pro-Collagen Rose Cleansing Balm. I rub this all over in circular motions to really let the product sink in and then rinse off with warm water using my hands.

3 Apply a rich night cream. As I mentioned, my skin is DRY, so I always opt for cream instead of lotion. I love Eve Lom Night Cream—it's very rich and clean.

4 Slather on a face oil. This is where I like to have fun and test new oils out. Herbivore Phoenix is a favorite for a glow, Vintner's Daughter Active Botanical Serum is great for when my face needs a renewed appearance, and Caudalie makes beautiful grape-based serums that are all natural. Basically, I like to go to bed looking like a greasy chicken!

5 Can't live without lip balm! I alternate between Summer Fridays Lip Butter Balm, Too Faced Hangover Pillow Balm, and a little something we are developing for + LUX UNFILTERED (coming soon!).

WHAT WOULD YOU SAY TO YOUR YOUNGER SELF ABOUT SKINCARE IF YOU COULD?

Don't forget to rub your skincare products on your neck and décolleté! I'm pretty sure a teacher once told the class to do this, but I obviously didn't listen because I find myself smoothing my neck wrinkles in photos more than my face! While you're at it, rub any excess product on your hands, too. Hands are such a telling sign of aging that SPF and creams are an incredibly easy way to keep them looking young.

WHAT IS AN UNUSUAL OR SOMEWHAT WEIRD PRACTICE YOU DO TO KEEP YOUR SKIN YOUTHFUL?

I apply my eye cream to my upper lip. Apparently, the skin there is the same thinness and texture as under your eyes, so it needs a little extra TLC. Learned that from this incredibly youthful-looking facialist I saw years ago, who was in her 50s at the time but looked maybe 30. I love finding ways to use excess product on other areas of my skin that could use the TLC. ♥

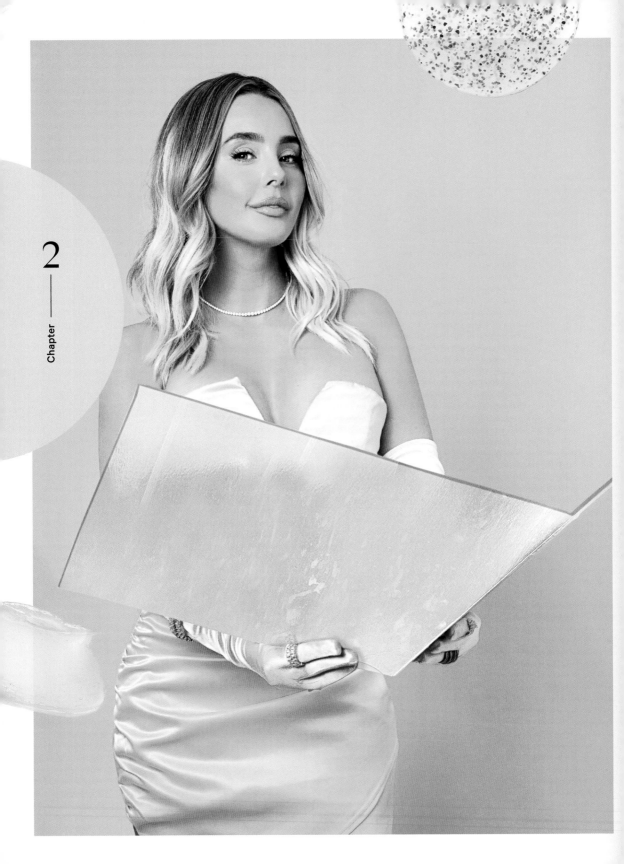

WHY YOU SHOULD GTFO OF THE TANNING BED & APPLY THE DAMN SUNSCREEN

O K, so the sun does have some benefits, like vitamin D, but staying out of the sun is, hands-down, the best way to keep your skin looking young and fresh. If you love the sun, by all means, lie in it! I'm not here to tell you what to do—you have to do what works for you. But please, oh please, consider learning from my mistakes—I've made a lot of them! Given my history, it's important to go over the importance of sunscreen, staying out of the tanning bed, and PROTECTING YOUR PRECIOUS SKIN AT ALL COSTS.

With that, let's get into our first HOT TIP. (If you're wondering, a HOT TIP is just what it sounds like—a quick but valuable tidbit, like a little Aperol Spritz to enjoy before your meal.)

HOT TIP 🤍 *Vitamin D is actually a hormone that is produced in your body when it's exposed to sunlight. It's essential for keeping your body functioning at peak performance, but getting it from the sun isn't always your best bet because (1) the sun sucks for your skin and (2) most people don't get enough D from the sun anyway because of where they live. So, while I do think it's important to be outside in nature, and I don't think the sun is the devil, I don't feel the need for the sun to touch my skin because I get my vitamin D from a supplement.*

CHEMICAL & PHYSICAL SUNSCREENS

There are two common kinds of sunscreen—chemical and physical. Let's break down the difference: physical sunscreen creates a—wait for it—physical barrier on the skin, protecting it from damaging, wrinkling, cancer-causing UV rays by deflecting them away. These sunscreens are usually called "sunblock" and have more mineral-based ingredients, like titanium oxide & zinc oxide.

Chemical sunscreens, on the other hand, contain chemical compounds that sink into the skin and filer out UV rays. These ingredients typically include oxybenzone, octinoxate, octisalate, and avobenzone.

Here are some of the pros & cons of both physical and chemical sunscreens.

PROS OF PHYSICAL SUNSCREEN:

🤍 Safe protection from UVA & UVB rays.

🤍 Safe for babies & to use during pregnancy. I didn't start using sunscreen on my daughter until she turned one. After talking to nurses & doing my own research, this is just what I decided was best in my opinion—you do you. Up until that point, I kept her out of the sun with lots of shade & hats.

🤍 The skin is protected as soon as a physical sunscreen is applied, so you don't have to wait.

🤍 Less likely to irritate sensitive skin (good option if you have rosacea).

🤍 Longer shelf life so you can keep it on your vanity looking all cute.

CONS OF PHYSICAL SUNSCREEN:

🤍 Prone to sweat off, rinse off, and rub off very easily.

🤍 Can cause a chalky film on the skin.

🤍 A lot of makeup artists don't like it because it creases makeup & makes the upper lip sweaty (thank god for Tinkle razors, because a mustache makes a sweaty lip so much worse).

🤍 Takes longer to rub in—not ideal when you have to rub it on your husband's back. SUCH an effort sometimes.

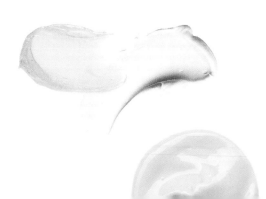

PROS OF CHEMICAL SUNSCREEN:

- 🤍 Way thinner & spreads like a moisturizer.
- 🤍 You can use less of the product.
- 🤍 Easier to use with makeup.

CONS OF CHEMICAL SUNSCREEN:

- 🤍 A lot of people get irritation (careful if you have rosacea).
- 🤍 Sometimes it can irritate your eyes. Nothing worse than sunscreen stinging your eyes.
- 🤍 This is a BIG CON: You have to wait 20 minutes for it to sink in before going into the sun.
- 🤍 Known to clog pores & cause acne.

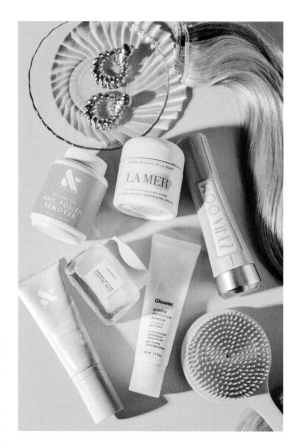

Personally, I like to mix it up. I have favorites from both arenas and choose one based on what I'm doing. If I'm lying out in the sun, which I RARELY, HARDLY EVER DO, or if I'm in Cabo getting incidental sun exposure when I walk from the bar to the pool, I'll opt for a physical sunscreen with a hat. If it's everyday use, I'll go more for a chemical sunscreen because I like how it lies under my makeup.

Recommendation time: I'm OBSESSED with Colorescience Sunforgettable, a tinted brush-on powder sunscreen. I also love a good caffeinated sunscreen, especially when I'm applying makeup. It's not fancy—I purchase it off Amazon and it comes in a random bottle, nothing special. Just search "caffeine sunscreen." The caffeine tightens your skin, which allows your makeup to appear all fresh, dewy, and tight against the skin (tight skin creates a nice canvas for makeup AND shrinks the pores), which we LOVE. The secret here is to apply it with a damp Beautyblender, a little pink sponge that is the best ever for applying makeup. (There's something about the way it applies products to the skin that just works. Trust me, you'll never go back to using dirty fingers.) Use the Beautyblender to pat the sunscreen all over your face, then treat it like a primer under your makeup.

For body, I love a mist spray—Supergoop! makes a good one. I particularly love it for touching up my SPF throughout the day (something I'll talk more about in a bit).

Speaking of body, I HOPE THIS WILL REMIND YOU ONCE AGAIN to bring the sunscreen situation down the body. So many women cover their faces but forget their chest! Hands! Neck! Arms! Boobs! I'm a big fan of applying sunscreen *everywhere*.

And for extra credit: A brand called TULA makes a sunscreen that also protects your skin from the blue light emitted by your computer, phone, TV, and/or indoor lighting. The more you know . . .

NO, BUT REALLY, BE A PSYCHO ABOUT IT

"A Sunscreen Role Model" will be on my gravestone. Like, think of me crying when you're baking in the sun. I'm like your mom but even *more* annoying. Why am I *so* psycho? Well, after picking so many experts' brains and seeing firsthand the damage tanning in beds or outside can do, I became very interested in the subject. And I learned that too much exposure can lead to:

- ♥ Wrinkles
- ♥ Skin cancer
- ♥ Aging
- ♥ Pigmentation
- ♥ Fine lines
- ♥ Sallowness (yellow discoloration of the skin)
- ♥ Benign tumors
- ♥ The destruction of collagen—buh-bye, youth!

HERE'S THE DEAL:

I'm a believer in wearing sunscreen every single day. If I'm riding my bike, walking the dogs, working on the patio, gardening, or even just doing outdoor chores—I wear my freaking sunscreen. Specifically, I use SPF on my body, face, neck, chest, and hands (by the way, the first places signs of aging appear are usually the hands, chest, and neck, so protect yourself accordingly). I'm ALSO a huge fan of wearing sunscreen . . . at NIGHT. Crazy, I know, but here's the deal: Artificial lights (especially fluorescent lights—you know, the cheap ones that bathe you like you're at the DMV getting your license renewed) are bad for your skin because UV lights cause premature aging. So even if it's nighttime, I wear sunscreen. I don't wear it to bed, but to happy hour? YES. You never know where there will be a harsh, DMV-esque (you know, like where you get your license?) light. (There's a reason your driver's license photos are never your favorite. I looked like a wet rat in mine last time I renewed my license.)

So, if you're meeting a friend for a hike, throw on sunscreen & a hat. If you're throwing a poolside boozy BBQ, pass the sunscreen. And if you're going to the grocery store, don't forget to slap some sunscreen on. Oh ya, and apply SPF 15–20 minutes before you go in the sun and be sure to use at least 1 teaspoon on the face and 2 tablespoons on each body part. It's very important to reapply every 2 hours, and obviously more often if you are swimming or sweating a lot.

Some weird sun-protection quirks that sound outrageous that actually work:

1 I paid to get my car windows tinted, but this isn't an I'm-too-cool-for-school situation. It's to protect my hands & chest area from the sun while I'm driving.

2 There's a trucker hat (or five) in my oversize purse. I use it daily when I'm getting out of my car to grab something from the grocery store; I wear it when I walk and take conference calls (passive multitasking), when I'm going to the bank, when I'm pumping gas, when I'm grabbing coffee. I wear it whenever my face and neck are vulnerable to incidental sun exposure.

3 I put SPF on my hands, fingers, chest, face, neck . . . every day.

4 My husband isn't allowed to open the sunroof.

5 I asked my vet if there's sunscreen for dogs. There's a life vest they can wear—it's on Amazon and it works. Try it before you judge.

6 So crazy that I even protect myself from the UV lights at the DMV, in underground offices, and at the supermarket.

7 I use an SPF protector mist on my hair. Because yes, the sun is harmful for hair, too.

8 Tanning beds are a no for me—those days are long gone after the tale of the hyperpigmentation mustache.

9 My sunglasses cover my entire face.

Dr. Anjali Mahto

/ @anjalimahto

DERMATOLOGIST AND AUTHOR OF
THE SKINCARE BIBLE

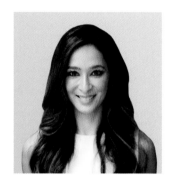

Before we even think about treatments or procedures and why we need them, we should be focusing on protection and prevention where possible. This is partly because it is possible to slow down the signs of premature skin aging, and partly because any effective "in-clinic" treatments are likely to be costly in comparison. About 80 percent of the signs we associate with skin aging—fine lines, wrinkles, and pigmentation—occur because of the effects of sunlight. Wearing a broad-spectrum sunscreen, ideally SPF 30–50 with protection against UVA, UVB, and visible light, can reduce premature skin aging as well as the risk of development of skin cancer.

HERE'S MY POINT:

If you want to age quickly, go lie out in the sun without protection! And then hit the tanning beds!

PUT SUNSCREEN ON YOUR EYELIDS … YES, ON YOUR EYELIDS.

If we're going to get hard-core on sunscreen, this is the place to do it!

Sunscreen. On the eyelids.

::crickets::

That's right, like, your eyeLIDS. Eyelids are the thinnest skin around your eyes—almost 10 percent thinner than other areas—so they are very susceptible to UV damage.

First, make sure you get a sunscreen that doesn't make your eyes sting. We all know there's *nothing* worse than applying sunscreen or CC cream & having your eyes water for hours. After trying about 42,957,234,587 sunscreens, I finally figured out that the magical solution for me is a caffeinated formula, which really tightens my skin. But remember: *Everyone is different*. It's kind of like marriage—you have to try things out yourself before you fully commit. Test a little of the sunscreen on your hand first, then move to your face & then go all in with the eyelids.

ANOTHER SIDE NOTE: I ALSO APPLY MY FAVORITE CAFFEINE SUNSCREEN LIGHTLY TO MY LIPS. AS YOU CAN SEE, I DON'T FUCK AROUND WHEN IT COMES TO SUNSCREEN APPLICATION.

BE SURE TO REAPPLY SUNSCREEN EVEN WHEN YOU HAVE MAKEUP ON, K?

HOW DO YOU APPLY SUNSCREEN WHEN YOU HAVE MAKEUP ON?

This is a hard question for me to answer. Especially because it screws up my makeup most of the time. However, recently I discovered sunscreen *mist*.

THAT'S RIGHT, *MIST*.

Doesn't something about the word "mist" make you feel whimsical & vibey? I love it.

Supergoop! setting mist is ideal for touching up your SPF throughout the day, especially later in the day, around 2 P.M. You can even mist your neck, chest, shoulders—you know I go crazy & even do my arms.

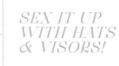

Wearing visors and other huge hats was inspired by a beautiful woman I met while running. We struck up a conversation and she showed me the side of her neck. There was a ton of sun damage. She told me the damage immediately made her feel older & even scared (because of skin cancer). Then she went on to say she had protected her face her entire life . . . but had failed to pay attention to her neck. And now her neck was a completely different age than her face. Not only does a massive hat or visor protect your face & neck, it protects your *chest*, too! Multitasking, man.

There's nothing I love more than to embarrass my husband by wearing the most obnoxious hat in the world. And I'm all about visors. The bigger, the better—WIDE-BRIM like your tenth-grade camp counselor or 92-year-old neighbor, mkay. So, instead of calling it "an old person's visor," how about we go ahead & call them "the antiaging visor of your dreams." Hats & visors are not expensive, and yes, maybe people *will* think you're odd, BUT you'll be protected from the sun, so who cares? I don't.

IF YOU DO HAPPEN TO GET A SUNBURN… ALOE VERA SAVES THE DAY

Once, when I was little, I went to Palm Springs with my mom and got the MOST horrific sunburn on the planet. It was a beet-red, skin-that-feels-hot-to-the-touch, painful, peeling kind of sunburn. The kind that makes you never want to go outside again. My dad has always been obsessed with aloe vera & keeps it on his bedside table to use on his cracked heels—your dad, too? Maybe it's a dad thing. And I remembered him telling me about its healing benefits. Boy, did they work on my Palm Springs sunburn—relieved the burn SO MUCH.

To get specific, aloe vera is the gel-like pulp from the inside of the leaves of the succulent aloe vera plant. You should know that it was used in Ancient Egypt, and it has some CRAZY healing benefits. While it heals, it also moisturizes, aka perfect post-sunburn. You could also use it for a rash or dermatitis—basically it's going to soothe any irritated skin.

THE ALOE OBSESSION IS REAL:

- ♥ **"THE SUNBURN CURE":** Applied topically, it naturally treats sunburns.
- ♥ **IMMUNE SYSTEM:** Drinking aloe vera juice enhances the immune system. It contains copper, iron, sodium, calcium, zinc, potassium, chromium, magnesium & manganese! Not to mention vitamins A, B1, B2, B6, B12, C & E, as well as folic acid. If you're stressed, tired, fatigued, whatever… BOTTOMS UP!
- ♥ **MOISTURIZER:** It provides oxygen to cells that build the skin tissues, so they give off a beautiful, healthy glow.
- ♥ **ACNE:** It's known to help cure acne.
- ♥ **WEIGHT LOSS:** The plant promotes energy & naturally cleans the digestive system. Los Angeles, add it to my wellness shot, please.
- ♥ **RASH-BE-GONE:** Aloe is known to alleviate itching, burning, and pain from allergic reactions on the skin, eczema, burns, inflammation, wounds & psoriasis.

BUT WHAT IF I WANT TO GET TAN?

We've covered sun protection, but now it's time to discuss what the fuck to do if you want to tan that ass. Enter: spray tans. I might avoid the sun like I avoid jury duty, but don't get it twisted: I still like a pretty glow, which I achieve through spray tans about three times a month. And since I'm ALL about lookin' like a sun-kissed goddess, I've picked up some tips over the years that you have to know about—ones that will keep things looking natural.

HOT TIP ♥ *Personally, I always opt for violet tones because it pops the whites of the eyes & teeth. I always say NO to orange & red tones. They make the whites of my teeth and eyes look yellow. Check with your local spray-tan artist to see what works best for you.*

INSIDER SPRAY TAN TIPS:

1 Shave & dry brush before.

OK, this seems rather obvious, but we should go over it just in case: Shave everything you need to shave BEFORE you spray tan (I like to do it the night before). Then I always dry brush RIGHT before I spray tan to exfoliate & help ensure the tan goes on evenly. (We'll dive deep into dry brushing soon, don't you worry.)

Also, I wait 3 to 4 days after a spray tan before dry brushing again, which makes me cry because I love dry brushing SO much, but hey, beauty is pain and you don't want to fuck up your spray tan by brushing it off.

3 Put a towel underneath your feet.

This is my ride-or-die TIP! You will want to do this ESPECIALLY if you have cracked heels. If you're getting a spray tan in a booth, always request a little towel. Put it on the floor of the booth BEFORE you step in (because sometimes there's like, old spray tan residue, which is highly annoying), then stand on it during your tan. The tanning solution gets all over the floor of the booth and, without the towel, the solution will stain the bottoms of your feet, which is just not pretty, like HI, I JUST STEPPED IN ORANGE PAINT.

5 Wear a lightweight maxi & flip-flops (or shoes that won't cramp your toes).

You don't want to wear a tight sports bra with suffocating leggings & tennis shoes. Why? Because when you put those super-tight clothes back on after the tan, they'll leave marks. IT'S A REAL PAIN IN THE ASS. Trust me on this, because it's happened to me five million times. Wear something lightweight like a maxi dress (my personal pick) and opt for sandals so your toes can breathe OR shoes that aren't too tight.

2 Get a pedicure before & a manicure after, or do "the claw."

This one's a weird one: Get a manicure after a spray tan, but if you get a pedicure after, BEWARE. If you're getting a manicure, it's best to get it *after* a spray tan because you don't want your tan to get all over your beautiful white, pale pink, or burgundy nails. But here's the deal: If you're getting a pedicure after you spray tan only get a polish change. Otherwise, the leg scrub and massage will rub your tan off. My favorite is to get a spray tan, manicure, then a paint job on the toes. If I get a real pedicure, I like to do it far away from my spray tan appointment. If you do need to get a spray tan after your manicure, try "the claw". Just curl your fingers in toward your palm so your nails are hidden.

If you're getting a pedicure after, use a barrier cream to preserve your tan. I know, this shit is like quantum physics. But it works.

4 Wash your hands & feet off the second you get out of the booth.

Even if you have access to a sink or tub, I'm a fan of baby wipes. I use them to wipe off my hands, feet, and fingernails after exiting the booth.

HOT TIP **TANNING OIL IS NOT ONLY FOR TANNING.** *In fact, I DEFINITELY recommend that you don't use it for tanning. When I was in high school, I would use it all the time just to smell like a tropical vacation. Cat Marnell takes it to the extreme, naturally. The author of How to Murder Your Life says she uses dark tanning oil day or night. Anywhere and everywhere. She loves one with a dark tint so it looks like she has a fresh tan. Cat and I both like to wear it at night to make our legs look shiny.*

TO SUM IT UP: Avoid baking in the sun Madga-style, grab some driving gloves & an oversized visor, slap some sunscreen on your neck & nipples, and say sayonara to sloppy spray tans!

Now we're talking to Mandy Madden Kelley, Annie Lawless Jacobs, and Payton Sartain about LED masks, plus Summer Fridays co-founders Marianna Hewitt and Lauren Gores Ireland spill all their tricks.

Mandy
Madden
Kelley

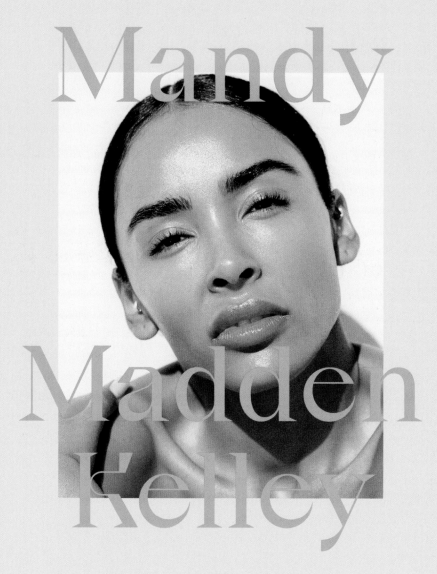

/ @mandymadd

BEAUTY INFLUENCER, CREATIVE
CONSULTANT, AND FOUNDER OF PAGERIE

WHAT HAVE YOU FOUND TO BE THE MOST EFFECTIVE SKINCARE PRODUCT UNDER $50, AND WHAT'S YOUR BIGGEST SPLURGE?

I'm so glad you asked! It really matters to me that good skin is accessible to anyone, and that includes at all price ranges. I have been enjoying the Biologi Bqk Radiance Face serums as a more affordable skincare product. They have the same effects as some higher-priced skincare products and create a near-immediate glow. These serums improve issues with pigmentation, texture, and hydration. As for a splurge, I prefer to consider it an investment in myself, which takes away any associated guilt! For higher-priced products, I love all things Biologique Recherche. I have used this brand for years, stocking up on my favorites: Lotion P50 1970, Masque VIP O2, and Masque Vivant, while on vacation in Thailand. The Complexe Iribiol is a magical holy grail–type product that is worth every dollar. It shrinks pores, heals imperfections, and truly creates an effortless perfection.

"Skincare to me is not just a routine, but a ritual for me to celebrate myself and to tangibly practice an act of self-love and wellness. "

WHAT IS THE MOST PRACTICAL, RELATABLE ADVICE YOU'VE RECEIVED FOR PREVENTATIVE SKINCARE?

The best advice I've received is to embrace aging as a part of life. I'll certainly do my best to prevent premature wrinkles or fine lines, and to maintain as flawless a complexion as possible. However, there is no need for me to stress over the inevitable—especially since stress causes infinitely more problems, including loss of elastin and more wrinkles! I do as best as I can to treat and love my skin, but I refuse to take issue with each and every new mark. Similarly, my grandmother taught me at a young age to do at-home beauty routines and to be

innovative in our skin care processes. This has been more helpful than I ever imagined. Honoring myself through these beauty routines offers a chance to honor my grandmother, which I intend to pass down to my daughter, Kaia, as well. We already have beauty rituals, and I cherish our time together. I hope that she remembers it fondly, and carries with her the confidence and self-worth tied to taking excellent care of herself. She deserves that, and so do you!

WHAT IS THE WORST ADVICE YOU'VE EVER HEARD WHEN IT COMES TO TAKING CARE OF YOUR SKIN?

I once heard that facials, aestheticians, and lasers were not only helpful, but

absolutely necessary for good skin. When I first moved to Los Angeles, I had some difficulty adjusting to the climate and my skin suffered greatly. In hopes to improve my situation, I followed this advice and spent a great deal of money, time, and concern handing the power of my skin to others. At the time, I felt there was no other choice. Although those are wonderful resources for our skin, and also amazing luxuries to enjoy, I really don't believe they are necessary at all for healthy, beautiful skin. My motto is, "Good skin is a matter of discipline," and that discipline is largely self-motivated and self-actualized. It's empowering to not depend on something or someone else, and to take matters into your own hands to heal and improve. It also means that you can achieve it without spending hundreds or even thousands of dollars on treatments, or doing anything too far outside your comfort zone. It is also an acknowledgment of how unique everyone is, and how what is wonderful for one person may not work for another. There's no "one size fits all" approach to great skin, especially not one that makes treatments from others a necessity.

WHAT IS A HABIT YOU'VE DEVELOPED OVER THE YEARS THAT MAKES A DIFFERENCE IN YOUR SKIN?

Since our skin is our largest organ, it is profoundly impacted by a wide variety of influences. In fact, almost everything we do or experience can change the condition of our skin. This makes just about every healthy habit you have ever tried to cultivate even more worth doing—it'll show on your face! I make sure to eat clean, stay active, get good sleep, control my stress as best I can, stay hydrated, and wear sunscreen, on top of my already comprehensive skincare regimen. My motto that "good skin is a matter of discipline" doesn't only apply to removing makeup and applying serums. It also reflects dedication to the overall healthy behaviors that impact healthy skin. Of course, there are factors that are hard to avoid, like being exposed to air pollution in Los Angeles. And there are times when finding life balance to stay consistent in these habits is more challenging, or even impossible. But for the most part, I am able to remain consistent because I know it's worth the extra effort. It's also a wonderful way to multitask, since there are so many health benefits beyond our skin for each of those, too!

WHAT STEPS DO YOU TAKE DURING YOUR DAILY SKIN ROUTINE?

I always like to double cleanse, and often with an oil cleanser to keep my skin as hydrated as possible. I like to use microfiber cleansing cloths to ensure my skin is thoroughly cleaned. Next up is a cocktail of serums that really depend on what my skin needs that day. The most important factor is that I always use time and care in my daily facial massage ritual. This promotes blood circulation and stimulates lymphatic drainage. It took me a while to really learn from various aestheticians and dermatologists what works best for my face, and I encourage others to study and apply this as well. I follow up with a moisturizer, eye cream, and, of course, sunscreen. I don't often wear makeup, so in the evening I usually follow a similar routine, minus the sunscreen. I'll also use face masks liberally as needed. Paying close attention to my skin's changing needs and adapting to address them on a daily

and weekly basis is the best way for me to maintain a consistent, healthy, and clear glow.

WHAT WOULD YOU SAY TO YOUR YOUNGER SELF ABOUT SKINCARE IF YOU COULD?

I grew up in a small town in Romania where I was bullied for the color of my skin. My father is Sudanese, but he wasn't ever a part of my life. My white, Romanian-Turkish family couldn't relate to my mixed darker skin tone, and neither could my community. I actually hated my skin, and would spend hours every day trying to scrub it to be white. Beyond the troubling racism, I started to blame any misfortune on the color of my skin, or any skin imperfections. My transformation from hating my skin to loving it, from having people criticize my skin to praising it, has truly become a huge source of pride and one of the largest obstacles I've overcome. I wish I could wrap my younger self up in a hug, provide her a sense of acceptance, and teach her the importance of self-love. Skincare to me is not just a routine, but a ritual for me to celebrate myself and to tangibly practice an act of self-love and wellness. I encourage my daughter, family, friends, and audience to take time every day to love and appreciate their skin.

WHAT IS AN UNUSUAL OR SOMEWHAT WEIRD PRACTICE YOU DO TO KEEP YOUR SKIN YOUTHFUL?

I have an extensive skin tool collection. It's quite vast, and I'm constantly searching and testing the next big thing: from ultrasonic skin scrubbers, red light eye masks, to high-frequency devices—I use everything. Most

skincare tools are gentle enough to use at home and are quite effective at keeping my skin glowy, buoyant & fresh. On a weekly basis, I use an Environ microneedling device to generate new skin tissue and collagen, and the Dr. Dennis Gross DRx SpectraLite FaceWare Pro to firm my skin's elastin and promote blood circulation. Every couple days, I do a microcurrent treatment such as NuFACE or ZIIP Beauty Device to lift my muscles and treat any wrinkles. I'll often use glass cupping devices to promote circulation and treat fine lines. Almost daily, I use a Lanshin gua sha tool to help with lymphatic drainage, which reduces toxins in the body. I could go on and on! ♥

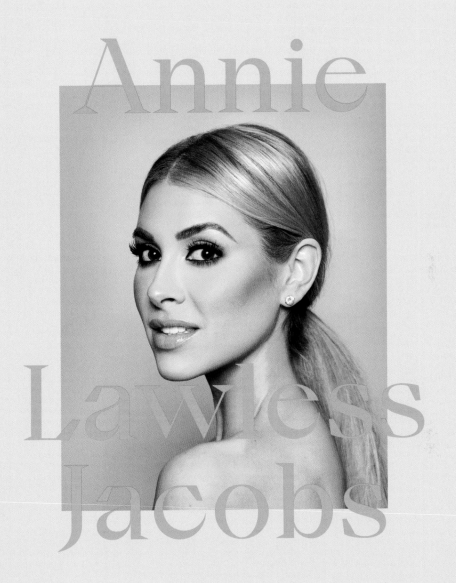

Annie
Lawless
Jacobs

/ @annielawless

FOUNDER AND CEO
OF LAWLESS BEAUTY

WHAT HAVE YOU FOUND TO BE THE MOST EFFECTIVE SKINCARE PRODUCT UNDER $50, AND WHAT'S YOUR BIGGEST SPLURGE?

At $33, the Sanitas Skincare GlycoSolution 15% toner is the most effective skincare product I've found under $50 that I have purchased time and time again. It has a high concentration of glycolic acid for deep exfoliation of dead skin cells, dirt, and oil. It visibly tightens my pores and gets rid of texture overnight. It also softens my lines and wrinkles, controls oil, and prevents breakouts. I have used this for years, and it is such a highly effective treatment that you only need to use it 2 or 3 times a week to see and feel results. My biggest skincare splurge, at $295, is the Joanna Vargas Super Nova Retinol Treatment Serum. This is an amazing retinol for me, because my skin is pretty sensitive to retinols, and they often irritate me and cause redness that lasts for days. This serum uses a type of retinol called palmitoyl oligopeptide that stimulates collagen without the traditional side effects of retinol. It really makes my skin glowy, bright, and smooth and is worth every penny for me.

WHAT IS THE WORST ADVICE YOU'VE EVER HEARD WHEN IT COMES TO TAKING CARE OF YOUR SKIN?

In high school, I had extremely oily skin—I could saturate at least two oil-absorbing sheets per hour. I began to experience mild to moderate break-outs and saw a dermatologist to learn the best way to care for my skin to minimize blemishes and manage my oil production. She advised me to use Proactiv in conjunction with Retin-A and an oil-free moisturizer. This combination was way too harsh for my skin and completely dried it out to the point of peeling and feeling raw. I thought this was part of improving my skin, so I continued with this regi-men for months until I saw a different dermatologist, who explained I was doing more harm than good with this combination. I stopped using those products and switched to a gentle cleanser and a deeply hydrating face cream. My skin balanced out pretty quickly, and I learned that oily skin needs hydration in order to regulate and balance its oil production and achieve equilibrium.

WHAT IS THE MOST PRACTICAL, RELATABLE ADVICE YOU'VE RECEIVED FOR PREVENTATIVE SKINCARE?

Get plenty of sleep! Sleep is one of the most underrated things we can do to benefit our skin. Our cells repair and regenerate when we sleep, and skin makes new collagen, which means fewer wrinkles. Blood flow to our skin increases during sleep, which helps our skin look more fresh and glowing. Getting adequate sleep also prevents puffy eyes and dark circles, making us look brighter and more youthful. While we sleep, our skincare products also penetrate better and are more effec-tive because our skin heats up and our pores open.

WHAT IS A HABIT YOU'VE DEVELOPED OVER THE YEARS THAT MAKES A DIFFERENCE IN YOUR SKIN?

Drinking 2 liters of water daily! It took me a long time to get into a consistent routine of drinking this much water throughout the day every day, but now it is second nature, and I don't even think about it. My skin is so much more hydrated, supple, and clear from doing this! I could not believe how beneficial this simple habit was in the overall appearance of my skin when I started doing this religiously. I always knew drinking lots of water was great for my skin, but I never saw amazing results until it became a real, daily habit—not just a sporadic water kick. Within a week or two of drinking a full 2 liters each day, I was so impressed by how much it helped my skin.

WHAT STEPS DO YOU TAKE DURING YOUR DAILY SKIN ROUTINE?

I love the Korean skincare regimen, so I have adopted many of those steps into my daily routine. It may seem like a lot, but I personally feel taking the time to care for your skin is one of the best skincare investments you can make. The first step in my routine is cleansing. In the morning I use a gentle cream cleanser, and at night I double

"Get plenty of sleep! Sleep is one of the most underrated things we can do to benefit our skin."

cleanse using an oil cleanser to break down my makeup, followed by a foam cleanser. Next, I tone. I use a hydrating toner in the morning and a balancing toner in the evening. After toning, I use a water essence to help my skin absorb my serums more efficiently and to plump my skin with hydration. Following my essence, I use serums. In the morning, I use a vitamin C serum and a hyaluronic acid serum. In the evening, I use a glycolic acid serum or a light retinol. Next, I use a moisturizer, and since I love very glowy, hydrated skin, I use a rich cream both morning and night to lock in all of the skincare I just applied. Finally, I use an eye gel in the morning to brighten and de-puff, and richer eye cream at night to hydrate and soften fine lines. Two or three times a week, I use a sheet mask as the last step over my moisturizer before bed, to seal in all of my skincare and help it deeply absorb.

WHAT IS AN UNUSUAL OR SOMEWHAT WEIRD PRACTICE YOU DO TO KEEP YOUR SKIN YOUTHFUL?

Three times a week, I set my alarm for 30 minutes earlier and lie in bed with an LED therapy light on my face. It's a little light dome that I place directly over my face while I go back to sleep, and it looks weird, but it is so relaxing and highly effective. Red and near-infrared wavelengths are proven to effectively generate more collagen and elastin in your skin to combat the signs of aging. I love using LED light because it is a way to actually improve my skin from the inside out, versus temporary injections, or more invasive solutions like surgery and intense peels. LED light may also be used for pain management, acne, and wound healing.

WHAT ARE YOUR FAVORITE BOOKS, WEBSITES, PODCASTS, OR OTHER RESOURCES YOU REFER TO FOR PREVENTATIVE SKINCARE ADVICE?

For podcasts, I love *Natch Beaut* because it is informative while being so funny and lighthearted, and *Fat Mascara* because they have interesting interviews with experts, and they really do their research on beauty topics. Two books I have learned a lot from are *The Skincare Bible* by dermatologist Dr. Anjali Mahto and *Glow from Within* by Joanna Vargas. 🤍

Payton Sartain

/ @paytonsartain

LIFE AND STYLE INFLUENCER AND BLOGGER OF *HUSTLE + HALCYON*

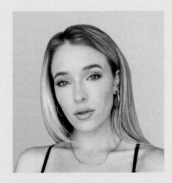

WHAT HAVE YOU FOUND TO BE THE MOST EFFECTIVE SKINCARE PRODUCT UNDER $50, AND WHAT'S YOUR BIGGEST SPLURGE?

I actually use a number of effective skincare products priced under $50, but in terms of the MOST effective, I'm going to have to go with my cleanser. I am obsessed with simple, affordable cleansers! Right now, I switch between the sensitive skin facial shampoo from my favorite skincare clinic in LA, Corrective Skincare, and Kate Somerville DeliKate Soothing Cleanser, though you can find plenty of gentle cleansers at your local drugstore (just make sure you check what's in them!). I have relatively sensitive skin, so using straightforward, gentle cleansers with none of the added fancy stuff, has been an absolute game-changer for keeping my skin calm while also keeping it clean. No one wants dry, irritated, inflamed skin, which is what is often left in the wake of more abrasive, do-too-much cleansers, in my personal experience.

My biggest skincare splurge is, hands-down, my vitamin C serum. I use SkinCeuticals C E Ferulic with 15% L-ascorbic acid. Now that I'm well into my mid-20s, protection and prevention have become a big part of my skincare routine. This product is NOT cheap, but I view it as the gold standard of vitamin C serums, as its patented (yes, PATENTED) technology is proven to reduce combined oxidative damage from free radicals generated by UV, ozone, and diesel exhaust by up to 41 percent. We love a good product proven to work by extensive research. If I'm spending over $100 on a skincare product, I need to be sure it's worth it. And of course, when using a vitamin C serum, I always seal the deal with a quality sunscreen!

WHAT IS THE MOST PRACTICAL, RELATABLE ADVICE YOU'VE RECEIVED FOR PREVENTATIVE SKINCARE?

The most practical preventative skincare advice that has been bestowed upon me is to be consistent with my routine! Instead of pushing intensive treatments or extensive, exhausting skincare routines, I've had a number of skincare experts explain to me that protecting your skin from signs of aging doesn't need to be so damn serious. And it most certainly doesn't need to be expensive. Instead, I've been told time & time again to be consistent with my routine. Small actions over time yield big results! I always make time for skincare, morning & night, whether I wore makeup that day or not. I keep my skin clean daily. I always make sure to exfoliate, and I protect my face & neck from the environment daily. I use good-quality products morning & night. I keep my skin hydrated from the outside and the inside, always. The not-so-secret secret to preventative skincare seems to be consistency, which isn't shocking; consistency seems to be the "secret" to basically everything else in life as well, right?

WHAT IS THE WORST ADVICE YOU'VE EVER HEARD WHEN IT COMES TO TAKING CARE OF YOUR SKIN?

I think the notion that you need to invest your life savings into keeping your skin its healthiest is extreme, to say the least. This is the trend I see in the influencer world, which has always rubbed me the wrong way. As influencers, we're lucky enough to receive high-end products that we otherwise wouldn't purchase for free. (And sometimes, we're PAID to use it! Wild.) Because of this, these excessively expensive products are constantly pushed by lifestyle & beauty influencers online. It seems like one's arsenal of beauty products has become as much of a status symbol as owning a nice watch, fancy car, or designer handbag. Of course, I'm all for a skincare splurge here and there (when it makes sense), but your entire skincare routine doesn't need to break the bank. I understand the desire to be on-trend, and I definitely relate to wanting that beautifully packaged product in an Instagram "shelfie" shot (I feel this one very deeply, HA). But *expensive* doesn't always mean *better*! I tend to find plenty of clean, high-quality, and effective skincare products that fall under the $30 mark. You can cut price corners in your beauty routine pretty easily, it just takes a little research!

WHAT HABIT HAVE YOU DEVELOPED OVER THE YEARS THAT MAKES A DIFFERENCE IN YOUR SKIN?

I really hate to say this, because I know it induces immediate-eye-roll syndrome, but drinking enough water on a daily basis has completely changed my skin both short term and long term. It's no secret that staying hydrated has an immensely positive effect on the health of your skin. It's repetitive (and almost *annoying*) to hear because it's TRUE. Throughout my 20s so far, I've learned that basically everything dehydrates your skin. The sun, pollution, an unbalanced diet, alcohol, caffeine, not drinking enough water, and on and on the list of things that dehydrate your skin goes. For me, there is nothing worse than waking up after a night of drinking to a dehydrated-looking face, as if I aged ten years and all the blood drained from my body overnight. NO THANK YOU. But it's nothing that a day of indulging in a little *extra* water intake can't alleviate. I start each morning with an XL lemon water (in a huge mason jar), and I refill my glass at least eight times per day. At LEAST. If I have an intense workout planned, or if I'm going to be outside the majority of the day, I drink even more water. It's a daily habit we all need to undertake for a number of skin-related & non-skin-related reasons, in my opinion!

WHAT STEPS DO YOU TAKE DURING YOUR DAILY SKIN ROUTINE?

It has taken me a while to develop a skincare routine I'm confident in and that works for my unique skin issues. In the A.M., I start with a gentle cleanser (Kate Somerville DeliKate Soothing Cleanser) to remove any oil or debris that may have gotten on my face while sleeping. I tone with a gentle face mist (Gya Labs Bergamot Hydrosol), and then it's time for the fun stuff. I apply a few drops of my favorite vitamin C serum (SkinCeuticals C E Ferulic) and wait a few minutes for it to really soak in. Then I moisturize with a light moisturizer (TULA 24-7 Moisture), sometimes adding in a few drops of hyaluronic acid if I'm feeling particularly dehydrated. Lastly, I finish off with a mineral sunscreen that's at least SPF 30 or higher. I haven't found my favorite sunscreen quite yet, so I'm always testing a couple out at a time.

In the evenings, I remove my makeup with a Face Halo and then use a gentle cleanser on my skin. I exfoliate my skin every other night with Dermalogica Daily Microfoliant, as I'm slowly building my skin's tolerance to being exfoliated daily (like I said, my skin can be very sensitive). One night a week, I use a retinol (Obagi Clinical Retinol 0.5 Retexturizing Cream), and I'm also working this into my routine more frequently as my skin permits. Then I finish with my moisturizer (I use the same product at night as I do in the morning), with the occasional touch of hyaluronic acid mixed in.

WHAT WOULD YOU SAY TO YOUR YOUNGER SELF ABOUT SKINCARE IF YOU COULD?

Basically, I would sum up all that I've talked about above, with a few added tips. I'd tell myself to drink more water, for starters. It wasn't until the last couple of years that I started paying attention to my water intake. I'd say don't sleep on protecting your skin, even at a young age! Always wear your sunscreen. I'd tell younger me to create a more robust skincare routine, even if it's a simple one, and to not be afraid to exfoliate my skin a bit more. Also, I'd say don't pick your pimples! When it comes to acne, step away from the blemish! A hands-off, treatments-on procedure is necessary and will help you avoid dark spots. Lastly, I'd tell myself to educate myself on better skin practices in general. I'm learning a lot about skincare in my mid-20s, but much of this information would have benefited me 5 years ago as well!

WHAT IS AN UNUSUAL OR SOMEWHAT WEIRD PRACTICE YOU DO TO KEEP YOUR SKIN YOUTHFUL?

Though I don't think either of these could be considered unusual, I think they could be considered *extra*, *excessive*, and a bit *weird*. First, I am obsessed with LED light treatments, especially LED masks. Many spas & skincare clinics offer LED treatments in-house, but as we know, consistency is KEY, so I've been incorporating light treatments into my routine at home when possible. LED masks can get pricey (like, *really* pricey), but I found one on Amazon that works wonders (it has a 4.5-star rating) and is leagues cheaper than every other quality LED treatment mask I've found. (If you want to check out my exact mask, it's the "LED Light Therapy 7 Color Facial Skin Care Mask" by a company called NEWKEY.) LED treatments can help with everything from stimulating collagen production to clearing acne to soothing your skin. It looks a little serial killer–esque while in use, but consistent use yields some pretty impressive results, in my experience.

Second, I love shaving my face, and not with a Tinkle razor, but with an actual razor. I'm very gentle and careful when doing so, of course, and I don't do this frequently. I first tried this after watching one of my favorite supermodels, Josephine Skriver, explaining how she does it via a YouTube video. I've found that straight-up shaving my face every so often makes my skin feel softer and appear glowier, and allows makeup to apply more seamlessly. It's also much quicker than using something like a Tinkle razor, and it irritates my skin a whole lot less. I just make sure my blade is new and completely clean beforehand! 💜

SUMMER FRIDAYS

@laurenireland / @marianna_hewitt

INFLUENCERS AND SUMMER FRIDAYS
CO-FOUNDERS LAUREN GORES IRELAND
AND MARIANNA HEWITT

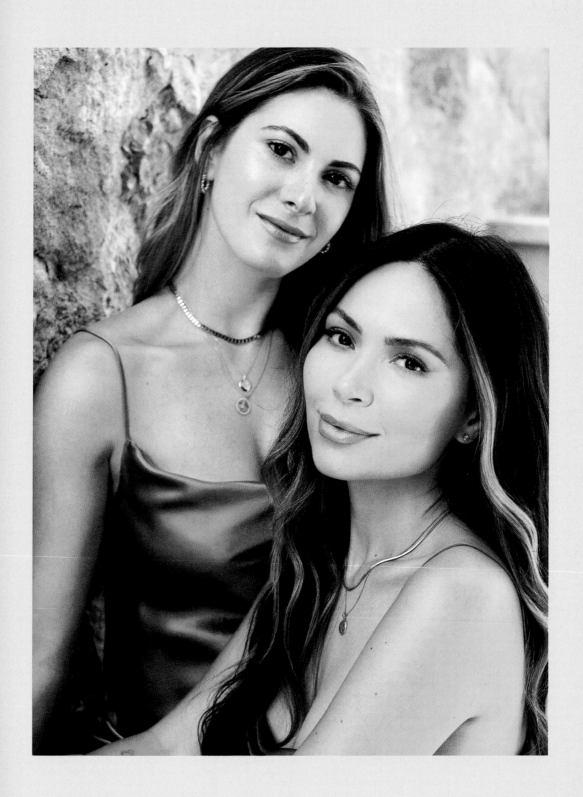

WHAT HAVE YOU FOUND TO BE THE MOST EFFECTIVE SKINCARE PRODUCT UNDER $50, AND WHAT'S YOUR BIGGEST SPLURGE?

MH: Summer Fridays Jet Lag Mask! It really is such a versatile product that does so much. You can wear it as an overnight mask, moisturizer, eye cream—people even use it on their arms and hands.

My biggest splurge is getting facials—they are definitely an investment, but it helps my skin so much to get treatments done by a professional, especially when I am breaking out. Seeing an esthetician really helped me to figure out what my skin type is and what products I should be using A.M. and P.M.

LGI: By far, my most effective skincare product under $50 is our Summer Fridays Jet Lag Mask. Of course, I am biased toward something we created . . . but it's truly a sleepy skin saver! Marianna and I formulated this product out of a personal need: She was constantly traveling, and I was newly pregnant—our skin was craving hydration from a clean, effective list of ingredients. Our jet lag mask is also incredibly versatile and can be used as an overnight mask, a 10-minute mask, an undereye cream, and a daily moisturizer, which makes it a can't-live-without product. We worked on the formulation for several months and used it to launch our brand in 2018.

As for my biggest splurge—my facials! It's pricey to keep up with regularly scheduled appointments and I admittedly fall behind, but the time and cost are really worth it for long-term results. Also, I believe in some personal TLC, and facials provide an hour off from mom/work life!

WHAT IS THE MOST PRACTICAL, RELATABLE ADVICE YOU'VE RECEIVED FOR PREVENTATIVE SKIN CARE?

MH: Wash your face every morning and night and wear SPF every single day. Oh, and don't pick at your pimples! Those are three things, but all equally important. Properly washing your skin morning AND night makes sure the products you are using can actually penetrate your skin.

I think people really understand the importance of SPF now, so I love that it is becoming a must in people's morning skincare routines.

And don't pick at your pimples— I know it is SO hard to resist, but the scarring and dark spots that come after are not worth it!

LGI: A few things:

♥ **Hydrate, hydrate, hydrate**
It sounds cliché, but drinking more water all day makes a noticeable difference in my skin—I have more glow and fewer breakouts, and my fine lines appear less stubborn.

♥ **Wash your face before bed**
My mom encouraged this from the time I was a tween, and even through high school, college, and late nights working in my early twenties, I rarely missed a night of washing my face. I think it has truly made a big difference for my skin long-term. Sleeping with makeup, dirt, and bacteria on can be really damaging over time.

♥ **Moisturize** | I think a common myth when breaking out is the belief that all moisturizers are bad—but choosing a clean moisturizer that you can apply day and night makes a mega difference, especially when thinking about aging both short- and long-term.

WHAT IS THE WORST ADVICE YOU'VE EVER HEARD WHEN IT COMES TO TAKING CARE OF YOUR SKIN?

MH: Everyone's skin is so different and personal. What may work well for others may not work well for you. There's a lot of information and misinformation online; some ingredients or products get a bad rep based on false information. I would recommend to always double-check with a professional like a dermatologist or esthetician before believing anything you hear.

LGI: When I would have breakouts as a teen, I was told to constantly exfoliate. The problem then was the lack of knowledge on good exfoliants—and they're not all created equal. A number of exfoliating washes were incredibly harsh on my skin, some even leaving small tears because they were too abrasive. It created more blemishes and red spots that took time to heal. Exfoliating can indeed be great for our skin, but I've learned it's important to find one with fine particles that don't damage your skin. This was something we spent a lot of time working closely with our lab on, when we created our Overtime Mask—which is an exfoliating face mask meant to be used a few days a week.

WHAT IS A HABIT YOU'VE DEVELOPED OVER THE YEARS THAT MAKES A DIFFERENCE IN YOUR SKIN?

MH: Drinking a lot of water and using chemical exfoliants in my nighttime skincare routine. It helps SO much with the texture of my skin and overall makes my skin GLOW. By removing the dead skin cells, my serums and treatments penetrate so much better.

LGI: Consistency seems to really be key for me—in both my routine and the products I use. I find that good daily habits make enormous positive changes long-term. The two most significant skin habits I have made are using SPF and a vitamin C serum daily (I use our Summer Fridays CC Me Serum). Sunscreen specifically has proved to be especially important—I notice my skin is hypersensitive into my early 30s versus my 20s, so I am grateful I adopted that habit early on! Plus, applying vitamin C daily has helped fight a lot of dark spots and hyperpigmentation I developed during my first pregnancy. That combination of products has been a game-changer. Oh, and one more! Lots and lots of water—drinking more water than I think I need really improves my skin's brightness.

HOW DOES YOUR NUTRITION AND WELLNESS PLAN AFFECT YOUR SKIN?

MH: More than you think—everything starts in the gut! When my friends ask me about breakouts, the first thing I think of is to drink more water, and try eliminating gluten, dairy, sugar, and alcohol. I know it sounds extreme, but what's in your gut really does show up in your skin.

For me, if I eat too much dairy, I will break out around my chin or jawline. Too much gluten? My cheeks flush red and pink.

But when I am eating clean and drinking a lot of water, that's when my skin feels its best. You can also try adding in a probiotic to see if that helps.

LGI: Nutrition and wellness play a significant part in my overall skin health. I started to develop really strong habits as I entered into my early adult life (aka, right after all the not-so-great health habits I developed in college). I started to really pay attention to how certain foods made me feel, both physically and emotionally. It's kind of wild what a huge difference nutrition can make when we pay close attention! Each person is different, but it's helpful to both track times that your skin is breaking out and try eliminating certain trigger foods (e.g., dairy can be one for a lot of us). Also, I think an allergy test and/or blood test can be super helpful in learning what nutrition is best for your personal body!

Wellness is also huge for me—and I notice a big difference in my overall skin health when I am taking care of my body. Everything is connected, so taking care of one thing within our bodies always has a positive impact on another part! Hence, positive wellness and nutrition habits tend to show up in my skin.

I will add that hard workouts usually mean a lot of sweat! So I work out makeup-free and wash my face immediately after so bacteria doesn't settle in my skin for too long. It's a simple habit that goes a long way.

WHAT STEPS DO YOU TAKE DURING YOUR DAILY SKIN ROUTINE?

MH: A.M.: Cleanser, vitamin C serum, moisturizer, SPF. Extras would be a hydrating mist or serum.

P.M.: Cleanser, chemical exfoliant or retinol, eye cream, moisturizer, then sometimes a few drops of a face oil.

LGI: I have a relatively set morning and evening routine, and I'm not one to make drastic changes that often. My skin works best with consistency, and so I try to keep up with my regular routine. That consistency also makes testing our products a lot simpler, because if I develop a breakout or negative reaction, I know where it's coming from. In the same way, I can also identify when a product is absolutely incredible, when I see a noticeable difference after trying it, because everything else in my routine is consistent.

A.M.: Cleanser, vitamin C serum, moisturizer, undereye cream, lip balm + SPF. I also love using an ice roller in the mornings for de-puffing.

P.M.: Cleanser, AHA serum or retinol (if not pregnant), moisturizer, lip balm + our Jet Lag Mask used as an overnight mask. I also love using tools at home for my neck and fine lines before sleeping.

WHAT IS YOUR WHY FOR TAKING CARE OF YOUR SKIN?

MH: I truly feel more confident. When my skin looks good, I feel good. And when my skin looks good, I wear less makeup. I still wear makeup, but I just don't need as much coverage from foundations.

LGI: Health, confidence, and longevity. *Health,* because I consider personal health and self-care a priority. I aim to treat my skin, soul, and body with the love and respect I know they deserve! Good skin starts with good nutrition, and so when I prioritize my health I am simultaneously prioritizing my skin.

Confidence, because I think we can probably all agree that we feel most confident when our skin is at its best. I think back to my tween acne meltdowns—all because a silly pimple impacted my confidence! But good skin really does boost my overall mood, and so by taking care of my skin, I like to think I'm also taking care of my self-confidence!

Longevity, because life is long! I feel good knowing that habits I develop today will have a direct impact on my skin for years to come—*well* into my future! It can be easy to dismiss good skincare when we are young, because we don't see a lot of the direct effects of sun, aging, sleeping with our makeup on, etc., in our youth. However, I know these habits make a huge difference long-term.

WHAT IS AN UNUSUAL OR SOMEWHAT WEIRD PRACTICE YOU DO TO KEEP YOUR SKIN YOUTHFUL?

MH: I LOVE beauty tools—if something is out there, I've probably tried it. It isn't so unusual now, but I live for LED lights. I bought a panel to have at home and try to do 30 minutes a day—it doesn't seem like it is doing anything while you are under the light, but after a few uses I see a visible difference.

LGI: I am all about that glow, so my friends laugh at my constant need for applying hydrating face masks, dewy skin mists, and multi-use balms everywhere. A glow makes my skin feel more youthful, so I am obsessed with anything that will keep me hydrated all day!

Also, I more recently learned a few sleep habits make a *huge* difference in how we age (it's kind of mind-blowing)! So I've made a few changes . . . sleeping on a silk pillowcase is a lot kinder on our skin and helps keep fine lines away. Harsh sheets can impact our skin in the long term. Also, the *position* you sleep in makes an impact—sleeping on your back is usually best for aging, since gravity can have its way when we side-sleep and belly-sleep!

YOU GUYS ARE THE MASKING GURUS. TELL US EVERYTHING AND ANYTHING WE NEED TO KNOW ABOUT MASKING.

MH: It is the best little moment for yourself—masks are great for addressing skincare concerns while pampering yourself. Is your skin dry? Soak in a layer of Jet Lag Mask. Love face oils? Indulge in our R+R Mask, which is exactly how you'll feel! Need help with dullness and texture? Our Overtime Mask works overtime to help address those issues.

LGI: Masking is my self-care miracle and the ultimate skin saver! I use our Jet Lag mask every night as an overnight mask, which always makes me look less exhausted than I typically feel between work and mom life.

Multi-masking is also one of my favorite skin hacks—meaning, I'll use an exfoliating or polishing face mask, rinse, and then apply a hydrating mask immediately after. It's a dream for my skin! The combination tackles dead skin cells and blemishes while also giving my skin the ultimate glass of water it usually needs.

Prioritizing that little time for yourself is also so important! For me personally, masking at the end of a long day is my "me time." It allows me to decompress, take a few deep breaths, and indulge in knowing I got through another day of imperfectly juggling my work, parenting, and home life. ♥

Dom Roberts

/ @domrobxrts

CREATIVE ACTIVIST AND HOST OF
THE UNCOMFORTABLE PODCAST

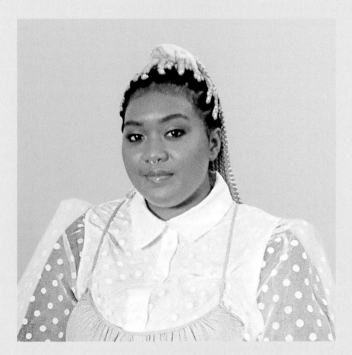

WHAT HAVE YOU FOUND TO BE THE MOST EFFECTIVE SKINCARE PRODUCT UNDER $50, AND WHAT'S YOUR BIGGEST SPLURGE?

My favorite skincare product is coconut oil. I use that instead of lotion, and my biggest splurge . . . well, I wish I spent more on skincare, but I don't. I do use The Ordinary AHA 30% + BHA 2% Peeling Solution, though. I just rub it all over my face, and it says to keep it on for 10 minutes, but I keep it on for 15. Just so it can really get rid of all my dark spots, because that's my biggest thing. Then it peels off your face. I have a lot of dark spots and I've been working on getting rid of them, so I use this three times a week, but if you just want your face fresh, use it one time a week. It's the chillest thing before getting a chemical peel.

WHAT WOULD YOU SAY TO YOUR YOUNGER SELF ABOUT SKINCARE IF YOU COULD?

Start washing your face and moisturizing your skin. Take off your makeup and stop popping your pimples. I would always pop my pimples when I was younger and started getting acne. I was the biggest acne-picker ever! Doing this creates dark spots, which is why I have some that I'm trying to get rid of now. I use spot treatments and Mario Badescu Drying Lotion, and I just try not to touch my face.

WHAT IS AN UNUSUAL OR SOMEWHAT WEIRD PRACTICE YOU DO TO KEEP YOUR SKIN YOUTHFUL?

I spread turmeric powder and lemon on my face and it creates this homemade face mask. Turmeric is really good if you have bad hyperpigmentation—it evens your skin out. So I'll just make this mixture of honey, lemon juice & turmeric powder, spread it on my face, and let it sit there for 2 hours. That might be too long, but it doesn't sting or anything. It totally evens out my skin tone.

WHAT ARE YOUR FAVORITE BOOKS, WEBSITES, PODCASTS, OR OTHER RESOURCES YOU REFER TO FOR PREVENTATIVE SKIN CARE ADVICE?

Usually it comes from a place of needing to get rid of my dark spots, so I just watch random YouTube videos, mostly from other Black women. It's really refreshing to hear from other Black women that they were struggling with dark spots or darker areas on their skin. And a lot of Black people know hyperpigmentation is one of the biggest issues that Black women have when it comes to skincare. ♥

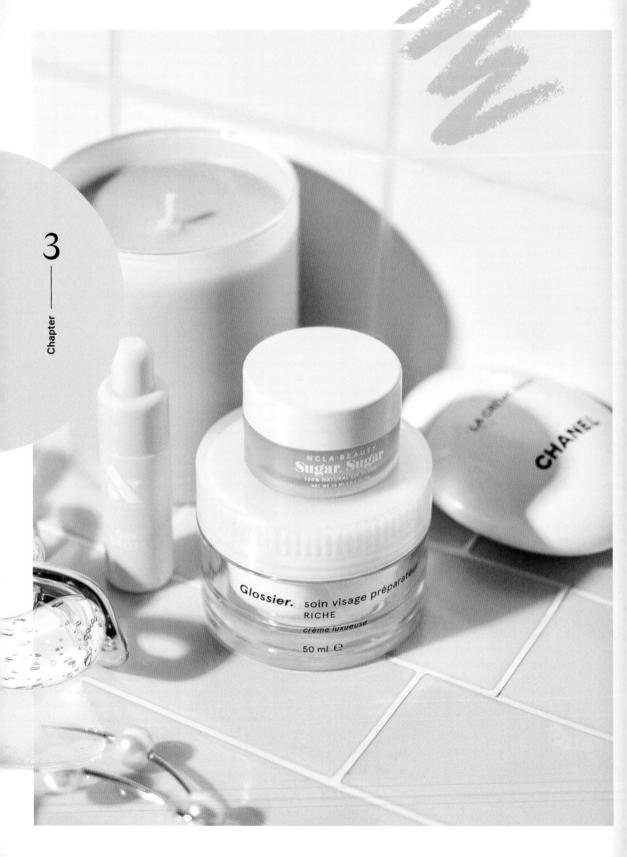

BEAUTY TOOLS & WELLNESS HACKS

Facial Massage, Lymphatic Drainage & Tips on How to Get Rid of "Wine Face"

I've had four surgical procedures in my life: an appendectomy in high school (my mom thought I had the flu . . . turned out my appendix ruptured & went gangrene. Hurt like a bitch), a boob job (two, actually), and wisdom teeth extraction (who hasn't?), but nothing was as gnarly as my fourth surgery: *corrective jaw surgery*.

When I was 13-ish years old, the dentist told me I had an INTENSE overbite, my teeth were crooked & my bite was off and I'd eventually need corrective jaw surgery to align everything.

And whelp, I was in my teens, aka too busy with butterfly Frankie B.'s, conference calling my girlfriends & boys (including Michael, my future husband, actually—we met when we were 12), so I just brushed off the dentist's warning. A year later, I got those nasty clear braces with rubber bands like everyone else in seventh grade.

High school came and I finally got the braces off, but my jaw always bothered me after that. The pain wasn't too bad, but there was a gnawing tenderness that made my jaw click when I opened it. And I felt like my mouth would never open as wide as it was supposed to. I tried banning gum (cinnamon Trident specifically) because it made the jaw click worse.

Then, after high school, I was involved in an AWFUL car accident that fucked up my neck. Lateral whiplash BIG TIME. The accident affected my jaw, too, adding more pain to the whole situation.

Then there was the grinding. Like a lot of people, I've been grinding my teeth for as long as I can remember. But not like, silent grinding . . . sort of a little like GNASHING SO LOUD it wakes people up. Accompanied with snoring. And the snoring has been described to me as sounding like "a dying wildebeest." It's not like a cute, girly snore. It's actually dreadful. Oh and hard plastic night guards? Tried 'em. I've ground THROUGH about 10 of those $500 suckers. Michael will tell anyone who listens that he's never heard someone so aggressive in their sleep. It goes something like this: *HUGE SNORE, grind, clap my teeth together, BIGGER SNORE, full-on mouth hanging open.* Chic.

Sleep is supposed to be restful, but instead of feeling rested, I would wake up every morning more fatigued than when I went to bed. Also, I firmly believe that half of my anxiety came from jaw clenching.

When my first semester at San Diego State University began, my jaw was REALLY ANNOYING. Full-on TMJ (temporomandibular joint dysfunction), grinding, neck pain (accompanied by cracking my neck 40 times a day for relief), snoring (my poor fiancé). I could chew on only one side of my mouth . . . and of course, my anxiety was worse than ever. I was working three jobs, pretty broke, and distracted by college, home life, and keeping my head afloat.

One day I went to a new dentist to get teeth-whitening trays. Right when he saw me, he said, "You're a candidate for corrective jaw surgery."

UGH.

He suggested I go see a jaw specialist, so I did. The surgeon told me the same thing: "You will get so much relief with this surgery. The overall process is intense but totally worth it in the end." Unfortunately, I didn't have health insurance at the time, so no cigar there.

I ended up trying resistance stretching (which helped A LOT), medical massage, chiropractor, yoga, the works. Nothing took the jaw pain away. Two years went by & basically I was uncomfortable every day of my life. So much so that I began to get used to jaw uncomfortableness and to accept the whole situation.

Then about a year ago, I went to my NEW, NEW dentist and he took X-rays.

Shocker, same outcome. He said I was a candidate for the corrective surgery. He explained that my bite was severely off, my teeth had micro-cracks all over them, and, without the surgery, my teeth would slowly deteriorate from the aggressive grinding.

At this point, my grinding was SO bad, Michael would have to wake me up to make it stop. And if I drank a glass of wine or 10? It was 20 times worse. It's kind of like this: Clench your jaw right now. Hold it for a minute. That's how I felt EVERY WAKING SECOND. My jaw was clenched every minute of every day, even when I was sleeping. The constant jaw clicking gave me anxiety, and the morning fatigue was getting old, too. And it was all because my jaw was crooked. I WAS FED UP.

I started to come around to the idea.

I had health insurance (that helped cover the surgery), was in a position to support myself financially & worked from home . . . So why not fix the problem? Instead of sweeping it under the rug, I decided to face it head-on.

Even so, I went into surgery SCARED. Scared not for surgery but scared because I hate IV needles. The surgery took 7 hours, during which the surgeons broke my upper & lower jaws, and moved them into the proper places to put my teeth in alignment. The doctor made all the incisions in my mouth so you couldn't see them and put my jaw back together with screws & plates. Afterward, I woke up DRUGGED AND VERY SWOLLEN. To be real, I looked like Sloth from *The Goonies*.

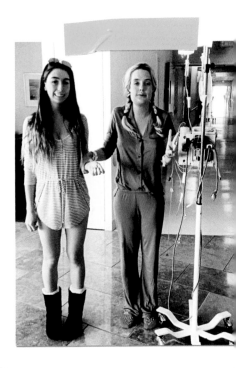

The second day, looking like Sponge-Bob SquarePants (literally), it was time to check out of the hospital.

And quite honestly, that whole first week was hell.

Basically, the second day I fainted and my eyes rolled back in my head. It was BAD. The whole week was verryyy uncomfortable. Each day got a little better, but bone surgery is just GNARLY. The whole ordeal tested my patience, discipline & mind—BIG TIME.

I was also still swollen as fuck.

And that's when I discovered lymphatic drainage.

IT. WAS. LIFE. CHANGING.

It's something that's not talked about a lot because the word "lymphatic" isn't exactly hot. It's kinda ugly & gross, in fact. But I'm here to tell you it's something you should pay attention to when it comes to skincare.

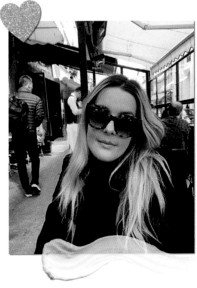

STIMULATING YOUR LYMPHATIC SYSTEM:

- 🤍 Reduces swelling.
- 🤍 Detoxifies the body.
- 🤍 Increases immunity & production of antibodies.
- 🤍 Promotes healing.
- 🤍 Reduces headaches.

Immediately, I was captivated and obsessed with the way the lymphatic system works. (This is why I dry brush, too; turn to page 79 for more on dry brushing). But at first, the thought of someone touching my lymph nodes really grossed me out.

To me, lymph nodes were sort of an "unknown" and were super tender, so the thought of a stranger touching them . . . FREAKED ME THE F OUT.

But I had heard so many unbelievable reviews about lymph drainage massages that I figured I should try one on an upcoming trip to Hong Kong. When I arrived, I wasn't feeling so hot. I'd been working nonstop, not sleeping well & definitely had a sniffle or ten. AND HOLY MASSAGE.

This massage was different. This massage was weird. This massage was amazing. Enter obsession. It wasn't a deep-tissue massage, but the aftereffects were so insane that it was worth every second.

Picture this: It was a couples massage. Michael was next to me getting a head massage. After massaging the lymph nodes in my legs and arms, the masseuse flipped me over & started on my undereyes. At this point I was so relaxed, I fell asleep, fully snoring. With four people in the room. Michael told me afterward that he couldn't relax because it sounded like a wildebeest was next to him.

MMMmm, SEXY.

So she gently massages under my eyes, by my eye sockets & at the sides of my eyes. I am dead asleep. ALL OF A SUDDEN, I AM WOKEN UP by a flush. There's a drainage detox throughout my body. It was an orgasm-like flush—kind of like endorphins running through the body. My sinuses immediately drained. It also felt like fluid drained from my eyes down into my body. I COULD NOT BELIEVE IT.

When the massage was finished, I had a full-on cough attack on the massage table. The masseuse must've known this would happen because she had a water bottle on hand. I drank the whole thing & then had to get up IMMEDIATELY to pee.

My face looked the tightest it had ever looked postjaw surgery. I could see contour. I was shocked after being swollen for SO LONG. The massage truly snatched my face.

After that, I asked the masseuse a billion questions:

"Why did I cough?"

"Why did I have to pee?"

"What was draining?"

"What are the effects?"

"HOW IS MY FACE SO TIGHT AFTER BEING SWOLLEN FOR SO LONG?"

Basically, she said the cough was a natural reaction after the lymphatic system drains. It's totally normal—it's the body releasing toxins. The immediate need to pee? Even more normal. When you get a lymphatic drainage massage, it cleans the toxins out from the underarms, legs, pelvic area & neck, and they release through the kidneys. The draining was built-up fluid. And the effects are clearing toxins out of the system while INSTANTLY de-puffing the undereyes. The massage is also known to relieve pain. The effects last for about a month. And as for how often you can get it done, she said once a month would be fine.

Afterward, I was SO relaxed in an energetic way & I felt detoxed. And get this: I did not have ANY puffiness under my eyes. You know how in the morning after you wake up, your eyes are puffy? NONE, ZIP, ZERO.

So naturally, the whole eye thing was mesmerizing because it was like a little balloon had been popped under my eyes, and the horrific swelling I'd had for FOUR YEARS had finally gone down.

BEAUTY TOOLS & TECHNIQUES

Suffice it to say, swelling and I have a long history. So in addition to getting regular lymphatic drainage massages, I'm armed with plenty of tools so I can have a home regimen, too. Actually, I spent two and a half years developing my own tools because there wasn't anything out there that I liked, and I saw a gap in the market for cute ones that you actually want sitting on your vanity. So, while products are awesome, tools and hands-on facial techniques are what really sculpt and contour your face. Here are my go-tos for overcoming a puffy (sometimes hungover) face:

ICE ROLLER

The first tool I created is an ice roller. Backstory: I was using the typical crappy ice roller that everyone else was using. It squeaked, had a slippery nasty-nat grip, broke, and only stayed cold for like 2 minutes—UNACCEPTABLE. I took matters into my own hands & decided to create a chic, solid, effective one that holds cold for HOURS (in fact, it even stays cold when it's not in the freezer). I also added a baby pink silicone grip and an indentation where the user can lay their thumb and know exactly how to hold the roller. And because I saw that girls were throwing their ice rollers in the freezer next to food, I included a pink bag for storing the ice roller so it has its own home in the freezer. (PS: The bag is also fun because you can wear it out for a night with your girlfriends, keep your ID, lip gloss, and credit card in it, then come home—maybe you're buzzed, maybe you aren't—and use your ice roller the next morning when you're hungover.)

Wait, wait, wait—we are getting ahead of ourselves: What exactly *is* an ice roller? An ice roller rolls cold all over your face. It tightens your face and energizes your skin, which gives you natural contouring. It will prime your face for makeup, freeze your wrinkles, AND shrink your pores. If you're a swollen mess from the night before, have no fear—an ice roller is here.

We've all been there: went overboard on the half-salt-rimmed margaritas, one too many slices of late-night spicy pizza, or a boozy mimosa brunch with friends.

The cure? A morning ice roll.

Here's the deal. I've been doing ice facials since Sonja Morgan from *The Real Housewives of New York City* recommended them after a brutal hangover circa 2014-ish when noble Countess Luann de Lesseps was yelling at Heather *Yummie Tummie* Thomson about being "uncool." And it was because of my brutal jaw surgery that I discovered *the best beauty tip ever.*

I'll set the scene: It's early 2014-ish, and I was actively perusing Amazon searching for a "jaw surgery book." Weirdly, an ice roller popped up.

So I was like, "Umm, yes. This will make life easier PLUS give me a little lymphatic drainage while I'm rolling it downward on my swollen jaw."

Adds to cart . . . and then shit, the rest is history.

Not only did I fall absolutely HEAD OVER HEELS in love with ice rolling, I also entered into a committed relationship with my ice roller. I use it every (EVERY) day, once, sometimes twice a day, for as long as it's cold (usually 2 to 3 minutes per time). In fact, I'm grumpy if I don't get to use it first thing in the A.M.!

If this hasn't transformed your beauty routine yet, let me to tell you why you NEED one:

- ♥ A cold massage that tightens up pores/wrinkles while giving you a kind of lymphatic drainage.
- ♥ Minimizes redness, swelling, discomfort & irritation while fighting fatigue.
- ♥ Prevents wrinkle formation & lifts your face.
- ♥ Roll it on your eyes: Puffy eyes are a bitch. This literally helps so much with any eye puffiness. If you just had an eyebrow wax? Use it on your eyebrows to fight any swelling or redness.
- ♥ I also roll it on my neck & chest. It seriously revitalizes & lifts EVERYWHERE.

(BOYS: You need this, too, *especially* after shaving.)

HOT TIP ♥ *And while we're talking about combating puffiness, for years insiders have been in on the secret of using hemorrhoid cream to get swelling out of undereye bags—and, I mean, ya . . . you can use it for hemorrhoids, too. So ice roll your face and add a little hemorrhoid cream under those eye bags and you're snatched & ready to conquer the day!*

HOT TIP ♥ *If you want some of that ice facial realness without an ice roller, just dunk your face in a bowl of ice water for 10 to 30 seconds up to three times in the morning. Models do this all the time before shoots because it de-puffs the eyes, eases redness, tightens the skin, fights wrinkles & keeps the face looking so fresh & so clean, clean.*

GUA SHA TOOLS

Gua sha is an ancient Chinese practice, and it just WORKS! If you haven't heard of gua sha yet, let me fill you in:

Facial gua sha is a massage technique designed to relieve tension in the muscles of the face, boost blood circulation and encourage lymphatic drainage to banish bloat. It helps break up fascia—the connective tissue that hugs muscles but can sometimes interfere with optimal circulation—and can even help to make your face look slimmer (albeit temporarily). Devotees swear by its ability to ward off headaches and jaw pain and brighten skin (due to the boost in circulation). Some even consider it a Botox alternative for its ability to unkink settled-in muscle folds.

—**Lauren Hubbard,** Fashionista

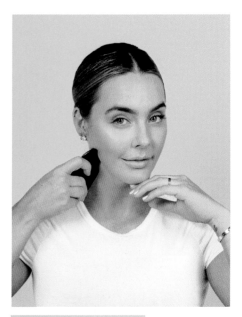

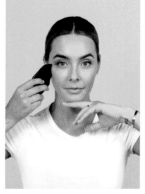

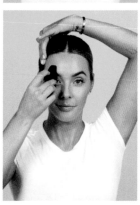

Gua sha tools usually come in jade and rose quartz. I prefer rose quartz because Cleopatra used to soak in a bath with rose quartz. Ancient Egyptians believed that rose quartz crystals had antiaging properties. Apparently the goddess Isis would gather rose quartz crystals by the Nile River and use them to keep her skin clear. Rose quartz is believed to lower stress, raise self-esteem, restore confidence, and balance emotions. It has minerals (including magnesium, iron & oxygen) that help reduce inflammation and support the renewal of skin cells. And, obviously, I'm going to copy Cleopatra, K.

To get specific, a rose quartz gua sha is different from an ice roller because the ice roller is more about bringing down inflammation. The gentle pressure and motion of gua sha also promotes circulation, reduces sinus inflammation, and is FAB for lymphatic drainage (aka getting rid of puffiness & bloat in the face). Sometimes it feels like I have lost 10 pounds in my face! When doing this at home, the key is to always work from the inside of the face outward. And ALWAYS scrape UP, never down. Don't ever pull the face down. This is so important, I can't say it enough. And don't forget the neck!! Make sure you use an oil with your gua sha tools, too. I like to keep mine in the fridge to reap all the cold benefits. WARNING: If you Google gua sha, DON'T GET SCARED! Facial gua sha is different from BODY gua sha. I like both, though.

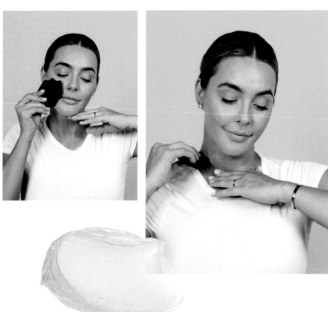

Melissa Wood-Tepperberg

/ @melissawoodhealth

WELLNESS EXPERT AND
CREATOR OF MWH METHOD

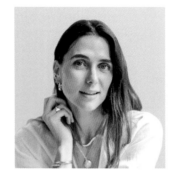

Daily gua sha. Holy. Game. Changer. This technique has made the biggest difference reducing fine lines and puffiness in my face. My face has completely transformed from this alone. I'm fully obsessed and make sure I fit it in daily even if it's while sitting on the toilet. #truth

PS Don't forget that little wiggle at the end of each stroke toward your hairline (using light pressure) to push the lymph out.

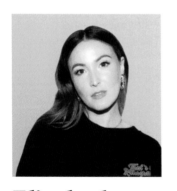

Elizabeth Kott

/ @elizabethKott

PODCASTER OF THAT'S SO RETROGRADE

Right now I am all about facial tools, and in particular facial cupping—you can find a set online for under $20. I suffer from major TMJ pain, and just working the fascia of my face releases the tension and results in increasing circulation and really activates the glow.

Danna Omari of NOY Skincare

/ @noyskincare

FOUNDER OF NOY
SKINCARE SPA IN NYC

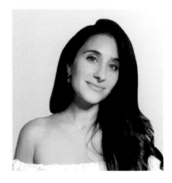

I hardly ever, ever pick at my skin. Even when I notice blackheads! It's a bad habit that often makes skin look worse because it is inducing inflammation. I would rather work on my lymphatic system to promote flow, which aids in optimal skin function and ultimately helps with the formation of blackheads. An easy way to do this is to incorporate gua sha into your routine!

DERMAPLANE/FACE RAZOR

I've shaved my face for as long as I can remember; my girlfriends and I did it all the time. First, you should know the hair on my face is pretty much blonde. Like I don't have a beard—not that there's anything wrong with that. My point is that I still shave my face even though the hair isn't super prominent. (Although my lovely husband sometimes points out a black hair on my upper lip when the sunlight is shining directly on my face . . . and then I tell him to get a hobby.)

You should also know I've tried every single thing on the planet.

Nair? Doesn't work on my face & smells too strong for the face.

Waxing strips? OH HELL NO. IT MAKES HYPERPIGMENTATION aka my sun mustache WAY worse. Really brings those brown spots to the surface.

Plucking? Who has time?

Threading? Meh.

I love shaving my face & I'm not stopping anytime soon. Have you ever wondered why men seem to age more gracefully with fewer wrinkles? I HAVE. My theory is it's because they shave their face practically their whole life. It exfoliates the skin, which increases cell turnover for smoother skin.

Want *another* reason to shave your face? It creates a smooth canvas for your makeup. Seriously, I can tell such a difference when applying makeup on a shaved face vs. unshaved. It slides on and helps you achieve that dewy glow. IT'S CRAZY HOW NICE OF A FOUNDATION shaving your face creates for your makeup to lie on. Just run the razor down the face with warm water.

Rachel Perry, author of *Reverse the Aging Process of Your Face: A Simple Technique That*

How to Fight Razor Burn

I feel like this is a question every girl has at some point in her life: HOW THE HELL DO I GET RID OF THIS RAZOR BURN?

But really, there's nothing worse than sliding into your one-piece bathing suit only to look down to see a red, spotty situation . . . Oh wait, there is something worse: when it's ingrown hair, too! UGHHHHHHHHHHHHHH.

It's such a *buzzkill*. I'm like, "Do I put foundation around my crotch area? Or do I opt for a simple cover-up? What the fuck should I do here?"

BUT! There is a fix for this—a fix that I discovered in high school, actually. All my friends got on board IMMEDIATELY. Seriously, my girlfriends passed this around like green apple Smirnoff.

It's called Tend Skin. AND IT IS REALLY, SERIOUSLY THE CURE TO RAZOR BUMPS, INGROWN HAIRS & RAZOR BURN. Whether you're a waxer or a shaver, this shit is the cat's meow. There's a full size to keep at home & a mini size for travel, perfect for those annoying hotel razors that give you the worst razor burn, you know?

You can use this on on your bikini line, armpits, legs, anywhere really! Guys can even use it on their face.

Another random fact: It also removes ink from your skin, which is great if you ever get random Sharpie stains.

As a natural option, you can also use chamomile tea bags. They always work well on shaving bumps, and I also put them on my daughter's eyes when they're puffy or if she has any kind of rash. Give both a whirl!

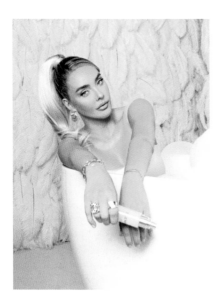

Works and founder of Rachel Perry Inc., a cosmetics company, made a very interesting observation when it comes to shaving faces:

"Men rarely get the fine lines above the upper lip that are frequently present on mature women's faces. Why? I believe it is because most men shave every day, automatically epidermabrading that area and renewing the skin tissue. Many of the world's top dermatologists now agree that epidermabrasion (or exfoliation) is an absolute must for achieving translucent, smooth skin. Excellent results are being obtained not only with the problems of dry and aging skin, but also with overly oily skin that is prone to blackheads and even with troubled, acne-prone skin."

So there you have it—no need to steal your man's razor—get your own and call it a day. Hello smooth, baby skin. Hope this inspires you to give it a try!

FACIAL STEAMER

I remember doing at-home facials with friends. We'd heat up a bowl of water & then stick our face above it to open our pores. Now this may sound nuts, but even as an adult when I'm cooking lentil pasta, I STILL DO THIS. Like the pasta is cooking & there I am sticking my face above a boiling bowl of lentil pasta. You know you've tried it, too.

I don't recommend this hack, by the way—I feel like it's very unsafe.

So now you don't need a boiling pot of pasta—just an at-home steamer. It's everything you love in one stop: hydration, skin priming, AND it helps with the effectiveness of beauty products.

The deets:

WHAT IT IS: Just what it sounds like—a way to bring the spa home and steam your face.

WHAT IT DOES: It helps clean out the pores while softening the skin, which makes blackhead extractions easier while plumping the skin. It also primes the skin for exfoliation and product application, helping them absorb more quickly. Dr. Dennis Gross has the best steamer.

HOW TO USE: Cleanse your face & then pat dry. Fill the water tank with distilled water (I use bottled water if possible). Turn on the device & STEAMY-STEAM.

NOTE: I like to add some eucalyptus or peppermint essential oils to open up the sinuses. In fact, eucalyptus is so great to use on your skin. It's good for soothing irritation, antiaging & cleansing because it's antiseptic, anti-inflammatory, antibacterial, antioxidant, antiviral & antifungal.

Now that we've gone over those must-haves, it's time to talk about one of my favorite subjects: FACIAL MASSAGE.

FACIAL MASSAGE

Facial massage is something where once you start doing it, you'll just keep coming back for more. It drains your sinuses, tightens your face, and really does give you the prettiest glow.

All muscles have the same properties. They grow when they're exercised and shrink when they're not. That's why facial massage keeps your skin so youthful. But you have to do it daily. Getting a deep tissue facial massage once a month isn't going to cut it. *Daily* to really see the difference, K?

Not only will it strengthen your muscles, but it'll strengthen your facial capillaries, too. And just an FYI: If you're worried about breaking your capillaries when you massage your face—DON'T BE. The reason you get them in the first place is that they're weakened from not being manipulated.

FACIAL MASSAGE 101

THE CRAZY AMAZING ADVANTAGES OF FACIAL MASSAGE:

- It increases circulation.
- You get a natural facelift.
- All skincare products will absorb better.
- It prevents fine lines & wrinkles.
- It will make skin appear more youthful/ younger!!!!

Jenna Rennert

/ @itsjennarennert

BEAUTY, FASHION, AND WELLNESS EXPERT, AND FORMER BEAUTY EDITOR AT *VOGUE*

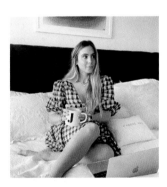

I try to give myself a mini face massage every morning while washing my face. Los Angeles–based master facialist Joomee Song (the hands behind Lady Gaga's sculpted face!) once told me that breakouts are often the result of the face holding on to excess fluid. According to the pro, daily deep face massaging and stretching can increase circulation, leading to a tighter and less clogged complexion.

Now, if facials aren't your thing, whether you don't want to spend money on it or you're not a fan of strangers touching you, I got you.

Enter the at-home facial massage.

WE ARE GOING TO GO OVER THE WORKS HERE: You can use tools, you can use oils, or you can just use your hands. Let's walk through this together.

First, I have to acknowledge one of my idols, Rachel Perry. Ever since I was little, I've looked up to her. She is the founder of cosmetics company Rachel Perry Inc. She has passed away, but her cantaloupe lip balm will live on forever (it was a favorite of my mom's), and so does her book, *Reverse the Aging Process of Your Face: A Simple Technique That Works.* I came across it in the library when I was younger. I'd sit with a stack of books around me and Rachel's was always on top. It just spoke to me. Eventually I found a used one on Amazon—torn cover and all—and I became even more obsessed with her age-reversal process. Naturally, I neon pink–highlighted the fuck out of her book, but of everything, my favorite advice was about facial massage. She talked about how, by contracting facial muscles and massaging the skin over them, you could improve both the skin and muscle tone. She also argued that good circulation is the most important factor for having a young-looking face, because it's what boosts oxygen supply to skin cells—a crucial antiaging factor. It also delivers essential nutrients to the skin, which nourishes healthy new skin cells, while also releasing any accumulated toxins that are gunking up skin tissue. But what really got my attention was when she described older ballet dancers whose bodies still looked young while their faces looked . . . less so. Basically, all that muscle toning they'd done for their bodies had kept them rejuvenated—so, if you could do it for your body, why not also do it for your face?

When You Want to Call in an Expert

If you're not into DIY, or you want to change things up, you'll want to bring in a facialist to help with your massage efforts. If you're like me, you're a huge enthusiast of getting facials. It's the most productive hour of my day when I get one. I can lie there uninterrupted while I get my face massaged and work at the same time. And personally, I would rather spend money on skin than clothes & handbags.

Find someone you vibe with. Meaning you need to find someone who has energy that you like. That's number one. They're touching your face and in your space. A facialist who doesn't want to talk your ear off and lets you have YOUR TIME is ideal—talk if you want, work if you want, be quiet if you want.

Once you find a vibey facialist, what you want to do is micromanage the situation in a polite way. There's nothing wrong with knowing what you want in life. That doesn't make you a bitch.

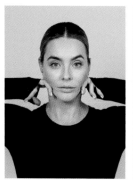
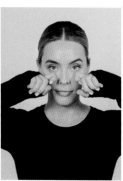
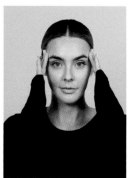
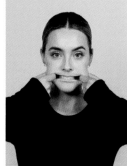

I travel a lot, and when I do, I tend to swell (thanks jaw surgery). So I'm constantly meeting new facialists and describing to them exactly what I need.

Here are some tips and tricks for perfecting your facial:

💜 Really emphasize *facial* massage to whoever is doing your lymphatic drainage or facial. You need to drive home this point because sometimes you can say it & they'll only do the face for 5 minutes. Sometimes it's fun to throw a little scalp massage request in there, too, if your hair hasn't been freshly washed.

💜 Tons of facial massage is the way to go—up the face & down the neck (it's really important to go down the neck because you want to drain all the fluid they're moving from your face).

💜 Ask for brightening & tightening products, please & thank you.

💜 Gua sha tools, a jade roller, or cups for facial cupping are always welcome if avail.

💜 Ask your facialist to use anything that's cold, too. Ice globes, an ice roller, or a cryotherapy facial really gets me going.

💜 It also feels so good when they heat your face up & cool it down at the end, but MOSTLY just ask them to focus on lymphatic drainage—that means under the eyes & all around the face to rid you of puffiness.

When you walk in with 5 pounds of bloat in your face and walk out looking like Kim K. circa 2019, that's an ideal facial lymphatic drainage massage.

It's a huge bonus if they have relaxing oils, crystals & nice music. It's important you like your environment, so scope it out.

BEAUTY TOOLS & WELLNESS HACKS

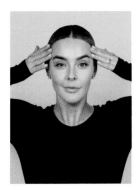 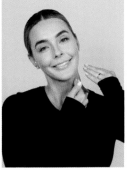

THE CASE FOR
SPEAKING UP

Mimi Bouchard

/ @mimibouchard

CREATOR OF MIMI METHOD AND HOST OF *THE MIMIBEE* PODCAST

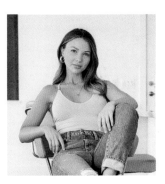

I once went for a facial somewhere in London and let the woman do whatever she wanted to my skin. I trusted her because it was an upscale spot, so I didn't really ask what she was doing. As an influencer, I was getting this facial for free, so it's not like I had booked something specific. She ended up doing two different peels and a hydro facial, then manually picking my skin and popping whatever she could find. My skin is pretty sensitive, so this was disastrous! I left the salon with red marks and intense swelling all over my face. I ended up having scarring on my chin and around my mouth area for over a year after the appointment. So the lesson here is always ask what your facialist has planned. Ask them what they're doing and why. Let them know if you have sensitive skin, and make sure they don't overdo it!

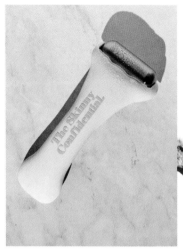

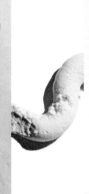

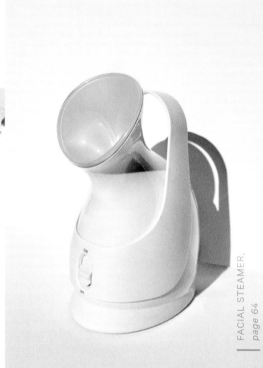

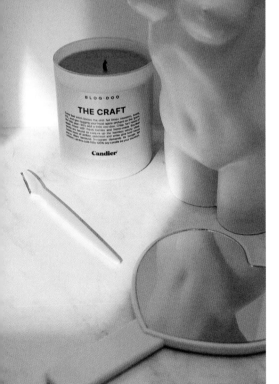

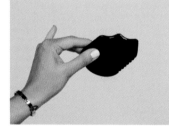

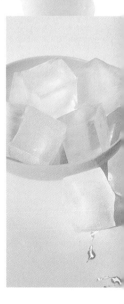

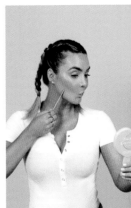

SHAVE YOUR FACE,
page 63

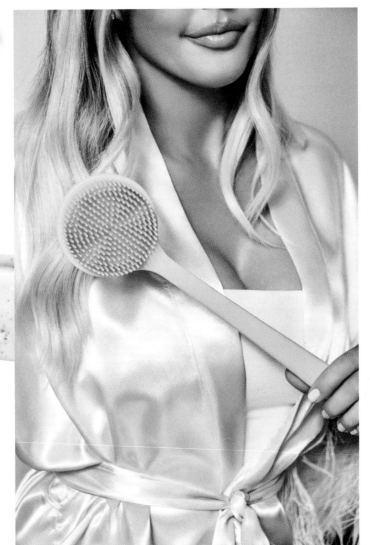

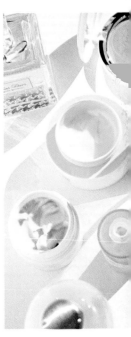

DRY BRUSHING,
page 79

5 AT-HOME FACIAL TIPS FROM MASSAGE GURU

Mo Trezise / @heal.thygoddess

Mo Trezise is a master holistic esthetician specializing in sculptural facial massage and lymphatic drainage. She is also my facialist in San Diego, and she is sharing all her secrets with you:

💜 Always start by cleansing your skin with your favorite cleanser, and also washing your hands with an antibacterial soap. To optimize lymphatic drainage during your facial massage, you can also exfoliate your skin with a physical exfoliant (aka scrub) before you massage. Exfoliating beforehand will slough off any dead, dry skin and stimulate new cell turnover; that way, the products you use following exfoliation go deeper into the skin's layers (instead of sitting on top of dry skin). Not to mention a light exfoliation will also encourage circulation, thus promoting lymphatic drainage, before you've even started massaging!

💜 Use an oil for your facial massage! Gone are the days of us using drugstore moisturizers labeled "oil-free" . . . Oils are your skin's BEST FRIEND. While moisturizers have their time and place, they are typically aqueous (water-based) so they absorb fast into the skin. Meaning they're not ideal for providing a nice slip and glide for massage movements. Oils speak the same language as our skin, and so our bodies are incredibly receptive to the healing benefits and nutrient content of oils (think about it, your skin naturally produces oil just like your hair!). So lather up your skin in some juicy oils before massaging. I recommend using jojoba oil for any skin type, rose hip for sensitive skin, sea buckthorn for acneic skin, and tamanu oil for dry skin.

💜 Massage movements should be upward & outward motions, always! Our skin can lose its sense of buoyancy and youthfulness over time, due to muscle weakness, gravity, and emotional stress. So our goal here is to work against gravity & massage away any stress! You'll want your massage movements to go in an upward fashion, for lifting muscle tone and sculpting facial features. Then, you'll want to focus on massage motions that move outward from the midline (center) of your face and toward the perimeter. This will help de-puff your complexion, as it will encourage any excess lymph to move and drain through the body. The end results will leave you feeling refreshed, contoured & oh so glowy!

💜 Don't forget the neck. EVER. Our neck contains one-third of our entire body's lymph nodes! So as you can imagine, our neck can act as a funnel. Excess fluid can get backed up in the neck if you don't massage it, too. If you massage your face and move around lymph, blood, toxins, fluids, etc., it has to go somewhere; otherwise, it will all just stay in your face (or even worse, cause a headache!). So I cannot stress enough the importance of massaging the neck before & after massaging your face. However, unlike the face, we want to focus our massage movements going down the sides of the neck only. This will help release any muscle tension in the neck and make way for proper circulation!

💜 Don't forget the décolleté, either! End your at-home facial massage with massaging the chest. This again promotes lymphatic drainage, proper circulation, and releases muscle tension. As we have such a vast, intricate inner network of lymph, blood & muscle, we can't overlook this area either for the best at-home facial massage results. You'll want these massage movements to start at the center of your chest and move toward your underarms. Making little circular motions with your finger pads or broad strokes with your whole palm—whatever feels best. As you finish loving on yourself with all the massage, take a deep breath and center yourself in gratitude, showing appreciation for all that your body does for you!

FACIAL MASSAGE ACCORDING TO CLÉMENCE VON MUEFFLING

THAT'S RIGHT, FACIAL MASSAGE IS FRENCH WOMEN'S BEST-KEPT SECRET

Excerpt from *Ageless Beauty the French Way*

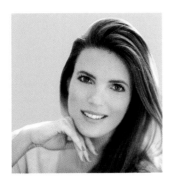

Clémence von Mueffling writes the blog *Beauty and Well-Being*. She also happens to be the megastar author of the book *Ageless Beauty the French Way: Secrets from Three Generations of French Beauty Editors*. She's truly an expert in the space when it comes to my favorite thing on earth: facial massage. Obviously, I had to get the best of the best to share all her tips and tell us why facial massage is a French woman's best-kept secret.

My friends in New York always ask me what it is that French women do to have such wonderful skin, and I tell them that one of our best-kept secrets is the face massage. This is without a doubt the single best noninvasive treatment you can do to improve the quality of your facial skin.

Facial massages tone and hydrate the skin and give you a great glow. Just as working out tightens the muscles of your body, facial massage tightens your skin. It is like taking your face to the gym! Regularly practicing these methods of molding stimulates the muscles of the face in areas that usually hollow with age.

French women love facial massages for a whole variety of reasons. First, they stimulate circulation, which awakens the complexion. Massages don't hurt; they actually make you feel wonderful. Massages are also completely manual, making them eco-conscious, and they don't need any special (or expensive) equipment. Results are guaranteed if you do it regularly and properly; and, of course, they are a beloved and well-kept secret! No wonder that the best facial-massage specialists in Paris are frequented by well-known French celebrities. They know that you'll look as if you had a mini natural facelift, and you'll need a lot less makeup because your skin will look so good.

I follow the *Pincement Jacquet* method, which is difficult to translate but basically means a light pinch around the oval of the face. Always with the motions moving upward toward the crown of the head and around the lines at each side of your mouth, an antiaging effect by massaging the skin, not pulling it.

Choose one of your moisturizers that has a smooth texture, as this will facilitate the massage and allow your fingers to slide easily. Avoid any creams that have a sticky texture or that could start to peel while you massage. Usually a hazelnut-size amount of a cream or oil is enough for the face, and another one should be used for the neck and décolleté.

A VIBRATOR...
FOR FACIAL MASSAGE

As in, a pocket rocket for my face. No, I'm serious. (This one is really for the babe on the budget, mkay!!)

I love my facial massagers almost as much as my husband, but when I was in college, there was NO WAY I would have been able to afford a skin-savvy facial massager. It just wasn't in the cards, you know?

SO I totally understand when my community direct messages me: *"I'd love to try this! Is there a cheaper version?"*

My response is always the same: *"Use your hands! They're free. A video is on my channel."*

BUT I was never fully satisfied with that response. It just didn't do it for me. Like sure, hands are great and everything, but there's something fucking fabulous about having a facial massaging device at your fingertips every day.

So I do what I always do when I'm not satisfied.

Nothing.

I sat back, waited—patience is a friend.

It's all about gaining perspective, right? When you step outside something, you can see it clearly.

So I meditated. I meditated on a facial massager hack for a month. Weird? Nothing's weird here. Me in meditation: What can I do as a facial massage hack? How can I find something that substitutes this $59.99 situation? OMMMMM.

And then? Well, I found the hack: a $9 vibrator.

Soooooo!!! Of course I did what I always do—I tried it on myself—AND SLAP ME SILLY, IT WORKS!

Not only does it work, IT RULES.

No, I'm not embarrassed to be using a vibrator on my face—in fact, I think it's a real hoot. Hilarious. I actually like it. Who cares what anyone thinks!

Here's how to use it—DIY, if you will?

♥ After you're all moisturized, grab some oils. Oils are amazing. Insane. So fab.

♥ NOW IT'S TIME TO VIBRATE. I like to massage after oils. Go around your eyes gently & all over your face with your vibrator. Go from your nose to your ear and then pull down the neck to get all that lymphatic drainage going. Easy. In the morning, use the vibrator for 2–5 minutes. (At night, I can go 10 minutes while watching *Housewives*).

♥ Then I love an eye cream if we're being real. A little more oil. And maybe even a lip conditioner, because we can't forget about the lips. Lip wrinkles are a thing.

NOTE: There are different caps for the vibrators. On your face: Use the rounded one (NOT the one with the spikes).

PHEW. It sounds like a lot of info, but once you do facial massage, you're never going back. I promise.

BUH-BYE DOUBLE CHIN

Your facial contour will lose its definition when lymph flow is lazy around your ears and neck. To prevent a double chin, I do this massage whenever I find the time:

Push the lymph fluids from the underside of your chin toward the ears by sliding your thumbs along your jaw. Firmly press the lymph nodes in the hollows behind your ears, then massage down the neck so as to drain the lymphatic waste toward the collarbones. MAKE SURE TO GO DOWN THE NECK! By continuing this technique, you will find that sagging decreases, and your face line will sharpen up in a few months.

MEGHAN MARKLE'S BEST-KEPT SECRET: BUCCAL MASSAGE

WTF is *buccal massage*, you ask?

Basically it's a facial for the inside of your MOUTH. The jaw-dropping part of the pampering involves a massage therapist or aesthetician kneading your inner cheek and jaw muscles—aka your new best friend if you get puffy easily.

It also happens to be Meghan Markle's best-kept beauty secret. That's right. It totally contours your mouth, jaw, cheekbones by increasing the production of collagen. *How do I know this?* Because I've done it 23,028 times. Typically, my facialist will do a 30-minute facial massage, then 15 minutes massaging the mouth & then ends with applying product. She gets super deep into the cheekbone area & drains the lymphatic system in the best way possible.

You can also easily do it yourself for free. Mo, my facialist, was kind enough to share her tips when looking for and getting buccal massage:

HOT TIP ♥ *If you suffer from TMJ, chronic clenching, etc., long strokes downward on the masseter (the big muscle that moves the jaw up & down) will help to release excess tension.*

> DOING BUCCAL MASSAGE INSIDE THE MOUTH IS AMAZING FOR DRAINING EXCESS LYMPH, MOVING TOXINS, DE-PUFFING THE CHEEKS, AND ALSO FOR RELIEVING TMJ.

HOT TIPS WHEN LOOKING FOR A BUCCAL MASSAGE:

♥ **Google & Yelp are your best friends.** It's hard to find aestheticians that offer this, so try finding someone who is dual licensed, meaning both an aesthetician & massage therapist! These types of aestheticians have extensive massage training. Alternatively, you may also find a massage therapist or chiropractor that offers this type of specialty massage.

♥ **Communicate.** Communicate openly with your practitioner beforehand. Express your concerns & explain what you want to work on (aka micromanage the situation); let them know if you have TMJ, or if you want to focus on lymph drainage, etc.

♥ **Tell them what you want.** Let them know if it feels like too much (or not enough) pressure, or if you want to focus more time on this dedicated area. Any good practitioner will want you to feel comfortable during the massage & ultimately satisfied with your experience.

HOT TIPS FOR DOING BUCCAL MASSAGE AT HOME:

♥ Use clean hands or even a glove to do the massage.

♥ Using one hand at a time, use your left hand for the right side of your mouth & your right hand for the left side. Enter the mouth with the thumb!

♥ Proceed to massage using thumbs on the inside of the mouth & your four fingers externally. Massage starting at the corner of your mouth & moving toward the corner of your jaw (circular motions feel best).

♥ Be gentle and slow! Take your time, start off lightly. If you apply too much pressure, you may feel sore the following day. So be mindful—a lot of stress & emotions are harbored in the jaw, so take it easy to start.

♥ If you really want to optimize lymphatic drainage, make sure to massage down the sides of the neck afterward. This way, any excess fluids/toxins/lymph that move, have somewhere to drain & flow down through the neck (instead of staying there & giving you hamster cheeks).

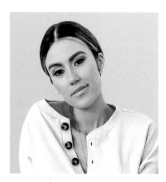

Christine Andrew

/ @christineandrew

FOUNDER OF THE BRAND
HELLO FASHION

I discovered face slapping skincare on TikTok last fall (aren't all the best life hacks on TikTok?) and have been hooked ever since. Cody always makes fun of me when he hears me slapping away in the bathroom, but it's an amazing K-beauty secret. It gets the blood circulating in your face, tones and firms your skin, and increases collagen. It is also a great way to help your skincare products absorb into your skin more effectively. After applying your serums and wrapping up your skincare regimen, lightly slap your skin in a circular motion, moving upward. Not only does it seem to wake up my skin every morning, a few face slaps help dust off the morning cobwebs, too. It might seem strange and will be sure to draw a side eye from your S/O, but add this to your daily gua sha and wait and see how it transforms your face.

Alexandra Potora

/ @alexandrapotora

DIGITAL MARKETING PRO, BEAUTY INFLUENCER, PUBLIC SPEAKER, AND ENTREPRENEUR

In Romania (I was born and raised there), there's an interesting technique of skin *slapping* that's pretty common. You're reading this right, hang in there with me! Women in my family would literally SLAP their faces after applying moisturizer (or just straight up oil in the communist days since that's all they had), in an attempt to increase blood flow. I remember looking at my mom doing it like she was a lunatic, but now I understand that there was something to it. While I don't slap my face (which I can't even say with a serious face right now) because I use facial massage, facial cupping, face rollers, and gua sha to accomplish that more gently, I do give myself a good neck slapping a few times a week. With upward movements to be specific, and never in a "harmful" way. It should not be painful or uncomfortable. Just a little slapping to increase blood flow, activate cells, and help product better penetrate the epidermis. I can laugh now; but seriously, I do do that.

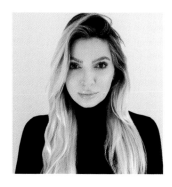

Sarah Lee

/ @sarah_glow

& Christine Chang

/ @christine_glow

CO-FOUNDERS AND CO-CEOS
OF GLOW RECIPE

SL: I prefer patting in skincare as opposed to rubbing to aid absorption. It goes back to the Korean skincare philosophy of being as gentle as possible. Fast movements cause friction, and over time it can cause micro tears in your skin. Tugging and pulling at the skin can contribute to wrinkles, so I always advocate patting in skincare. You can pat in toners, serums, and moisturizers all the way as it also minimizes downtime between steps or the wait time for the product to dry.

One example of the patting philosophy taken to the next level is the "7 Skin Method," where you pat in a hydrating toner or mist seven times in a row. It may sound excessive, but your skin drinks up all the moisture as patting helps drive the product deeper into skin's layers and skin is plumped with hydration from within.

CC: My mom taught me to gently pat the face after cleansing with the fingertips until skin was damp but no longer dripping wet. This way, I'm not using a towel that has been hanging near my toilet and my skin feels plumper and bouncier afterward.

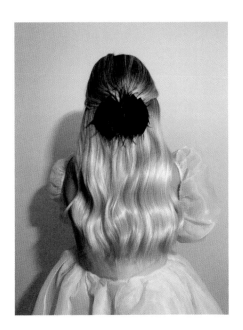

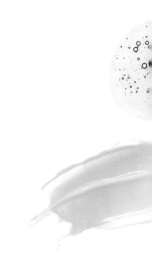

FACE YOGA

Another thing becoming very popular (thank God) is face yoga. Yes, you heard that right. Face yoga.

If face yoga doesn't go hand in hand with facial massage, I don't know what does . . .

In Japanese culture, many people are big advocates of facial massage. My husband is a quarter Japanese, so I started to get really into it. It's kinda like kegels, but for your face.

Because face yoga is SO very effective, I'm going to give you some facial exercises to do wherever you are—AND LIKE, IT'S FREE, sooooo. I mean shit, you could do them at your desk, in bed, or in the shower. It requires 1–2 minutes of your time each day, and it makes all the difference in the tightness of your skin.

But wait, what exactly is face yoga? Well, it's what it sounds like:

Danielle Collins created the Danielle Collins Face Yoga Method after a couple years of teaching yoga.

According to her, "Clients were enjoying the health benefits of yoga for their bodies & minds. I was getting more & more requests for a similar natural way for the face to look & feel healthier, too. As well as my drawing on my training [in Pilates & yoga], I spent many years researching & trialing face techniques from ancient Eastern medicine, the latest studies on facial composition & renowned well-being strategies & created the Danielle Collins Face Yoga Method, which is now enjoyed by millions of people worldwide."

Basically, face yoga is a completely natural alternative to antiaging remedies. It just works. I've been trying it. Wrinkles essentially are the end result of your face muscles stretching and becoming very soft. And your face muscles become soft when they lose their tightness, which is why facial exercise and face yoga is so important.

Anyway, here are five face exercises you can do at home.

FACE YOGA EXERCISES TO TIGHTEN & TONE

THE V

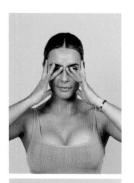

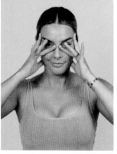

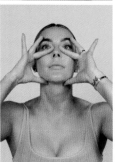

GOOD FOR: drooping eyelids, crow's feet, eye bags & puffiness.
ALTERNATIVE TO: Botox & eye surgery.

HOW TO:
- ♥ Press both middle fingers together at the inner corner of the eyebrows; then, with the index fingers, apply pressure to the outer corners of the eyebrows.
- ♥ Look to the ceiling & raise the lower eyelids upward to make a strong squint & then relax.
- ♥ Repeat 6 more times & finish by squeezing eyes shut tightly for 10 seconds.

HOT TIP ♥ *Your scalp is your skin, so don't forget it. A very famous Hollywood actor once told me that the reason his locks were so luscious is that he massaged his scalp every single day. I'm really not a fan of washing my hair (I probably do it every 10 days), but I am a big fan of scalp massage. Sometimes I make my husband do it & you can bet your ass I massage his head every day. I make sure to really get into the cul-de-sac area to keep his locks growing. While we're talking about the scalp, you should know that hairstyles can cause hair loss, so make sure your ponytail or updo isn't so tight that it's pulling your skin back.*

GTFOH, TURKEY NECK

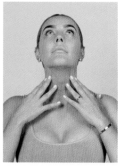

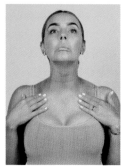

GOOD FOR: lines & loose skin on the neck.
ALTERNATIVE TO: neck lift & jowl lift.

HOW TO:
- ♥ Looking straight ahead, place the fingertips at the bottom of the neck & lightly stroke the skin downward with the head tilted back.
- ♥ Bring the head back down to the chest & repeat twice more.
- ♥ Finally, stick the lower lip out as far as possible to pull the corners of the mouth down & place fingertips on the collarbone with the chin pointed upward (hold for 4 deep breaths).

THE SMILE LINE SMOOTHER

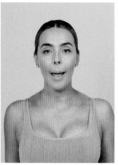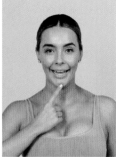

GOOD FOR: cheek lines & sagging skin.
ALTERNATIVE TO: lower facelift & fillers.

HOW TO:

- Hide the teeth with the lips to make an "O" shape with the mouth.
- Smile widely while keeping the teeth hidden & repeat 6 times.
- Hold the smile shape while placing one index finger on the chin. Then start to move the jaw up & down as the head tilts gently back. Relax & repeat twice more.

THE FLIRTY, FEISTY EYES

GOOD FOR: deep eye hollows & dropping eyebrows.
ALTERNATIVE TO: eyebrow lift.

HOW TO:

- Place an index finger under each eye, pointing toward the nose.
- Hide the teeth & tease the top lip & bottom lip away from each other at the mouth.
- Flutter the upper eyelids while gazing at the ceiling for 30 seconds.

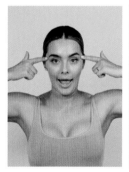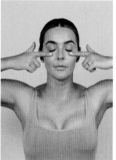

RELAX THAT NUMBER 11 BROW

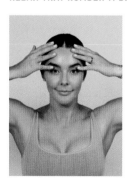

GOOD FOR: horizontal forehead lines.
ALTERNATIVE TO: Botox.

HOW TO:

- Place both hands on the forehead facing inward & spread all the fingers out between the eyebrows & hairline.
- Gently sweep the fingers outward across the forehead, applying light pressure to tighten the skin.
- Relax & repeat 10 times.

BENEFITS OF FACE YOGA

- Noninvasive alternative to Botox, filler & surgery.
- Increases blood circulation—so you get that post-sex flushed look.
- Allows more oxygen & nourishment to reach the cells of the skin.
- Stimulates elastin & collagen production: YES PLEASE.
- Creates a beautiful, dewy bitch glow.
- Tightens & smooths the skin.
- You can do them at home . . . for free. So like, no excuses, you know.
- Meghan Markle is a big fan.

Katie Maloney

/ @musickillskate

CAST MEMBER OF *VANDERPUMP RULES* AND FOUNDER OF BEAUTY BLOG *PUCKER AND POUT*

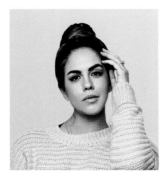

I recently have started practicing face yoga. And I feel incredibly silly doing it, but I swear it works! The one I do every night is I stand with my shoulders back and let my head up. And then I make duck lips and hold for 5 seconds. I then repeat, but this time I stick my tongue out and hold for 5 seconds. My husband makes fun of me, but it has strengthened the area under my jaw, almost eliminating a double chin. I was convinced after seeing some before and after pictures. And again, it's just a little bit of time each day that can make a major difference!

LYMPHATIC DRAINAGE BODY MASSAGE

Now that we've talked about the face, we need to dissect the body. I'm a bigger fan of the face because of jaw surgery, but body massage is very relaxing and makes a huge difference when it comes to bloating. As I said at the beginning of this chapter, I became a huge fan when I went to Hong Kong & had my very first lymphatic drainage massage.

I find the lymphatic system so interesting because there are so many different elements, and it feels like people forget about their poor little lymph nodes.

So I'm going to tell you how you can stimulate your lymphatic system. AHEM:

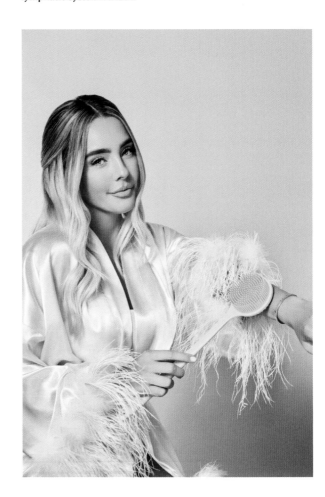

DRY BRUSHING

I'm addicted to dry brushing.

And no, I'm not talking about brushing your teeth/hair/brows/whatever.

I'm talking about your body.

This amazing, simple, and completely free practice has incredible benefits, including:

Stimulates Lymphatic System

We talked about this earlier, but when your lymphatic system is not working properly, waste and toxins can build up and make you sick. Lymphatic congestion is a major factor leading to inflammation and disease. By stimulating your lymphatic system and helping it release toxins, dry skin brushing is a powerful detoxification aid . . . YES PLZ.

Exfoliates

Dry skin brushing removes dead dry skin, improves appearance, clears your clogged pores, and allows your skin to "breathe."

Increases Circulation

When you dry brush your skin, it increases circulation to your skin, which encourages the elimination of metabolic waste.

Reduces Cellulite

Dry skin brushing may help to soften hard fat deposits below the skin while distributing fat deposits more evenly. This may help to diminish the appearance of cellulite.

Relieves Stress

The act of dry brushing has been described as meditative (especially if you do it in a quiet space) and may reduce muscle tension, calm your mind & even relieve stress. Many people who dry brush compare it to a light whole-body massage.

Improves Digestion & Kidney Function

Dry skin brushing may go even deeper, helping to support your digestion and organ function. ALSO: bloating—it helps so much with keeping the ass, thighs, and belly tight.

It's Invigorating AF

Many people become "addicted" to dry skin brushing (in a good way, LIKE ME) because it simply feels so good. Along with glowing and tighter skin, regular dry skin brushers report feeling invigorated after a quick session.

After dry brushing, I like to apply a body cream and really focus on my elbows, heels & hands because they tend to be drier areas. Then I let my skin dry before getting dressed.

Here are specific instructions for you:

1 Start on dry skin pre-shower. Go in gentle circular, upward motions, then longer, smoother strokes. You can use an exfoliant, too—have fun with it. Something like a nice eucalyptus scrub would be good because it gives you that tingly sensation.

2 I like to begin at the ankles in upward motions—think: toward the heart—the lymphatic fluid flows through the body toward the heart, so make SURE that you brush in the same direction.

3 When it comes to the back: Brush from the neck down to the lower back.

4 When you're done with the ankles, move up to the legs, thighs, stomach, back & arms. Obviously, be gentler when it comes to the sensitive skin around the chest & boobs, and avoid inflamed skin, sores, sunburns, or skin cancer. Lastly, make sure you shower afterward to wash away the dead skin cells.

FREEZING COLD SHOWERS

COLD showers are worth a mention here, too. They're another amazing way to get your circulation going.

I am not like one of those people that zings out of bed with a huge smile on their face, you know? In fact, I actually prefer not to talk in the morning. I like to think of myself as a delicate morning butterfly.

When I moved in with my husband (fiancé at the time), I discovered a little something about men: They're loud as FUCK.

I don't even know if loud is the way to describe it? It's more like HEAVY? HEAVY ENERGY? Lumbering, maybe?

For instance, is it absolutely necessary to wake up, stomp around, turn on the coffee machine like a savage wildebeest, play rap (LITERALLY RAP? I MEAN IT'S 7 A.M., ARE YOU KIDDING ME?) & put on boots that sound like 400 pounds against tile?

SO. Enter this shower trick.

This is an easy, quick, FREE (well, I guess water isn't free, but you get it) trick. AND it wakes you up so you're not a zombie.

I changed it up and made it a habit to shower in the morning—BUT MAKE IT A FREEZING COLD SHOWER.

Anyway, I came across Wim Hof. Wim Hof is also known as The Iceman. His body can withstand super cold temperatures & he is the definition of an extreme athlete. As my research into Wim went on, I found out that his wife had died by suicide after a long depression & Wim had developed this meditation to help people live happier, healthier, stronger lives. What he ended up with is a method that has amazing benefits.

Once you've finished your normal cleaning ritual, crank the nozzle as cold as it goes and stand under the water for about 30 seconds. Feel free to gasp or scream if it helps (some say it does).

After 30 seconds, turn the water up as hot as you can stand for another 30-seconds. This opens up the capillaries, increases blood flow, and provides an all-around sense of stimulation.

Finally, cap it off with one more cycle of icy cold. Always end in cold.

You might be asking, "Why would I put myself through such discomfort first thing in the morning?" Because it works.

Hot and cold hydrotherapy has been used for thousands of years. In Finland, the sauna isn't a luxury—it's a necessity. The country is home to 2 million saunas (for a population of 5 million) with 99 percent of Finns enjoying the stress-relieving benefits of the sauna at least once a week.

This little tippity-tip is also known to reduce stress, build the immune system, improve blood circulation, burn fat & aid depression.

Maybe it sounds crazy, but it works for me.

Sometimes I just say "fuck it" and do only cold. Like FREEZING cold for 3 straight minutes—this is really for when I want to shake my ass into gear. I will do Wim Hof's 10-minute breathing exercise and do a FREEEEEEEZING cold 3-minute shower while I listen to a podcast, brush my teeth (in the shower) & dance around all cold. Afterward, I feel like I did a line of crack cocaine—LMFAO. Finish it off with a slather of body oil—I love coconut—and you're good to go.

THE "THAT'S SO SABOTAGE" GIRLS

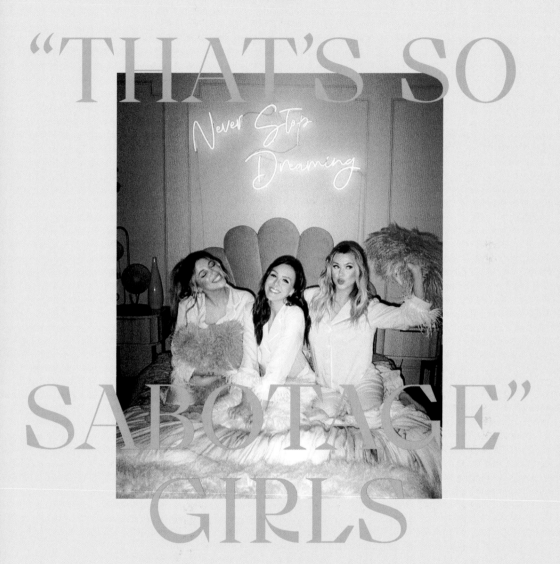

NITSAN RAITER, SOPHIE SUCHAN,
AND EMMA ROSE LEGER: A GIRL GANG
OF THREE HOTTIE INFLUENCERS

Nitsan Raiter

/ @nitsanraiter

ISRAELI FASHION, BEAUTY, AND LIFESTYLE BLOGGER BASED IN TORONTO, ON, CANADA

Sophie Suchan

/ @sophiesuchan

FASHION, BEAUTY, AND LIFESTYLE BLOGGER

Emma Rose Leger

/ @emmaleger

FASHION BLOGGER AND YOUTUBER BASED IN VANCOUVER, BC, CANADA

WHAT IS THE WORST ADVICE YOU'VE EVER HEARD WHEN IT COMES TO TAKING CARE OF YOUR SKIN?

NR: The worst advice I've ever received when it comes to taking care of my skin is that washing it with water is enough . . . Absolutely. Not. So much gunk and dirt and oils build up on our skin throughout the day, it's imperative to cleanse it properly. I always double cleanse my skin to make sure I get every last bit of makeup and dirt off before I go in with my skincare because otherwise, what's the point? Other than that, I haven't received any "bad" skincare advice but rather a lot of "don'ts"—don't touch your face, don't pick your skin, don't forget to wear sunscreen . . . These are all still things I need to improve on, haha.

SS: "Toothpaste will clear up your skin." I think this is a quote we've all heard at least once or twice. In my early teen years, I didn't have much of a skincare routine, so I would turn to Google for fast, immediate relief on problem areas. If I didn't have the proper products at home at that very moment, I would often use whatever was lying around the house. Toothpaste seemed to be the "magic cure" for blemishes. I would go to bed with a huge glob of toothpaste on a forming pimple and pray it would be magically gone in the morning, but that was never the case. Looking back, this method never worked for me or did anything for that matter, so it's safe to say you can't trust everything you hear or read on the Internet. I quickly learned that over half my daily "tips and tricks" I was including in my skincare routine at the time were more harmful than helpful. Nowadays, there are so many great options that work wonders.

ER: "Your skin is oily, so don't moisturize your face." WRONG! Not adding moisture will actually make your face create more oils and result in more acne. Another piece of advice that I don't agree with is "expensive" skincare is the only skincare that works. WRONG! Some of my favorite skincare is under $30. You can find some hidden gems at drugstores and they can work just as well.

WHAT STEPS DO YOU TAKE DURING YOUR DAILY SKIN ROUTINE?

NR: The first step I take when it comes to my skin routine, aside from taking off my makeup, is washing/cleansing my face. I'm obsessed with the iS Clinical Cleansing Complex. Morning and night, this is my absolute must-have step. I also *love* a good eye cream. I got into eye creams pretty early on while I was in high school, but now that I'm 26, it's a critical step in my routine. Right now, I'm using the Eye Concentrate by La Mer, which is a little more on the pricey side, but have also used some amazing, more affordable eye creams such as the one by CeraVe. Let's not forget moisturizer and SPF, of course. Once a week I try to go in with a detoxifying mask as well to give my skin a little TLC—I swear by Kiehl's Rare Earth Deep Pore Cleansing Masque.

SS: I like to keep my daily skincare routine simple while making sure that I am covering all areas to give my skin the most love & attention it deserves. I start my morning routine off by using the SkinCeuticals Simply Clean Gel cleanser or iS Clinical Cleansing Complex before anything! I love these cleansers because they cater to all skin types and they leave my skin feeling fresh and clean. These products don't dry out my skin or cause any unwanted problem areas, which previous cleansers have done in the past. After cleanser, I move over to my serums, which is something I am not shy about. I have many different serums that range from various benefits and price points. Some of my favorites include C E Ferulic by SkinCeuticals, which was mentioned before; Banana Bright Vitamin C Serum from Ole Henriksen; The Ordinary Hyaluronic Acid 2% + B5; Charlotte's Magic Serum Crystal Elixir by Charlotte Tilbury & many more! After applying my serum, I moisturize. I have been using the Ole Henriksen Banana Bright line of products and have found it has done wonders for my skin. I love how gentle his products are and feel they work really well with my skin type.

ER: **STEP 1:** Remove makeup.
STEP 2: Cleanse face.
STEP 3: Apply toner.
STEP 4: Use a face mask.
STEP 5: Use moisturizer (occasionally).

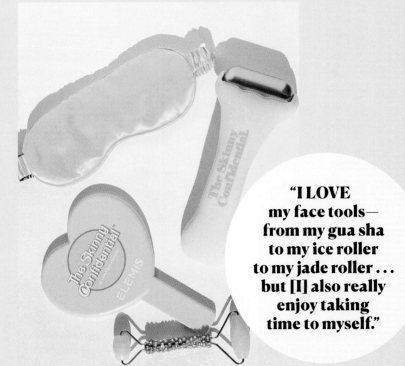

> "I LOVE my face tools— from my gua sha to my ice roller to my jade roller . . . but [I] also really enjoy taking time to myself."

WHAT IS AN UNUSUAL OR SOMEWHAT WEIRD PRACTICE YOU DO TO KEEP YOUR SKIN YOUTHFUL?

NR: I LOVE my face tools—from my gua sha to my ice roller to my jade roller, I'll try every tool in the book. I love the feeling they each give but also really enjoy taking time to myself. The method and technique behind all face tools is basically a facial massage to release tensions, circulate blood flow, and de-puff. I'm all about that! I've also really wanted to try those lymphatic drainage facial massages and have had my eyes on FACEGYM for the longest time. Oh, and I've tried a few sessions of FORMA facials, which use heat and radio frequency to increase collagen production in the face, ultimately lifting and tightening your skin. You name it, I'll probably try it ;)

SS: A couple years ago I was experiencing more breakouts than usual, and nothing seemed to work. I did some research online for some natural at-home remedies and came across the combination of lemon and baking soda. I combined the two ingredients and made a paste, which I then put on the problem areas. I noticed immediate results after washing off the paste. While I was doing the research, I learned that this combination not only helps banish breakouts but also claims to lighten blemishes, prevent and clear blackheads, and lightly exfoliate the skin. If I'm having a week of blemishes, I will only do this once or twice a week as I would a face mask and really became obsessed with the results. I typically steam my face before to open up my pores with a face cloth,

then proceed to apply all over my skin. I leave it on for about 10 minutes as it begins to tighten and flake off. Next, you can begin to wash the mixture off, and as it's slightly wet, you can do a light exfoliation from there. Some may not agree because there are conflicting opinions on this combination, so use at your own discretion.

ER: I love a good ice roller. I keep it in my freezer and try to use it almost every day! I also love to sleep on a silk pillowcase. It's super comfortable and also looks cute. Another unusual practice I do to keep my skin youthful, is I avoid frowning unnecessarily. ♥

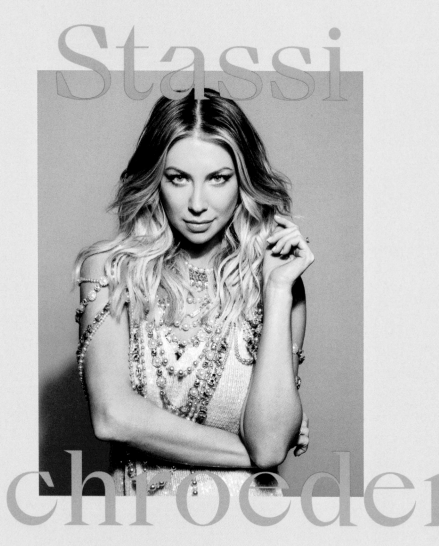

Stassi
Schroeder

/ @stassischroeder

AUTHOR, ENTREPRENEUR,
AND CAST MEMBER OF
VANDERPUMP RULES

YOU'RE THE STAR OF VANDERPUMP RULES. WHAT HAS BEEN THE LATEST & GREATEST MAKEUP TIP THAT HAS KEPT YOU SANE WHILE BEING ON THE BIG SCREEN?

Contouring my face is my number-one priority when I'm filming. I think of my face like it's a sculpture—like I'm Michelangelo & my face is *David*, no joke.

It truly all starts with foundation. HD television isn't my fave, because everyone can see every single wrinkle, every blemish, every discoloration of your skin. On top of that, I have psoriasis and rosacea—so I swear by airbrush can foundation (I love Dior Airflash and Sephora Airbrush Foundation) so even when I cry or swim in the water, that shit stays put.

Next, highlighter and bronzer. So, highlight . . . is my favorite thing in the world. I mean, I get off on seeing my highlight on camera: my cheekbones, nose, the bow of my lips, the inner corners of my eyes—I'm all about that freaking highlight. I love to use Becca Cosmetics Champagne Pop, Rihanna's Fenty highlighter, or RMS if I want a cream highlighter. As far as bronzer, I like Becca Cosmetics Sunlit Bronzer in Bronzed Bondi and I will use Kevyn Aucoin Neo-Bronzer 'til I die.

IS THERE ANYTHING YOU PREP YOUR SKIN WITH BEFORE YOU PUT MAKEUP ON?

I use a whole lot of moisturizer because my face is always really dry and I always make sure to use a green primer to tone redness, like Makeup Forever and Smashbox.

As far as moisturizers, I love Drunk Elephant, La Mer, First Aid Beauty Ultra Repair Cream, and I just bought this Origins Drink Up Intensive Overnight Hydrating Mask that I'll sometimes use during the day. In all honesty, I rotate between all of them because I never know which one is actually working the best!

I just began using Tatcha products, and it has been an absolute game-changer. My pores have gotten smaller, the redness has gone down, and my skin feels like baby skin. I start with the Deep Cleanse Exfoliating Cleanser and follow it with the Rice Polish Foaming Enzyme Powder. I splash on the Essence Plumping Skin Softener and then finish with the Indigo Cream Soothing Skin Protectant.

5   After that, I do my eyebrows just using a brow powder (Anastasia Beverly Hills) with a brow brush.

6   And then I decide what type of eye makeup I'm going to do . . . typically, I keep it simple with a creamy brown eyeshadow and I blend it.

7   I do lots of mascara and take the Ardell eyelashes (cut in half) and just put them on the edges.

8   I finish up with my lips—I line them with Whirl by MAC or Edward Bess lip liner and fill them with Heartspring's Tinted Rose Lip Balm.

And that's it. Simple as fuck.

"Here's my secret to at-home tanning: The only tanner that doesn't make me blotchy is bareMinerals Faux Tan."

WHAT IS YOUR MAKEUP APPLICATION PROCESS?

1   I rinse my face with water, no soap in the morning, and then I overmoisturize my face.

2   I apply green primer to get rid of any redness.

3   I spray my foundation on a tin mirror and then wet a makeup sponge and use that to apply it, then use Japonesque Velvet Touch Finishing Powder to set it.

4   I layer bronzer (Becca Cosmetics Bronzed Bondi) and blush bronzer (Kevyn Aucoin Neo-Bronzer—Siena) and then I highlight my face (Becca Cosmetics Champagne Pop).

WHAT IS A RANDOM BEAUTY OR MAKEUP THING YOU DO OR USE THAT NO ONE WOULD KNOW ABOUT?

If I want to look really pretty the next morning, I put self-tanner on my face the night before. Ha ha—for real, it always lifts my mood, and I wake up feeling a little more supermodel-y than I did the day before. Really. Try it.

WHAT IS YOUR FAVORITE DRUGSTORE FIND?

Hands down, Ardell eyelashes!!! I will never understand people who buy eyelashes that are so expensive. It is the biggest waste of money, in my opinion. They always look so fake because they're so thick—and, I mean,

I'm not going to reuse them! I know a lot of people are into reusing them, but that life is not for me. Seriously, all you need is cheap-ass eyelashes from Rite Aid, cut those suckers in half, and you're set.

I KNOW YOU'RE A BIG SPRAY-TAN FAN. GIVE US ALL YOUR SPRAY-TANNING SECRETS.

Here's my secret to at-home tanning: The only tanner that doesn't make me blotchy is bareMinerals Faux Tan. When I do it myself with a mitt, I'm never blotchy from that.

BUT, I will never master the spray tan. I am always blotchy afterward. It's just, my boobs sweat, and I hate to shower it off because I like to stay orange/brown as long as I possibly can (I don't care if I smell like cat piss or not). I do have two secrets, though, when it comes to spray tanning:

1   Exfoliate before you spray tan no matter what, and moisturize CONSTANTLY when you have one.

2   If I'm blotchy and I need to film or go somewhere, I just use any body shimmer cream and put that all over it so it just kind of blends and looks like a healthy faux glow. ♥

Amber Fillerup Clark

/ @amberfillerup
@daehair

YOUTUBE BEAUTY EXPERT, HAIR STYLIST, AND FASHION BLOGGER OF *THE BAREFOOT BLONDE*

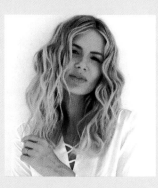

WHAT IS THE MOST PRACTICAL, RELATABLE ADVICE YOU'VE RECEIVED FOR PREVENTATIVE SKINCARE?

Two things: Wash your face every night and wear SPF. Most of the wrinkles, dark spots, saggy skin is from sun exposure, so SPF alone will help so much. It is also just really great to get in the habit of washing your face each night—not just for skincare—I also just think it feels so refreshing to get in bed with a clean face.

WHAT IS THE WORST ADVICE YOU'VE EVER HEARD WHEN IT COMES TO TAKING CARE OF YOUR SKIN?

In my 20s, I remember reading an article about exfoliating and it said to exfoliate every day. So I did. Until I learned that is actually not great for your skin to be exfoliated so frequently. Two or three times a week with a gentle exfoliator is plenty.

WHAT STEPS DO YOU TAKE DURING YOUR DAILY SKIN ROUTINE?

A.M.: Cleanse really well, use a serum (usually a vitamin C, brightening, or hyaluronic acid serum), and then either my night cream or my retinol cream. Then I apply the La Mer neck cream to my neck.

P.M.: I quickly cleanse or sometimes just use a toner pad (I love the Arcona Cranberry Triad Pads) and then I apply a serum (again usually a vitamin C, brightening, or hyaluronic acid serum). For SPF, I use either a tinted moisturizer or something with SPF as the base, or I love to use the Colorescience SPF Powder Brush over my makeup. I also keep the powder brush in my purse and car so I always have it on me. ♥

GET THE F♥CK OUT OF THE SUN

Jackie Schimmel / @jackieschimmel

COMEDIAN AND HOST OF
THE BLOG-TURNED-PODCAST
THE BITCH BIBLE

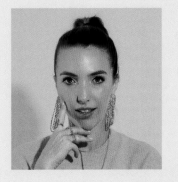

BEAUTY TOOLS & WELLNESS HACKS

WHAT STEPS DO YOU TAKE DURING YOUR DAILY SKIN ROUTINE?

I typically wash my face in the shower (I use Rhonda Allison Citrus Gel Cleanser, it is the best for sensitive skin), then spray my face with Le Mieux Iso-Cell Recovery spray (helps repair damage from cellphone blue light), steam my face for a couple minutes, apply a Rhonda Allison toner, Le Mieux hyaluronic serum, and will use either a gua sha tool or roller to de-puff. If I have somewhere to be, I will also use the NuFACE microcurrent device to give me a little contour lift! Then I apply First Aid Beauty's Eye Duty Niacinamide Brightening Cream. I then let it sink into my skin, shit gets slippery! And then I apply sunscreen and makeup while my face is still warm from steam. Extra dewy!

WHAT HAVE YOU FOUND TO BE THE MOST EFFECTIVE SKINCARE PRODUCT UNDER $50, AND WHAT'S YOUR BIGGEST SPLURGE?

My favorite inexpensive skincare product is a dry oil by First Aid Beauty that literally changed my fucking life. It's only $30! My biggest splurge is probably a very frightening LED light therapy mask from Dr. Dennis Gross that I wear every single night and terrifies my husband.

WHAT IS THE MOST PRACTICAL, RELATABLE ADVICE YOU'VE RECEIVED FOR PREVENTATIVE SKINCARE?

Don't be a crusty bitch and wash your face. No matter how many martinis you have consumed, how late it is, how beautiful your makeup looks. Get it OFF YOUR FACE.

WHAT IS THE WORST ADVICE YOU'VE EVER HEARD WHEN IT COMES TO TAKING CARE OF YOUR SKIN?

This is very controversial to say, especially in written form (Lauryn, don't kill me). People say that the sun is the devil when it comes to aging. Call me batshit crazy, but I disagree. I think a little sunshine on the face gives you vitamin D. With sunscreen, of course! If I look like an 87-year-old woman in 10 years, forget I said anything.

WHAT IS A HABIT YOU'VE DEVELOPED OVER THE YEARS THAT MAKES A DIFFERENCE IN YOUR SKIN?

Botox has really done wonders on my forehead. Beyond that, I look at my skincare routine as a stress-release ritual morning and night and milk the fuck out of it. I think taking the time to nurture and clean your face is really soothing. I love a face steamer—this is something I do religiously every day—I think it plumps your skin, cleans out pores, and helps all your products absorb. ♥

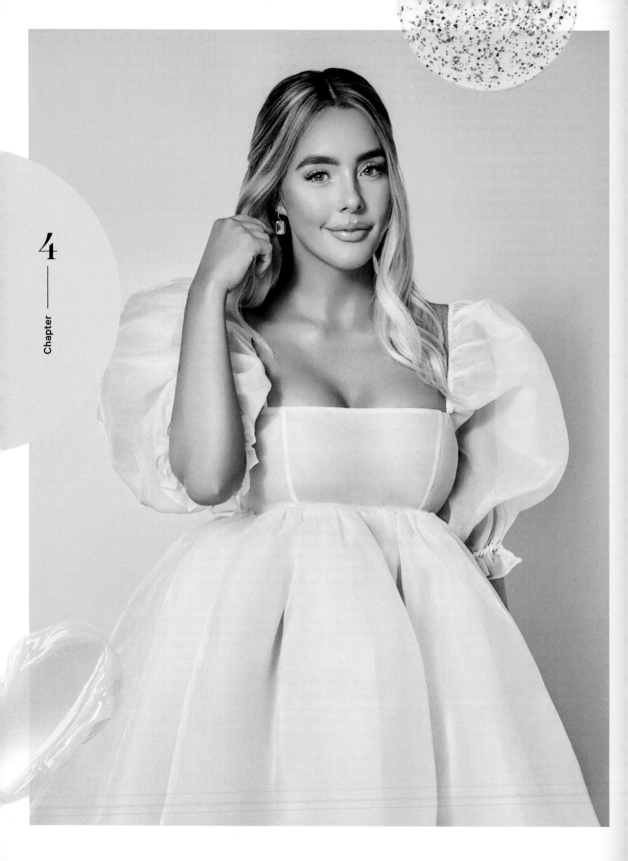

4

Chapter

I'M 30— SO LIKE, WHERE DO I START?

One of the main things I hope everyone gets out of this book is the importance of being proactive instead of reactive. After speaking with some of the world's top beauty experts and influencers, I've realized preventative skincare is the way to go. As in taking action before the problems start.

This means—not to be a mom here—*not* falling asleep drunk with makeup on, protecting your skin from the sun, dealing with discoloration, wearing hats, and other little tips & tricks that we'll get into.

Alright, now it's time to get into the nitty-gritty of how to tackle preventative beauty like a badass.

SEQUENCE MATTERS

After picking Dr. Dennis Gross's brain, I've realized that sequence very much matters. For instance, you don't want to apply a serum after a moisturizer.

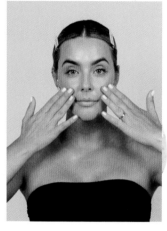
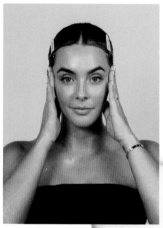

1 CLEANSE

This is going to get rid of all your makeup. I like to cleanse with an oil & right after cleansing, I like to rub more oil on my eyes to get rid of any residue.

2 MIST

I like to mist right when I wake up or after I cleanse at night. You could also use an essence, which will hydrate and nourish the skin, too.

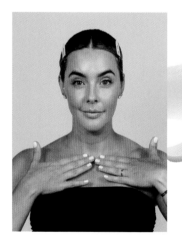

HOT TIP *Buy yourself two lazy Susans for your bathroom. On one side of your sink, fill your lazy Susan with all your A.M. skincare. On the other, your P.M. skincare. Everything will be seamlessly organized, so if you come home buzzed off wine, it'll be easy (& you'll remember) to take off your makeup.*

3 SERUM

You want to apply serum before moisturizer and eye cream so it really sets in and nourishes the skin.

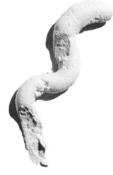

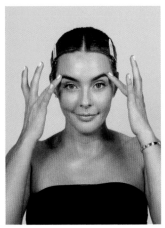
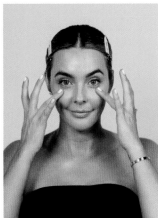

4 EYE CREAM

Always apply your eye cream with your ring finger. Here's the deal: The ring finger is the weakest/softest finger, so you want to use it under your eyes for very delicate movements. Always go in an upward direction, because you never want to pull your skin down. I am very, very psycho about this (just on a tangent here: so much so that I don't even like to lay my face in the massage hole when getting a massage. That's right: I ask for them to lay me on my back for the entire massage).

5 MOISTURIZER

Moisturizers are thicker and heavier and most likely to be designed to absorb over the course of several hours, so that's why you want to end with them. During the day, I like to use a moisturizer with SPF in it to keep things super simple. Think of a moisturizer like a protective coating on the skin. Kind of like frosting for a cupcake.

6 OIL

This is the thickest product. If you end up putting it on before your serum, your serum won't absorb as well into the skin. Apply oil after moisturizer for that glowy look we all want.

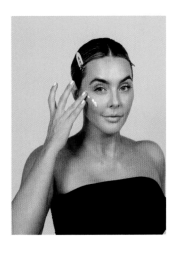

7 SUNSCREEN

Again, you can mix your moisturizer with your sunscreen, and if you don't want to do that, just apply a thin layer after you moisturize. I like to apply mine with a damp Beautyblender. It creates this perfect, dewy look & you'll never go back to a dried-up crusty makeup sponge.

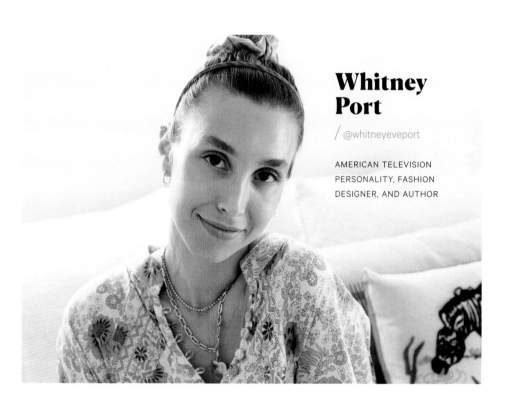

Whitney Port

/ @whitneyeveport

AMERICAN TELEVISION
PERSONALITY, FASHION
DESIGNER, AND AUTHOR

GET THE F♥CK OUT OF THE SUN

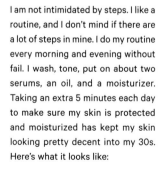

I am not intimidated by steps. I like a routine, and I don't mind if there are a lot of steps in mine. I do my routine every morning and evening without fail. I wash, tone, put on about two serums, an oil, and a moisturizer. Taking an extra 5 minutes each day to make sure my skin is protected and moisturized has kept my skin looking pretty decent into my 30s. Here's what it looks like:

1 CLEANSE & EXFOLIATE TOGETHER
2 TONE
3 SERUM
4 OIL
5 MOISTURIZER
6 EYE CREAM
7 MIST

Charlotte Cho

/ @charlottejcho

ESTHETICIAN, AUTHOR, CO-FOUNDER OF SOKO GLAM, OWNER/CREATOR OF THEN I MET YOU

Most people know me for coining the viral term "the 10-step Korean skincare routine," which was a great way to educate people on the steps in a routine and what they do. It became viral because people started doing multi-steps in their routine and saw their skin become glowy, dewy, clear, and bouncy. While there are no rules about using 10 steps, investment in consistent core steps in your routine works—and the results really speak for themselves.

The idea of the Korean 10-step skincare routine is to carefully pick and choose products that are going to give maximum benefit, and every step has a purpose—cleanse, prep, treat, and protect. It's about having the right products that are doing the right things and using them in the right order.

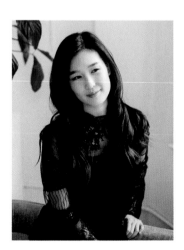

CLEANSE
1 OIL CLEANSER—Then I Met You Cleansing Balm
2 WATER-BASED CLEANSER—Then I Met You Soothing Tea Cleansing Gel

PREP
1 TONER—Then I Met You Birch Milk Refining Toner
2 EXFOLIATOR—Klairs Youthful Glow Sugar Mask (physical exfoliation) or Dr. Oracle Peeling Sticks (chemical exfoliation)

TREAT/NOURISH
1 ESSENCE—Then I Met You The Giving Essence
2 SHEET MASK—#17vDerma PibuWang Mask
3 SERUM/AMPOULE—Neogen Real Vita C Powder Lemon
4 EYE CREAM—Acwell Brightening Licorice Eye Cream

PROTECT
1 MOISTURIZER—Good (Skin) Days On the Bright Side Moisturizer
2 SUNSCREEN—Thank You Farmer Sun Project Light Sun Essence

HOT TIP *If anyone balks at the idea of a multi-step skincare routine, ask them how many steps they have when putting on their makeup. Even for a light makeup user like myself, I use about 6–7 makeup steps. General rule of thumb: We should invest the same amount of time that we put on our face to take it off.*

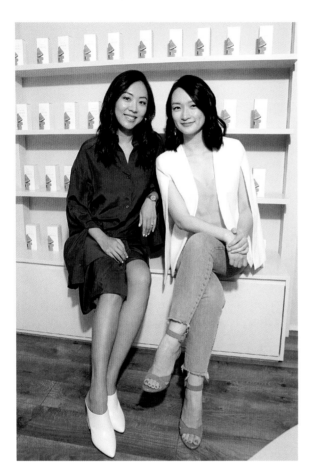

Sarah Lee
/ @sarah_glow
Christine Chang
/ @christine_glow

CO-FOUNDERS AND CO-CEOS OF
GLOW RECIPE

SL: Rather than focusing on the number of products used to layer in a skincare routine, what's important is to listen to your skin and to customize your routine based on how your skin feels that day. It's all about empowering yourself to pick & choose the right routine from your "skincare wardrobe" to treat and pamper your skin every day—because no one day is the same. "Skincare wardrobe" is a term we use to refer to a range of products that you can mix and match with your skin's "mood" that day.

CC: Korean women don't rigidly adhere to a set routine or count skincare steps. It's more about having an open dialogue with your skin and feeling empowered to pick & choose the treatments that you need that day from your "skincare wardrobe." On some days, I will double cleanse my face, then use a toner, then a cocktail of two serums and a moisturizer. On other days, I will foam cleanse, then slather on a sleeping mask and go straight to bed. Growing up in Korea, I loved watching my mom sometimes take some green tea powder, honey, and yogurt and whip up a DIY face mask, just because she felt like it. Her fluid, easy approach to skincare has always inspired me, and I firmly believe that your skincare routine ultimately has to work for your personal needs and lifestyle.

Erika Costell

/ @erikacostell

MODEL, SINGER/
SONGWRITER,
AND YOUTUBER

The steps I take, NO MATTER what, every day are cleanse, ice, tone, hyaluronic acid, serum, moisturizer, and sunscreen. If I'm feeling a little extra, I will add in more serums, masks, and a nice steam. I really enjoy doing skincare, especially at night—I easily spend 20–30 minutes on it, and there is NEVER a night I miss my skincare routine . . . I can be out until 4 A.M. and will STILL come home and act like I'm in my own little spa.

Some of my favorite serums/extra fun products are:

Glow Drops/Calming Serum from Dr. Barbara Sturm, Pollution Defense Booster from 111Skin, and literally ANY of the 111Skin face masks . . . they are a little pricey compared to other masks, but they literally save my skin, especially during traveling.

I have also recently discovered a new brand called Aloe Attiva, and I SWEAR its Waterless Face Serum and 3D Power Hydrator Waterless Face Cream have changed my life—that face cream at night is the absolute best.

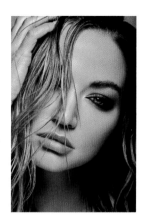

Jill Dunn and Carlene Higgins

/ @breakingbeauty

CO-HOSTS OF THE PODCAST
BREAKING BEAUTY

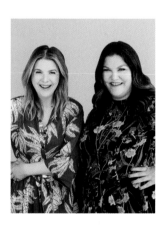

JILL: I believe a thorough cleansing routine is the foundation of a great and effective skincare routine—because when you have clean skin, you'll have fewer breakouts, and the active ingredients in your serums, moisturizers, etc., will actually be absorbed into the skin and do what they're designed to do. Double cleansing your skin at nighttime is truly game-changing. I started making it part of my routine about 10 years ago, and I believe everyone—any age and any skin type—can benefit from it. I personally saw a huge difference in my skin. The oil-cleansing first step makes a lot of sense because like attracts like, so the oil is able to dissolve dirt, long-wear makeup, and sunscreen so much more effectively—it almost "pulls" it from your pores. A couple of oil cleansers that I really like are the DHC Cleansing Oil and the Dermalogica Precleanse. To apply, just pump a few drops on dry skin and massage it all over your face for at least 60 seconds. Then wet your hands and continue to massage your face to melt away the dirt and oil, then fully rinse. The second

step should be a low pH cleanser; because I have oilier skin, I tend to like a gel-based cleanser—two that I love are Dermalogica Special Cleansing Gel and the CosRx Low pH Good Morning Gel Cleanser. Typically I reserve double cleansing for my nighttime routine, and in the A.M., I'll simply use a micellar cleansing water.

CARLENE: A habit that's made a big difference in my skin is using toners, and I'm not talking about the alcohol kind. (The old-school ones stripped away every speck of oil and were terrible for skin.) When I first learned about skincare "essences" and "waters" that came out of the Japanese and Korean skincare wave several years ago, I thought they were gimmicky. But these toners have smaller molecules that penetrate skin to deeply hydrate. My skin feels dewier and softer instantly. Shiseido and Clé de Peau are my ultimate favorites. In Japan and Korea, they believe hydration is the key to beautiful skin no matter what your skin type is, and I've pretty much adopted that approach.

SPRITZY SPRITZ. MIST IT UP.

Do you mist? IF YOU DON'T MIST—WHAT IS HAPPENING?! WE NEED TO GET EVERYONE ON BOARD WITH A MIST. Why? Because there's nothing better.

Mists are underrated. Mists tone the skin, set makeup & act as an on-the-go serum to hydrate the skin. Everyone in Korea sprays mists on their faces—I'm telling you, girls on the street do this ALL THE TIME. When your skin is lacking moisture, the protective barrier becomes weaker—this essentially means collagen is breaking down faster. With the extra moisture in a mist, you slow that breakdown. It's the best when you're traveling. I keep one in my purse. It's a coconut rose mist—super refreshing. Also makes the skin shiny in the best way possible.

HOT TIP *SPRITZER LIFE! Wanna make a quick, easy spritz? Simply fill a bottle with chilled chamomile tea. The chamomile helps calm the skin while the water keeps your skin hydrated. Cindy Crawford's secret trick is to mix a bottle of equal amounts of milk and water to use throughout the day. Even celebrity facialist Sonya Dakar RAVES about milk on the face because it balances the pH. HOW FUN!*

It's so my thing.

It smells good & is SUPER refreshing.

Misting yourself midday while you're walking to grab coffee—there's something excessive about it. But like, excessive in the best, bougie way—and you're getting hydration, so it's a real win-win.

I mist after my skincare routine every night. But I also mist midday when I have makeup on. Either works.

That's the great thing about a mist, you know? You can use it whenever you want. Carry it in your handbag or display it proud next to your perfumes.

After a while, your boyfriend will start misting, too—I'm telling you, he will become jealous. So just expect it & embrace it.

EVERYONE wants to mist! Just close your eyes & SPRAY AWAY.

But don't forget your neck. And hands can be fun.

A lot of mists contain rosewater, which has anti-inflammatory properties that can help combat red or irritated skin, acne, dermatitis & eczema. It is cleansing and aids in removing oil & dirt that accumulate in the pores.

TO USE: Simply close your eyes & spritzy spritz a couple of times . . . but don't forget your neck, or your tits.

MEET SERUM.
YOUR OTHER NEW BF:

When it comes to serums, I tend to reach for clean beauty—products without parabens, sulfates, and phthalates—because you put a serum on your face every single day & it's what's really going to nourish your skin. It's made up of these cute little molecules that penetrate into the skin and deliver a VERY high concentration of active ingredients, aka great for preventing wrinkles—which we love. Find a good one that's made with vitamin C— which keeps your skin looking radiant—plus collagen, and maybe even some amino acids. It's worth the hype & the investment.

Since I had Zaza, I've realized the number-one thing I'd add to her skincare routine when she's older is a good serum.

HOW TO APPLY:
- Wash or exfoliate (I like to exfoliate about three times a week) before you apply serum.
- THIN SERUM: 1 drop before applying.
- THICK SERUM: 3–5 drops before applying.
- Gently tap skin for 30–60 seconds until the serum is absorbed.
- Wait about a minute before applying your moisturizer.

I use a couple drops at night before using a night cream. In the morning, I hardly ever cleanse my face so I can keep on the oils, serums & moisturizers from the night before.

GET THE F♥CK OUT OF THE SUN

OILS. LOAD IT UP.

Oils are the secret to youth, if you ask me. As you read in chapter 1, I became OBSESSED with putting olive oil all over my body after reading an article on Korean skincare when I was young.

. . . And so began a love affair.

You should know that I've been known to order a side of olive oil from room service when I travel to remove makeup & cure dry airplane skin.

But I have to say, one of my favorite oils is organic grapeseed oil.

Every girl should have it on hand, and you can easily find it at the supermarket. I like to source mine from Italy or France if I can; if I can't, no big deal, I just go to Vons. You want to get one that's organic, cold-pressed, and in a huge-ass bottle. You can put it all over your body for that glow; it makes your spray tan look amazing (people think it makes your tan come off, but I always use oil after day 2 of my spray tan); you can put it on your collarbones for a pop, your stomach for stretch marks. On your face— it kind of does everything. It's one of the best makeup removers you can get and has so many benefits: It's moisturizing, contains vitamin E, doesn't clog pores, is great for sensitive skin, tightens pores & reduces the appearance of scars. And it smells good!

HOW TO APPLY: Put a few drops of oil in your hands and rub them together to warm them up. Then, gently pat them on your face. Make sure you aren't rubbing products on your face—a nice PRESS works great.

TO REMOVE MAKEUP: Pour some on a cotton pad & wipe your makeup off. Sometimes I just use my hands without a cotton pad. To be honest, it's usually just my hands, but if you insist on being bougie, do the cotton pad. Do what works, but OIL IT UP.

HOT TIP *If you do use an eye makeup remover, always look for one that's oil- or water-based and gentle. Your eye area is really sensitive, and some removers cause stinging. Oil ones tend to be better around the eyes. As I said, I like to use straight-up grapeseed oil or any other cold-pressed oil to remove all my makeup.*

GET A FACIAL. OFTEN.

We got into my deep facial love in chapter 3, but I'll say it again: Facials (and the massage that comes with them) are essential for keeping up with youthful, plump, dewy skin. I don't think they're a luxury—shocking, I know. Like, not at all really. In fact, to me—they're a necessity. I like a facial once a week.

Hear me out before you judge.

I like them once a week because I don't really care about spending money on shoes, handbags, or belts. I care about spending money on *my skin*. Your skin is with you for your entire life. That handbag that goes out of style in a year BORES me. Do I care about having the latest shoe if my skin looks dry? Oh & the latest belt? YAWN—BUT LIKE, how does my skin look?

PRIORITIES.

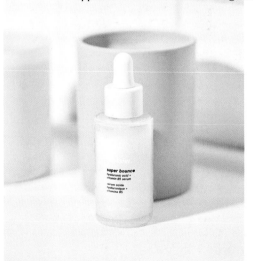

HEAR IT FROM A BOSS B:

Sonya Dakar

/ @sonyadakar

MEDICAL ESTHETICIAN AND
FOUNDER OF SONYA DAKAR
SKIN CLINIC

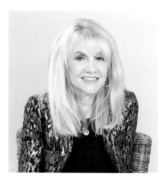

WHAT'S THE BIGGEST MISTAKE YOU SEE PEOPLE MAKING WITH THEIR SKIN?

I see people try to be their own esthetician and dermatologist. I am all about empowering my clients to be their own skin expert. I teach them how to identify and treat skin issues when they are not with me.

But I am simply referring to people in general—trying to pick at their skin, extract their breakouts and blackheads, and then slap on a cocktail of over-the-counter, overactive harsh products that strips, burns, and even overprocesses their skin. No one would dare think of doing their own dental work, so why would they do their own extractions and facials at home?

WHAT'S THE BEST TIP THAT PEOPLE CAN DO WHEN IT COMES TO FREE, AT-HOME SKINCARE?

Stay consistent with A.M. and P.M. This means using a routine and sticking to it morning and evening. It's like being on a diet and working out: It only works if you're consistent with it. You can't work out and eat a hamburger and expect your body to change. Same with skincare: You can't skip three days out of the week washing your face and thinking that your routine and your products are going to work the same.

Give yourself a home facial 1–3 times a week. I don't mean extractions by home facial. But there are a lot of wonderful exfoliators, pills, and masks available today that you can use to create your own facial at home. We get so many tips on our website/blog on how to recreate your own home facial. And you can even ask your own facialist what she personally recommends for you to use on your skin if you want to create a facial at home. But using these types of professional products a few times a week will really help improve your skin and take it to the next level. Cleansing and moisturizing is just not gonna do the trick and transition your skin the way we all want to these days. We're all looking for real results.

Never wash your face with hot water. Hot water can really deplete and irritate your skin, as well as even expand broken capillaries. It's a nightmare for eczema and rosacea as it's a trigger for the skin as well. Use cool to warm temperature water to wash your face. Also, squeaky clean is not the answer. You want to use detergent-free cleansers for your skin as not to strip it.

Change your towels daily. This one is really inexpensive and easy to do. Go online on Amazon/Target or anywhere to buy a dozen inexpensive face towels. Just make sure they are 100% cotton. And you're going to want to switch out your face towel every time you wash your face. Yes, every single time—that means twice a day. What happens is that when you wash your face and dry it with a towel, you leave it damp just like a towel when you walk out of the shower and dry your body with it. When the towel is wet and moist, it becomes the perfect breeding ground for bacteria. You don't want to use it again later that day or in the morning, as you don't want to spread that bacteria over your face again. I find that if you have a stack of face towels ready to go, especially if they're inexpensive, you could just stock up on 15 or 20 of them. It makes switching out your face towels really, really easy.

Change pillowcases every day. When you sleep at night, you sweat. Your scalp, your body, and even your face and your skin also produce oil; those oils and bacteria get absorbed into your pillowcase. It's really important to change your pillowcase daily, especially if you're prone to breakouts.

Massage skin while you apply the products with a firming facial massage. We have so many tutorials on our website, and I'm sure you could look some great ones up on YouTube to give yourself a facial massage with a jade roller, gua sha, or even your hands. It's really effective just for a few minutes for lifting, tightening, and firming. Massaging using upward strokes can be really beneficial to your skin. It helps the product absorb better, and it actually really does work to tone your skin.

IF YOU HAD TO PICK ONE HOLY GRAIL PRODUCT, THE BEST PRODUCT EVER, WHAT WOULD IT BE AND WHY?

How can I pick one? That's like telling me to pick my favorite child. I'll start with my top three:

ORGANIC OMEGA OIL: Because oils are my first love. I can't imagine a skincare routine without my liquid gold face oil.

BLUE BUTTERFLY BALM: Lauryn, I feel like I speak for both of us when I say this is the holy grail of skincare products. I developed this in mind for my rosacea clientele that was increasing. I needed something that not only was hydrating and soothing but also can protect your skin from the environment and boost its own barrier function. I discovered that the blue butterfly pea flour was a miraculous natural ingredient that was so healing to the skin. I knew I had to incorporate it into this face balm. It's super hydrating, seals all the moisture in, reduces any kind of irritation and inflammation, but most of all leaves your skin buttery soft.

JADE ENERGY: This is the sister product to the Blue Butterfly Balm. Everyone was obsessed with how it made their skin feel that I wanted to create something that would give a similar effect to the eye area—an area on your skin that craves hydration and naturally gets depleted throughout the day, and where we show the first signs of aging. We used green coffee & CBD and it really took this product to the next level. We have sold out multiple times since we launched it.

WHAT'S A SMALL HABIT THAT PEOPLE CAN DO EVERY DAY THAT MAKES A BIG DIFFERENCE IN THEIR SKIN?

Apply eye cream correctly. Because the eye area does not have any oil glands, it will naturally show the signs of aging first on your face—from expression lines to loose and saggy eyelids, etc. It's a place where we really need to focus on our skincare. I teach my clients how to really maximize their eye cream and serum and how to apply it properly. I call this "eyeglasses and sunglasses." Typically, people would apply cream right under the eye area in one quick swipe and that's it. But that doesn't really cover all the area around your eye that really shows all the signs of aging. Instead, start with some product using your ring finger and start at the inner corner of your eye on the bottom and apply it all the way out toward your hairline. Then apply again on the inner corner of your eye above your eyebrows, meeting at that hairline: one big circle like a big pair of Jackie O sunglasses. This is going to cover the area called your 11s in between your eyebrows, as well as under the eye and the outside area of the eye where you see expression lines. The next step is eyeglasses: You're going to go in again at the inner corner of your eyes, right underneath the eyes, and then take some more product and apply it to your eyelid and give yourself a massage. This is going to treat the dark circles under your eyes, the puffiness, the bags, as well as the droopy skin on your eyelids. This simple technique takes just 30 seconds, and you'll see a huge difference in how your eye products work so much better for you.

IF YOU WERE ASKING FOR A FACIAL AT A RANDOM SPA, HOW WOULD YOU MICROMANAGE IT, AND WHAT WOULD YOU ASK FOR? BE AS SPECIFIC AS POSSIBLE!

You must know me so well. Can you imagine me lying in another spot getting a facial? I love teaching aestheticians and guiding them and being their mentors, but it's hard for me to lie down and actually receive the treatment myself. But here goes . . .

First of all, I would inspect all equipment. I want to make sure that I am familiar with all the equipment they have in the room and what they're about to use on me. If I have any questions, I want to be able to ask them before I lie down, and also if I have any tips, tricks, or techniques with any specific equipment, I'd love to show them ahead of time. It's not about putting anyone down, it's just about teaching them how to make their equipment work even better and helping improve their own skills with some great techniques.

I would kindly and respectfully ask that they use my own products because I don't want to risk any reaction. I would ask for a mirror to see what they are doing. I would teach them how to do extractions before they start—being gentle is the key.

No strong peels—I don't believe in strong peels, and my skin doesn't react well to them. I don't like harsh acids that overstrip the skin. I would bring my own just in case and ask that they use it.

I would ask for a hydrating calming facial and LED lights. I'm a huge fan of LED red and blue and amber. I think they're so incredibly healing, and I would definitely request that treatment.

I also love a good lymphatic drainage massage, specifically focused on the neck and jawline.

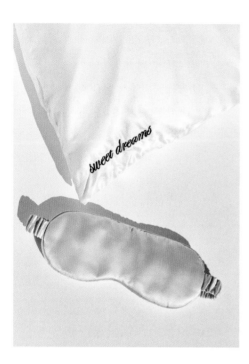

SUNSCREEN

We went over this in chapter 2, but I can't talk about it enough. A quick TSC checklist for you:

- 💜 Do you have a hat in your car or handbag?
- 💜 Did you order pink driving gloves?
- 💜 Did you mist sunscreen all over your body?
- 💜 Did you remember your eyelids?

BONUS: Tint your windows and close the sunroof.

HOW TO APPLY SUNSCREEN LIKE A BOSS:

- 💜 Instead of a huge glob on your hands, try a few dots of sunscreen directly on your face.
- 💜 Apply at least 30 minutes before going back into the sun.
- 💜 Like I said in chapter 2, apply with a damp Beautyblender. Just do it.

SILK PILLOWCASE (AND SILK EYE MASK IF YOU'RE FEELING BOUGIE)

Silk pillowcases have been my jam for a while. But last year when we moved, somehow my silk pillowcase disappeared. I went without one for a couple months and, you guys, it was like night & day—I could not believe my skin & my hair was more dry (like waaaaaaay drier), and I wasn't sleeping well anymore. My hairstylist even mentioned that she noticed I wasn't sleeping on a silk pillowcase.

If you're unfamiliar with a silk pillowcase, the benefits include:

- 💜 Hypoallergenic, naturally—resistant to the accumulation of mold, dirt & other allergens that could be playing a role in any skin problems.
- 💜 Smooths the face—you'll wake up looking fresh instead of having pillowcase marks imprinted on your face.
- 💜 Doesn't absorb moisture—this prevents bacteria & odor on your pillowcase & also keeps hydration in your skin.
- 💜 Good for your hair—see ya later rat's nest & split ends.
- 💜 Great for any climate—Aspen or Palm Springs, you'll be good.
- 💜 Silk is natural; it's spun by silkworms—the fabric contains 18 amino acids (which are amaze for your skin).
- 💜 Looks & feels super elegant & luxurious.

Silk pillowcases are recommended by plastic surgeons, hairdressers, dermatologists, all beauty experts & I'm here to tell you . . . IT'S NO JOKE!

The silky, delicious, buttery fabric is something everyone needs in their bed.

AND HOW YOU SLEEP MATTERS . . . I BRING YOU THE IMPORTANCE OF SLEEP POSITIONS.

Some people try to act like sleep isn't a big deal. Well, I disagree.

It's literally the foundation of youth & effectiveness. This means putting some thought into the way you sleep—like the vibes you create while you sleep & how long you sleep.

Personally, I need at least 8 hours—but like 8 & a half if I'm being a greedy bitch. And let's face it, I usually am.

I have a whole obnoxious nighttime routine (think oil diffuser is on, the salt rock lamp is glowing, my TWO noise machines are going, the lights are dim, the special blankets are out, my head is on a silk pillowcase & my books are ready to read), but I've started to pay attention to my sleep position.

If you're like me, you've woken up on certain days & seen a huge crease in your face. And if you think about it, getting a crease on your face night after night, day after day, can't be good for your skin. Ya feel me?

After doing some major research, I found that skincare experts really recommend lying flat on your back while you sleep, which I'm totally fine with because I love that position. HOWEVER, in the middle of the night I roll onto my side and I can totally see a loss of collagen in this side of my face opposed to the other side.

In fact, even the American Academy of Dermatology is a fan of people sleeping on their backs to avoid facial aging. But not only facial aging! Have you guys ever noticed that when you sleep on your side you wake up with deep creases in your chest? I feel like it also really sags the boobs & neck.

Just a side note here: We usually wake up looking puffy—that's because when you lie down, all the fluid goes to your face. I learned this after jaw surgery, so I started to sleep elevated. Two pillows instead of one does the trick.

OK, back to sleeping on your back. If you sleep with your face down or to one side, all the fluid is going to go to that area & will make you puffy in the morning. It's also going to bring out wrinkles on that side of your face.

I'm a big fan of small habits that add up to big successes, but small habits can also add up to things like aging, too. So, if you're constantly sleeping on one side & it's a repetitive habit, that side of your face is going to age way quicker.

What's even more wild is that many dermatologists & doctors have said that when they look at their patients, they can tell what side they sleep on. Which gives me even more of an incentive to sleep on my fucking back.

Also, if you have acne, many derms recommend sleeping on your back even more so, because you don't want to spread the bacteria. Sometimes, even when you sleep on your side & drool, that drool can cause bacteria to get on your face.

It's worth a mention that even Lisa Rinna from *Real Housewives* knows all about this. She never gets a massage facing down, she always lies facing up. It totally inspired me because it's so true.

INJECTABLES

We'll be getting into this in chapter 6, but for now, just consider it another option on the aging-prevention menu. Just remember: Don't go overboard. We all want Angelina Jolie's luscious lips but like, we need to be realistic. I am never going to have her exact lips. I always say I want to look like me, but an enhanced, slightly prettier version.

MICRONEEDLING & PRP

Let's get bloody!!! So bloody, I'm telling you—this isn't for the faint of heart.

Microneedling is one of those things you can do that ACTUALLY makes a huge difference. Basically, microneedling induces a controlled injury into the skin's dermal and epidermal to stimulate healing and rejuvenation, stimulate fresh new collagen for fine lines, and stimulate elastin to tighten the shit out of the skin.

Where I see the biggest difference with microneedling is with hyperpigmentation. This is one procedure that is worth every dime if you have sun spots on any part of your body or the linea nigra from pregnancy (the brown line that runs up your stomach, which in most cases is temporary).

Kourtney Kardashian even utilized microneedling for the hair on her head. She was balding in certain spots & used PRP (platelet-rich plasma) & her hair started to grow back. (We'll get into PRP in a minute!)

I've tried microneedling multiple times, with & without numbing cream. I've found that it's more effective without numbing cream. Not a lot of doctors will let you do this, but I've found that when there isn't that barrier between the microneedles & the skin, it's more effective.

People say you can't leave your house for a couple days after microneedling or PRP, but I

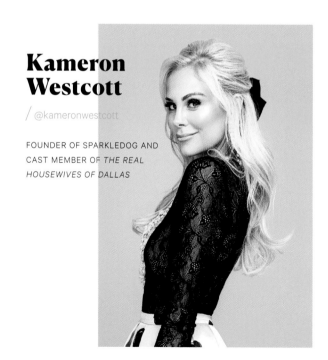

Kameron Westcott

/ @kameronwestcott

FOUNDER OF SPARKLEDOG AND CAST MEMBER OF *THE REAL HOUSEWIVES OF DALLAS*

Microneedling has kept my skin texture smoother, kept my pore size smaller, and helped me build more skin elasticity. I try to do microneedling at least every other month. Now, this is when my schedule allows this. If my schedule does not allow this . . . I find myself going to the Beauty-Bio GloPRO Microneedling Facial Rejuvenation Tool. This is an at-home device that does the same thing. It just is a bit less invasive. If you do this, I would also suggest getting the GloPRO Clarifying Prep Pads that prep the skin before using the roller.

don't agree. After my PRP treatment, I walked across the street & had a lemon, olive oil, artichoke salad & a chilled glass of rosé and I was fine. You can go outside—you're not going to look like roadkill.

My first experience with microneedling actually didn't hurt too much, but I have a pretty high pain tolerance, so it wasn't a big deal & I ended up going back for more treatments. If you're sensitive, you're going to feel it more.

If you're going to try microneedling, I recommend at least four treatments, because it makes a huge difference. Your makeup is going to glide on smoother, your skin will be plump & you'll notice a better overall complexion.

It's worth mentioning that a friend of mine did microneedling herself, at home. After, she went on the subway in New York City & ended up with a staph infection. SO, if you are going to do microneedling at home, I HIGHLY recommend doing an INSANE amount of research, but your best bet is to go to a professional.

Another thing I have tried that was totally wild is microneedling my arms. I met a jazzy aesthetician at a party and within 2 minutes of meeting her, she told me that she loved microneedling so much that she even microneedled her vagina! Yes, you read that right . . . you can microneedle your vagina lips if you want to plump them up or make them softer & smoother. This also might be a good thing to try if you have any ingrown hair scars around your vagina area.

ANYWAY! Because she told me that you can microneedle any area of your body, I immediately became interested in doing my arms. I had little sunspots on them & it was one of those things that I could do during Thanksgiving & no one would notice.

So, off I went to see this aesthetician. I didn't use any numbing cream, like a boss, because I didn't want that barrier there. She did her thing, wrapped my arms in plastic wrap & the next day I wore a huge sweater to Thanksgiving dinner & no one could tell.

After just one treatment, I noticed a HUGE difference. It's not something I'm going to do all the time right now, but it's great to know the option is there as I get older for when I want to microneedle my arms, legs, chest, hell even my vagina. Throw in a butthole & I'll be microneedled all over.

Another thing I've tried, because I'm in the beauty industry & I think it's important to be on the pulse with everything, is PRP. As we said earlier, this stands for PLATELET-RICH PLASMA.

This procedure involves your own blood. I'm deeply scared of needles (vasovagal syncope) so I went to the best—Dr. Jason Diamond.

He took my blood, spun it & not only microneedled it into my face, he injected it into my face. That time I used a thin layer of numbing cream. PRP was even more effective than just microneedling because my blood was being put back into my face. This is also known as the vampire facial.

PRP essentially helps new blood vessels grow. Lucky us, because it's great for collagen production & is great for promoting hair growth, which we love.

CLEAN, CRUELTY-FREE PRODUCTS

I balance my skincare like I balance my bank account. Sometimes I use things that are stronger and maybe more medicine-based, and other times I use things that are cleaner, as in free of chemicals and additives. When I got pregnant with Zaza, I was very careful about everything I put on my skin. It turns out that personal care companies are basically allowed to do whatever they want to do. This means they can sell us products with ingredients that are toxic & carcinogenic and disruptive to our hormones. Ever heard of "greenwashing"? This is when companies use words like *all-natural*, *eco*, and *green* to describe their products, but most of the time it's all a marketing scheme and the "selling points" on the front don't match what's really in the bottle.

If you're into clean beauty, do your research and be your own advocate and guru. Ingredients to avoid if you're looking to keep it clean are parabens, sulfates & phthalates. Some of my favorite clean beauty brands are Drunk Elephant, Lawless Beauty, and Summer Fridays.

I think clean beauty can be really effective, especially oils. But sometimes, for hyper-pigmentation and acne, you need to take a more aggressive route. You have to do you & listen to your body. Knowledge is power, but applied knowledge is more power. SO, go get all the knowledge, apply it & see what works.

KEEPING IT SIMPLE

Think of skincare like dieting. You can't hop in all at once. Just start, then add and modify as you go. My advice if you're wanting to keep it super simple is to grab some grapeseed oil, have a nice mist in the morning & be sure to apply sunscreen. Just those three little things are a big step in the right direction. And again, the lazy Susan idea of having everything to grab for A.M. and P.M. makes things so much easier.

STRETCH MARKS & PREGNANCY

Most of us have been there with stretch marks. However, I do have to say, I didn't get them very bad while pregnant. I attribute that to:

Camellia oil

What I like about this Japanese oil is that you can use it all over your body, face included. I've really realized how important it is to oil up your whole body, pregnant or not. It's just good for you, plain & simple.

This oil:

- ♥ is rich in vitamin E & sweet almond oil.
- ♥ is rich in plant collagen.
- ♥ is good for stretch mark prevention.
- ♥ maintains skin's elasticity.

What is camellia oil? Allow me . . .

Camellia oil is also known as tea seed oil. It's rich in antioxidants and is used for its nourishing & conditioning properties. In fact, Japanese women use it to care for their dry skin, nails, hair & scalp. It just leaves your skin so silky & supple.

Start with the face, then slather it on your whole body. I was stretching out big time, so I really slapped this on. I would do about six good shakes & put it everywhere—face, neck, chest, arms, tits, belly, legs. I looked like a wet rat going to bed, but who fucking cares because I didn't get stretch marks!!!

It smells so good and helps with fine lines, wrinkles, stretch marks, the works. Also, the bottle is pretty & you'll want it on your vanity. When looking for a product to help with stretch marks, opt for something with vitamin E & other antioxidants because they carry oxygen to the cells & keep the skin tight so stretch marks are less likely to occur.

As you'll see on the next page, Dr. Lancer says that oils will not prevent stretch marks in someone who is prone to them genetically. BUT, for me, oils worked like a charm (again, do you!).

Dr. Harold Lancer ON STRETCH MARKS

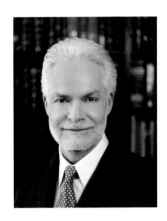

There are some people who have stretch marks that result from growth patterns. I saw a woman once who had about 6 inches of stretch marks from her kneecaps to the mid-thigh from rapid growth as a teen. There are other people who've gained 35–40 pounds with pregnancy and have no stretch marks. There are people who get stretch marks just thinking about getting pregnant. There's genetics to it. The oil may help reduce the amount, but it won't prevent them. If you're prone to getting them, they will develop to some extent, but they're treatable.

Stretch marks always require treatment medically first, so there's a retinol involved topically. There's going to be some mechanical polish, cleanse, nourish—and a mechanical home care part for maybe 2–4 weeks to prime it. Then it usually involves some in-office repetitive treatment—whether it's some sort of radio-frequency microneedling or whether it involves ultrasound or it involves some heat-based or energy-based device. With enough repetition, you can do incredibly well in removing the majority of stretch marks.

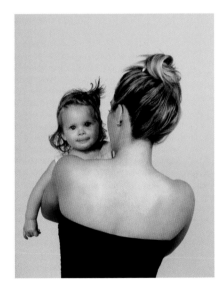

HYPER-PIGMENTATION DURING PREGNANCY

Speaking of pregnancy, we should talk about hyperpigmentation, aka "pregnancy mask." Most pregnant women know between the very swollen ankles, the weight gain & 27,389 trips to the bathroom to pee, there's another fun thing that happens in pregnancy . . . and that is the MASK.

Before we get into this, hyperpigmentation isn't something that happens ONLY to pregnant women. It's something that happens to everyone. Since the age of 17, I've had a pregnancy mustache, so I know this firsthand. In fact, I'm a pro at it.

SO, TA-DA, on the next page are my top 3 tips to deal with pregnancy mask. (If you're wondering about the science behind it, it's because of hormones. Basically, hyperpigmentation is caused by a surge of estrogen & can come out anywhere from your cheeks to your upper lip. Fun shit! There's nothing like waking up, looking in the mirror & seeing a bunch of new brown spots you never knew you had!)

TOP 3 TIPS FOR DEALING WITH PREGNANCY MASK:

DRUNK ELEPHANT C-FIRMA VITAMIN C DAY SERUM

I got this serum after Tiffany Masterson, the founder of Drunk Elephant, came on *The Skinny Confidential HIM & HER Podcast*. She said that it is THE BEST product when it comes to hyperpigmentation. Not only is it a superpotent vitamin C day serum, it's also mixed with vitamin D, so it contains tons of antioxidants & VERY MUCH brightens the skin.

This serum stays activated on the skin for 72 hours & it's not irritating. Like, no synthetic ingredients, dyes, or silicones & there's nothing drying in it, so it's ideal for pregnancy.

To get super specific, at night I like to mix this with another amazing product. I like to use a dime-size amount of this & a dime-size amount of the Kiehl's serum (we'll go over that next) & then finish off with a mist. For daytime, I like to use the Drunk Elephant serum alone. As I mentioned, it stays active for 72 hours on the skin, so there's no need to apply it again at night, but I do it anyway. I'm extra sometimes—so sue me.

This serum is really going to improve the signs of photoaging (premature aging because of the SUN), so this means it will improve uneven skin tone, dullness & firmness.

Trust me, this is one that you'll keep buying over & over again. It won't be sitting in your back drawer collecting nasty cobwebs. If you're skeptical, just check out the reviews on Sephora's website. I'm such a big fan of reading real, true reviews from all types of people before I buy a product. Anyway, people rave about this & say that it's helped with their melasma (a skin condition that causes dark, discolored patches on the skin) so much.

KIEHL'S CLEARLY CORRECTIVE DARK SPOT REMOVER

This is a magical facial serum containing Activated C, and it really zones in on correcting dark spots. At the same time, it brightens the skin, so you'll feel brighter, tighter, plumper skin. When you're pregnant you already feel radiant, but put this on top of your skin & it'll look even better.

Specifically, this serum is for dark spots & dullness. It's filled with:

ACTIVATED C: A vitamin C derivative that reduces the appearance of dark spots & prevents new dark spots from forming. It's quick absorbing and will even your skin's tone & clarity.

WHITE BIRCH EXTRACT: Derived from sugar and can restore hydration & nutrients in your skin. It's a potent, active ingredient that works with Activated C to even out your skin tone.

PEONY EXTRACT: An antioxidant that fights free radical damage. (Free radicals are responsible for the breakdown of collagen. It can give us wrinkles, pigmentation & saggy skin.) It works with Activated C to improve skin clarity.

Not only is this going to decrease the melasma, it's going to prevent it. We love a preventative measure over here. This is one of those products that you need to implement into your routine—it's not just a one & done type of thing. Use a dime-size amount every night & rub it in upward motions (never pull your skin down) on your face. This is usually my last step in my skincare routine before I mist. Also, it comes in a little dropper so you won't overuse the product.

You should also know that this can help reduce the appearance of acne scars. So if you have scars & brown spots, this is a great multitasker.

AVOID HOT YOGA

You're not supposed to really do anything hot when you're pregnant, which means no hot yoga, and saunas & hot tubs are basically out of the picture. But if you have hyperpigmentation, you should avoid these things anyway. The heat can really bring out the brown spots—I totally noticed this when I was doing a lot of hot yoga.

I love to steam my face, but pregnant or not, I only do it about once a week. BUT ICE. Bring on the damn ice. My ice roller is always in my skin fridge because it really helps even out your skin tone over time.

SWITCHING THINGS
UP TO DISCUSS
SOMETHING MANY
PEOPLE EXPERIENCE . . .
A LITTLE BITCH CALLED MILIA.

MILIA. What a fucking little bitch.

It sneaks up on you when you least expect it. There you are, living your life, you head to a bathroom, glance in the mirror & all of a sudden, to your horror, there are little bumps under your eyes.

And these aren't bumps you can pop. I mean, you can't pop them like a pimple. Milia are here to stay & they're like a long, drawn-out relationship that you don't want to be a part of.

WHAT IS MILIA?

Milia are small white bumps that appear on the nose and cheeks. They tend to cluster and happen when keratin gets trapped under the skin. It happens to all ethnicities and ages, even newborns.

There are tons of different kinds of milia, and things that cause it (as I said, it's very common), so let's get right into how to deal:

THE SKINNY CONFIDENTIAL GUIDE TO MILIA

Cryotherapy / cold plunges

You can get liquid nitrogen that freezes off the milia, but I think just being cold does the trick. Lately I've been doing a freezing cold shower for 3 minutes every day & I find it really gets rid of milia.

Even just a cold rinse on my face keeps it away, whereas I've noticed a hot shower makes it way worse. So get cold, do cryo, step into a cold shower. Freezing cold showers for life.

Lancing

Lancers are tiny little needles that can prick the milia. This is not my favorite & would be my last resort. I've only had milia around my mouth lanced & haven't done it around my eyes. If you're going to go this route, I would go see a professional & not attempt it yourself.

Any cream that contains vitamin A is going to exfoliate the skin in a gentle way without being too rough. If you have milia, I recommend looking for products with vitamin A.

Lasers

This is recommended by a lot of facialists. They do some laser around the milia and that helps shrink them. Apparently, this is very effective.

Chemical peels

Not a huge fan of peels because I had one when I was younger, then went out in the sun & it really fucked up my skin (hey, hyper-pigmentation mustache). So personally, this option is not for me, but people do it & it helps peel the skin off & get rid of milia.

Some people recommend surgically removing them, but no thanks. Also, diathermy is extreme heat that destroys the cyst, but again, this isn't for me. Cold all the way, PLZ. Can't be doing all that heat on my face.

All in all, though, I think the main trick to dealing with milia is two tips. The first one is staying out of extreme heat. Avoid hot yoga; if you're going into a sauna, get into some cold after; also, try to keep lotion or cream off your face if you're doing something hot like that, & try to use a sunscreen only, not a moisturizer if you're going out in the sun. Moisturizer makes milia worse because it makes your skin kinda sweat.

The most effective way to do something DAILY to combat milia is to find a legit eye cream. When I had a lotion-based eye cream, it made my milia worse. Now, I love a balm, and am obsessed with Sonya Dakar's Jade Energy Energizing Eye Balm because it's full of caffeine & doesn't clog your skin like cream or lotion does.

THINGS I AVOID LIKE MY EX-BOYFRIEND:

MAKEUP WIPES

I hate makeup wipes & I have a theory about them. We discussed this earlier, but here's a refresh for you:

THEY PULL THE FACE DOWN.

Makeup wipes also have unnecessary chemicals, which is why, since I was 16, I've been removing my makeup with oils. They're gentle, you have more control & they're more nourishing. Makeup wipes put chemicals on your skin every single day, sometimes twice a day.

If you travel and think makeup wipes are the shit, then try getting a little vial & filling it with grapeseed oil. You could even keep a vial of oil in your clutch so you can remove your makeup after a one-night stand. Seriously, though, get on board with oils.

If you're not a fan of oils, a cleansing balm is really good, too. (More on this in a bit.)

ANYTHING TO AVOID PULLING THE SKIN DOWNWARD, AM I RIGHT?

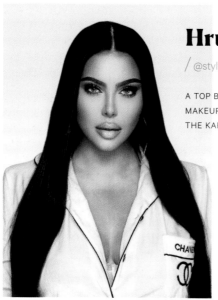

Hrush Achemyan

/ @styledbyhrush

A TOP BEAUTY INFLUENCER AND CELEBRITY MAKEUP ARTIST WHOSE CLIENTS INCLUDE THE KARDASHIANS

Makeup wipes are disgusting if you're ONLY wiping your face. I have a friend—she'll stay unnamed—who has really, really bad skin. She's a beautiful girl but just has really bad skin. I've looked at it, it's not cystic acne, but we haven't been able to figure out what it is. Then I said, "Can I just ask you what you wash your face with? What's your skin routine?" She said, "Oh, I use makeup wipes to wipe it all off." I said, "And then?" She said, "No, no, no. That's it." Houston, we have a problem. We switched up her routine with some hypersensitive face washes & creams & now her skin is much clearer.

So how about we all skip the makeup wipes. They leave a residue, pull your face down & it's just a lazy bitch thing to do. There are oil cleansers you can use on your face, or I like to use First Aid Beauty's Skin Rescue Deep Cleanser. I've been using it for years. It literally takes off mascara and anything and everything off your skin.

HOT TIP ♥ *Wash your ears. When you wash your face, give your ears a little TLC. Dry, dull ears make you look older than you are. I like to do a little horizontal massage so I'm not pulling them down.*

Molly Sims

/ @mollybsims

BLOGGER, AUTHOR,
ACTRESS, AND MODEL

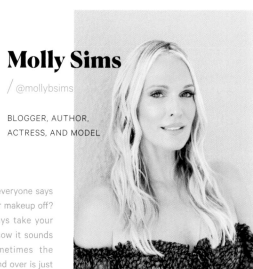

You know how everyone says always take your makeup off? Well, don't always take your makeup off. I know it sounds weird, but sometimes the stripping over and over is just constantly beating your skin in terms of taking your makeup off. I love how now everyone makes these cleansing balms that just melt your makeup off. There's a new product out called Face Halo that I'm obsessed with trying. It comes with this mitten that you dampen and it takes all your makeup off.

Claudia Sulewski

/ @claudiasulewski

LIFESTYLE INFLUENCER AND YOUTUBER

Every morning, I run a cotton round soaked in micellar water over my face. This washes away any product that didn't absorb overnight without shocking my skin from a deep cleanse. I spray my hydrating toner from BIBA, apply whatever serum I'm loving at the moment (currently Summer Friday's CC Me Serum) and lastly SPF moisturizer to finish it off!

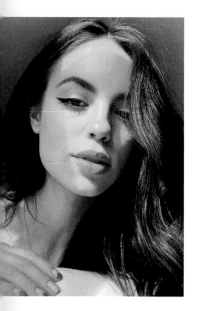

OVERCLEANSING

This is another thing that I've adopted that's worked really well for me. I only cleanse five nights a week. I exfoliate about once a week and I don't really cleanse in the morning. The reason being: I like to let the serums, moisturizers, and balms from the night before penetrate my skin throughout the day. Cleansing too much wastes the product and strips my skin.

When you wash your face too often you're stripping off a layer of the skin, which results in dryness and redness. It's unnecessary. I also like the natural oils of my skin to get comfortable—kick up their legs for a bit. SO GO AHEAD—hit that snooze button for an extra 2 minutes every morning (thank me later). If I do wash my face in the morning (which, to be honest, is hardly ever), I like to use a cleansing balm. There are tons you can buy, and they really cleanse your skin without making it feel tight and dry. You just take a dime-size amount, rub it in your fingertips, then gently massage it into your face. It literally melts away all your makeup. Then, take a baby washcloth (we get into it in chapter 11) to pat it off your face.

HOT TIP *Micellar waters were invented in Paris in the 1990s because of the harsh tap water. It's basically tons of itsy-bitsy cleansing oil molecules that act like a magnet for impurities on the skin. You could use this as a makeup remover or after a day of sweating. I like to keep mine in my workout bag. Just put a little on a cotton pad and tap it onto your face.*

WHATEVER YOU DO, TAKE OFF YOUR MAKEUP

Riawna Capri

/ @riawna

Nikki Lee

/ @nikkilee901

FOUNDERS OF NINE ZERO ONE SALON, IN COMMON BEAUTY, AND RAINDROPS

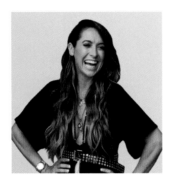

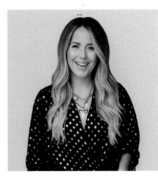

RIAWNA: I think the best skin tip that I actually ever received was from Steven Tyler. I asked him, "What do you do to your skin to look as amazing as you do?" And he had two answers. Number one: "Always wash your makeup off at the end of the night, no matter what. Don't ever be too tired to wash off your makeup. You have to wash it." Very strict about that. Number two: "Oil your entire body, head to toe, every single day." Coconut oil at Whole Foods. Doesn't matter. You need to add the moisture back into your entire body every single day. And if you look at this guy up close, he looks freaking amazing for 72.

NIKKI: I agree with Riawna that washing your face every night and oiling up is the best way to go. You have to wash your face. This is disgusting, but if I had to choose between washing my face and brushing my teeth, I would choose washing my face. I can deal with teeth in the morning, but I have to get that makeup off.

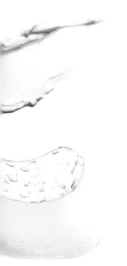

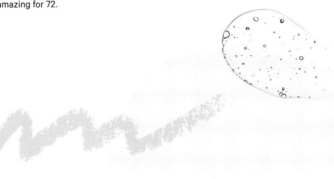

GET THE F⬤CK OUT OF THE SUN

INDY BLUE IS A YOUNG HOT INFLUENCER WHO NEVER FOLLOWS THE STATUS QUO, WHICH IS WHY I WAS SO EXCITED TO INTERVIEW HER ON HER SKINCARE. SHE'S A MOM, BLOGGER, AND SERIAL TRAVELER. AND SHE'S A BADASS. MEET INDY.

Indy Blue

/ @indyblue_

TRAVEL BLOGGER, INFLUENCER, AND SOCIAL MEDIA PERSONALITY

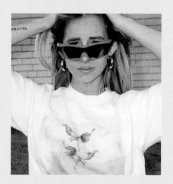

WHAT IS A HABIT YOU'VE DEVELOPED OVER THE YEARS THAT MAKES A DIFFERENCE IN YOUR SKIN?

I'm brand-new to this skincare world. I'm embarrassed to admit I haven't even cared about my skin long enough to have years of tricks and habits developed. But the one thing I have stood by since seventh grade . . . baby oil. Baby oil when you shave. Baby oil after every shower. Baby oil when you're having a panic attack about your wedding ring that's on too tight. BABY. OIL.

WHAT IS THE WORST ADVICE YOU'VE EVER HEARD WHEN IT COMES TO TAKING CARE OF YOUR SKIN?

"I don't have a skin routine, because I already have good skin."—India Blue Severe. Yep. The worst advice I've ever heard when it came to taking care of your skin came from myself. Fortunately for me, unfortunately for everyone who got to listen to me brag in middle school, I have always had clear skin. "Clear" meaning I rarely, if ever, had acne growing up. To me, that meant I had good skin. So what was the point in spending all this money and time and energy into something I already had? But then . . . I got pregnant. And getting pregnant forces you to get your shit together. So I finally decided to start taking care of my skin. And what I once thought was "good" skin is now actually healthy, hydrated, radiant, and GLOWING skin. Now I have REAL good skin. And I'm not kidding when I say diligently taking care of my skin has changed the entire look of my face. More than that. Diligently taking care of my skin has changed my entire LIFE.

WHAT STEPS DO YOU TAKE DURING YOUR DAILY SKIN ROUTINE?

I've been very into a dramatic beauty routine lately. I think it's my way of apologizing to my skin for neglecting it for so long. I start with a gentle cleanser and then TONE. Toning is my favorite step of my skincare routine. The Indie Lee COQ10 is my go-to. Then I ice roll, lay on some serums, and finish with an ultra hydrating moisturizer. OK, maybe it's not so dramatic. But for someone who used to wash her face twice a year . . . it's pretty elaborate, alright?

WHAT ARE YOUR THOUGHTS ON PLASTIC SURGERY, BOTOX, FILLERS, LASERS, AND OTHER COSMETIC MEDICAL PROCEDURES?

Listen. I loved myself before, but I'm not going to lie and act like I don't love myself WAY MORE with a nose job. But HEY, what's so wrong with that anyway? Isn't that what life is all about? Loving ourselves? Becoming the highest versions of ourselves? Well, my highest self has a ski slope nose, damn it. So unless you've never had extensions, colored your hair, microbladed your eyebrows, had braces, whitened your teeth, or done ANYTHING to change your appearance (permanent or temporary), you're no better than Becky down the road who likes herself better with a ¼ syringe of Juvéderm in her lips. I hate to break it to you . . . but we all care about how we look. So if a cosmetic procedure is going to make you feel better about yourself, do it. But the key is to do it for YOURSELF. Don't get cheek filler because Bella Hadid did it. Don't get laser hair removal because Tyler Smith called you hairy in ninth grade and you haven't been able to let it go. Changing yourself for others' approval will never fulfill you. So instead, do it because YOU want to. Do it because you get one life, and you deserve to love every inch of your one life. Even if it is a little superficial sometimes. Do it because you deserve to feel good about yourself. Do it because feeling good about yourself outweighs looking good, every time. ♥

Candice Kumai / @candicekumai

CLASSICALLY TRAINED CHEF, FORMER TV HOST, AND FORMER-MODEL-TURNED-JOURNALIST

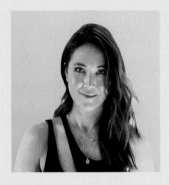

WHAT IS THE MOST PRACTICAL, RELATABLE ADVICE YOU'VE RECEIVED FOR PREVENTATIVE SKINCARE?

My Japanese mother taught me: greens + green tea daily + my Koko brand matcha and relaxing Japanese onsen baths work just as well as any beauty product. And you've also got to eat one big green salad daily—its totally cool to skip one once in a while, though!

My mom is from Kyushu, Japan—the onsen mecca of Japan (onsen = Japanese hot springs)—and her, my grandma, and my auntie Takuko all aged beautifully & gracefully and are pretty freakin' chill. My mom has so much natural collagen in her face still and has never been touched by a dermatologist or spa—she says it's also staying out of the sun, and using less is always more.

WHAT IS A HABIT YOU'VE DEVELOPED OVER THE YEARS THAT MAKES A DIFFERENCE IN YOUR SKIN?

I quit coffee! I love my Koko matcha powder and collagen every morning vs. coffee! The combination of these two powerful ingredients helps to fight aging & fine lines and perks up my skin with a matcha glow.

And these products *actually* work in emergencies: I use them in a pinch before set, shoots, or hot dates!

- ♥ Kate Somerville ExfoliKate (There's a gentle version, too!)
- ♥ Goop Beauty GoopGlow Microderm Instant Glow Exfoliator

HOW DOES YOUR NUTRITION AND WELLNESS PLAN AFFECT YOUR SKIN?

Every A.M. I drink matcha + collagen and eat fresh fruits like berries & my berry smoothies. I add greens like spinach—don't be fooled by the in-store smoothies—FULL of nasty sugar . . . I make my own smoothies, from my own books: low sugar, high on nutrition.

Generally, I eat as little sugar as possible; this means mostly only water and not too much alcohol. I cook for myself and loved ones each day, always. I eat out VERY LITTLE.

You'll find in my cookbooks—*Clean Green Eats*, *Kintsugi Wellness*, etc.—I follow a variety of my mom's Japanese recipes + fresh and traditional eating habits of my ancestors, like my grandma from Japan!

WHAT STEPS DO YOU TAKE DURING YOUR DAILY SKIN ROUTINE?

Most def—I love to treat my skin like I'm at a spa, daily:

First I'll drink one tall glass of lemon water, then wash my face gently with Indie Lee Brightening Cleanser, I'll put on my Drunk Elephant sunscreen daily, followed by a Kosas face oil or Juice Beauty CC Cream with SPF. Both Kosas and Juice Beauty give incredible natural, glowy, dewy coverage that looks so, so natural!

I use Aether Beauty for cheek glow and eyeshadow. I love natural brands on my skin. Always before leaving the house: Protect that décolletage with a COOLA SPF. I use it on my hands, too! I remove ALL of my makeup at night with coconut oil and a steamy clean cloth. I don't wear much makeup in the daytime anymore; when in a rush, I fill my brows and wear a lip tint.

I cleanse with Indie Lee Brightening Cleanser at night, then use a squalene by Indie Lee . . .

You always want to use a vitamin C serum every evening on clean skin; I love my vitamin C drops by Obagi or vitamin C serum by Drunk Elephant.

I sleep with plant therapy essential oils in my diffuser and read Buddhist books before bed (that's after some dirty TV shows). Sleep as long and as much as you possibly can.

GET THE F★CK OUT OF THE SUN

WHAT IS AN UNUSUAL OR SOMEWHAT WEIRD PRACTICE YOU DO TO KEEP YOUR SKIN YOUTHFUL?

I am a major hippie and Japanese wellness chef at heart so always believe in making my Koko brand matcha daily, with my matcha bowl and whisk (a chawan and chasen). I practice a ritual outside with my matcha and meditation each A.M.: I breathe deeply for at least 5–20 minutes daily, with the intent to set the tone of the day and to try to stay in peace daily.

I try my best to workout 5x a week. Crank the heat if you really want to sweat with Tracy Anderson—it feels like a cleansing detox after each of her classes! ♥

Ingrid De La Mare-Kenny

/ @ingriddelamarekenny

FOUNDER OF THE METHOD AND THE GANGSTER CHIC BRAND

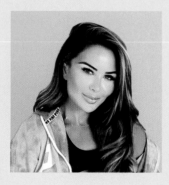

WHAT HABIT HAVE YOU DEVELOPED OVER THE YEARS THAT MAKES A DIFFERENCE IN YOUR SKIN?

Microneedling. It has changed my skin forever. I buy microneedles online and I microneedle my skin twice a month. Microneedling is used as a procedure to treat aging skin and wrinkles, imperfections, and pores. The needle length I like is 1.5 mm because it creates micropunctures.

I use numbing cream in sensitive areas like around my eyes or around my lips. I've gotten rid of wrinkles and imperfections successfully over the years. Microneedling is a skin rejuvenation procedure that uses tiny, sharp needles to create small holes, called microchannels, in your skin. These microinjuries trigger your skin's natural healing process, including the production of collagen.

WHAT STEPS DO YOU TAKE DURING YOUR DAILY SKIN ROUTINE?

I wake up, lather my skin with FUCKING BEAUTIFUL rose oil (my own brand) and I then walk to the window & soak up sunlight or daylight for about 5–10 minutes.

Then I add on a moisturizer être belle carotene aloe vera. I use Embryolisse Crème as a primer before putting makeup on.

In the evenings I wash my face with Charlotte Tilbury Magic Night Cream, I use alpha glycolic liquid gold and lather FUCKING BEAUTIFUL rose oil again to massage my face. I massage with my gua sha tool or with Lauryn's recommended face massager. My skin routine is simple. I don't like to overwhelm my skin with too much.

WHAT WOULD YOU SAY TO YOUR YOUNGER SELF ABOUT SKINCARE IF YOU COULD?

Don't buy into hype. I spent a lot of money on very expensive products like La Mer and La Prairie without questioning or researching what I was putting on my skin. Today I spend less on skincare and make more educated and effective choices.

WHAT IS AN UNUSUAL OR SOMEWHAT WEIRD PRACTICE YOU DO TO KEEP YOUR SKIN YOUTHFUL?

I give my skin makeup breaks once a week. I believe it's good for the skin to breathe at least once a week. So usually Saturdays or Sundays I wear no makeup at all. ♥

Kenzie

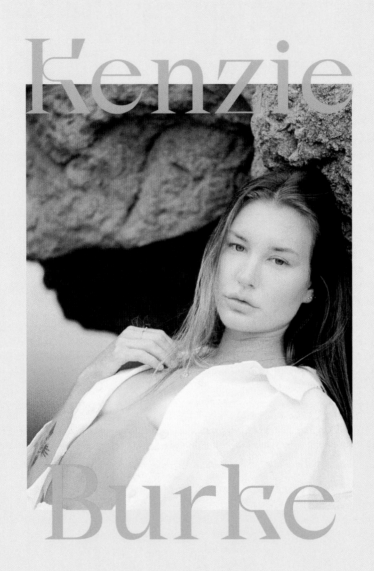

Burke

/ @kenzieburke

INFLUENCER AND HOLISTIC
HEALTH COACH

WHAT IS THE WORST ADVICE YOU'VE EVER HEARD WHEN IT COMES TO TAKING CARE OF YOUR SKIN?

Stay out of the sun completely. I know, I know, you may be thinking, "WHAT is this girl saying?!" But I truly swear by 20 minutes of sun each day (and my skin is REVERSE aging, so I am here to debunk that myth). By now, we have all learned about the damage and risks associated with over-exposing and frying your skin in the sun; this is not what I am suggesting. What I do stand by is the fact that there are some exceptional benefits and healing qualities that come from direct sunlight.

Sunlight is extremely healing, disinfecting, and energizing. The sun is capable of killing bacteria and bringing you wellness, energy, and light. The sun strengthens our bone health and immune function, decreases risk of cancer, and helps with circadian rhythms. We also receive the most vital source of vitamin D when our bodies are exposed to sunlight. Vitamin D is not a vitamin at all, but instead it's a hormone that works closely with cholesterol in the liver and in alliance with other hormones. Exposure to sunlight encourages every important function of the body to work at its best. Our nerves take the energy that they receive from the sun and transmit them throughout our entire body!

By spending 20 minutes in direct sunlight per day, without chemically filled sunscreens, our body receives the sun's health benefits. Not to mention, you will FEEL the glow throughout your entire being. Just a little bit of sun on my face each day keeps my face glowing, youthful, and full of life!

WHAT IS A HABIT YOU'VE DEVELOPED OVER THE YEARS THAT MAKES A DIFFERENCE IN YOUR SKIN?

Taking care of my overall well-being and making that my primary aim in life, while maintaining my natural state of being. I eat well and concentrate on an abundance of fruits and vegetables. I am mindful of how I combine my foods. I move my body. I spend time outdoors. I try to only consume content that enhances my life. I make sure the company I keep also keeps me at my highest self. I ensure that I sleep. If I don't feel happy, I sit with my emotions and figure them out. I feel what I need to feel and I pivot when it's time. I am always eager and thirsty to do better, be better, expand, and elevate.

"Just a little bit of sun on my face each day keeps my face glowing, youthful, and full of life!"

I let go of what no longer serves me. Adding this practice into my life—my well-being, my mental, physical, and emotional health—is something I work on Every. Single. Day. This makes a difference on my skin, which honestly used to be terrible. I had acne. I had lines and deep creases, and I was unable to look others directly in the eye. I was so insecure. I saw every facialist you could think of. I bought every product. I tried diet change after diet change. I even went on birth control and antibiotics (BRIEFLY). It wasn't until I changed my LIFE—my food, my thoughts, my outlook, my QUALITY of living—and that has taken YEARS off of my skin. My skin now is vibrant, glowing, and youthful. Taking care of it and more directly of myself physically and mentally has become my daily well-being practice. And that has made all the difference.

WHAT WOULD YOU SAY TO YOUR YOUNGER SELF ABOUT SKINCARE IF YOU COULD?

To relax. To look within. To go deeper with yourself. I was so worried and focused on how "awful" my skin was, it was only making my acne worse. I feel for that girl. She stayed home because she felt her bad skin couldn't be seen. I would tell myself that it's OK. It will get better. Your skin is reflecting how you are feeling on the inside. Look within, have patience, and LEAN into YOU. Oh, and DON'T PICK YOUR PIMPLES! ♥

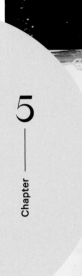
DR. BARBARA
STURM

MOLECULAR
COSMETICS

GLOW RECI

WATERMELON G
PHA + B
PORE-TIGHT TO
HYDRATING + PORE-REF

TONIQUE RESSERRANT LES

LA ME

the replenishing oil
exfoliant-huile régéné

E N
CLE

MADE

CRÈME SOYEUSE DE LA MER

LA MER

the moisturizing soft cream
la crème soyeuse régénération intense

MOISTURIZING & OILS & EXFOLIATORS, OH MY!

This chapter is for everyone. Let's be honest, we could all use a little more moisture, exfoliation, and more sheet masks. Hopefully this chapter is a gentle nudge-nudge and reminder to oil up before you hop into bed. I look like a total greaseball when I get into bed, but hey, I didn't get one stretch mark when I was pregnant, so it's important. You'll find out why Koreans aren't big on over-exfoliation, why oils should be your last step, and how to mask and multitask.

MOISTURIZER

Moisturizing is an essential when it comes to skincare. This shouldn't surprise anyone though, right?

Dry skin promotes acne, and moisturizer works great to prevent it. You just need the right one. Bad moisturizers = more acne. Good moisturizers = less acne. And Mrs. Right is hard to find. Choose wisely.

My jam is lightweight hydrating moisturizers. Lately I've enjoyed starting with a good mandelic serum and then adding some moisturizer. Mandelic serum is made of crushed almonds that are turned into an acid. Acids on the skin can be life-changing. They tighten, lift, and shrink pores. Even my husband wears it. A lot of people are unfamiliar with acids, but I'm here to tell you they're so beneficial because they tighten and tone the skin while exfoliating and lightening brown spots. Moisturizers provide a barrier function and are going to seal all the moisture deep into the skin.

HOW TO APPLY MOISTURIZER LIKE A BOSS:

1 Place a dime-size amount of moisturizer on your hand.

2 Carefully dab dots over your face with your finger (dot your nose, forehead, each cheekbone & chin).

3 Using your fingertips, gently press (not rub) the moisturizer into your face.

When it comes to your under-eyes, be sure to use your ring finger. (Remember: It's the weakest finger and gets the most blood flow so it's warmer for your product—we love this.)

ALWAYS remember to let your moisturizer dry a little bit before applying makeup or you'll get that cakey, flaky look that no one wants.

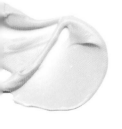

OILS

For me, as you can see, oils are queen. I apply them morning and night and like to put 4–5 drops in the palm of my hand. Dr. Dennis Gross says that applying oils should usually be your last step. There's nothing better than putting oils on before your makeup. It gives you the perfect primer for dewy skin. (For more on oils, head back to chapter 4). Again, I like to press the oil onto my face and neck using my palms. I even take it down to my tits if I'm being honest. When I was pregnant, I took it all the way down to the belly and would rub it all over in a clockwise direction. It smells so good and helps with fine lines, wrinkles, stretch marks, the works.

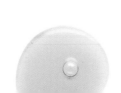

EXFOLIATORS

Just like I'm not an overcleanser, I am not an over-exfoliator. I exfoliate once, maybe twice a week. My sister went to South Korea and noticed that they aren't big on exfoliation over there and obviously they have the most beautiful skin.

If you over-exfoliate, you're going to create little cracks in the skin's barrier, which will leave your skin feeling dry, dehydrated, and possibly inflamed. Obviously this is just my hot take and you should talk to your dermatologist.

A good exfoliator is a star—I use it not only on my face, but my neck, chest, and shoulders, too! Never forget those areas—they're infamous for sun spots and wrinkles. A brush is amazing if you're looking for a lot of exfoliation. For me, I prefer a facial massager (if you need to choose between the two, I'd for sure get the massager). But the brush is a great hack for exfoliation, especially when used along with an exfoliator by Kate Somerville

You should also be very careful of certain exfoliators because some are full of microbeads or particles that are too hard and rough for the delicate skin on your face.

EXFOLIATE TO GLOW:

1 Put a dime-size amount of product on your fingers and apply exfoliator with tiny circular motions.

2 Massage face for about 2 minutes—listen to a podcast while you're doing it!

3 Rinse your face with cool water and pat, pat, pat with a microfiber towel.

4 If you're doing a mask, apply it now, girl. Otherwise, finish with your serum, moisturizer & an oil. And then, of course, sunscreen it up. Never forget your sunscreen.

HOT *Use a baby washcloth/microfiber tiny*
TIP *towel to dry your face. Because there's*
✔ *nothing worse than using the same white towel that you just used on your butthole (or that your husband used on his ball sack), on your face. That's going to put bacteria & nasty-ass germs all over your face.*

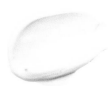

THE KONJAC SPONGE FOR ALL YOUR GENTLE EXFOLIATING NEEDS:

The konjac plant is native to Asia, is naturally alkalizing so it helps balance your skin, and is rich in vitamins A, B, C, D, and E. This little sponge is made from natural konjac root and was actually created for Japanese farmers to clean their babies' skin. It's soft but is a good and gentle way of exfoliating dry skin. It's great to use if you're prone to clogged pores, breakouts, and acne. And it helps your makeup stay on because your skin won't be all dry and flaky underneath your makeup. These sponges are inexpensive on Amazon and something to add to your collection if you're a ride-or-die skin babe. Most of the girls in Asia say this is their answer to exfoliation.

MASKS

Oh me oh my. I love myself a mask. Face masks have always been an important product for the skincare segment. Currently, there are different variations in this category:

SHEET MASKS

- Originally from South Korea.
- Tailored to certain skin issues.

PEEL-OFF MASKS

- Amazing for tightening pores & acne.
- Peeling it off will give you a bit of exfoliation.

CLAY OR MUD MASKS

- Absorb toxins! YES YES YES!!
- Good for acne-prone or oily skin because it balances.

HOT TIP *Aztec Secret Indian Healing Clay is an affordable product you can find anywhere and is a good option if you don't want to spend a lot of money on masks. This clay reduces acne scars, shrinks pores & provides a tightening sensation. And not only can you use this magic mud to beautify, it can be used on skin irritations & bug bites, too. All you do is mix this powdered clay with equal parts of raw apple cider vinegar &/or a bit of water. Use a bowl & spoon (preferably non-metal) & stir the mixture well so it turns to paste. Apply the clay to your face & allow it to harden for 10 minutes (sometimes I even leave it on for 20 minutes). Remove by washing it off with warm water. It's totally normal to have some redness.*

CREAM MASKS

- Use a cream mask if you have dry skin.
- Can be used as a spot treatment, too!

GEL MASKS

- Usually cooling & tingly.
- Good for dry or sensitive skin.

SLEEP MASKS

- Get yourself some sleep masks if you're into ULTIMATE hydration.
- Kind of like a hangover cure for your skin & you'll wake up radiant.

CHARCOAL MASKS

- Usually contain activated charcoal, which will detox the F out of your skin!
- Good for oily or acne-prone skin.

HOT TIP *Celeb facialist Sonya Dakar said that for my post-pregnancy hyperpigmentation I should mix yeast, lemon juice & milk, then spread it all over my face while I sleep. Sure enough, it worked very well. Basically, yeast is full of organisms loaded with B vitamins, proteins & other skin nutrients that have a stimulating effect on the skin.*

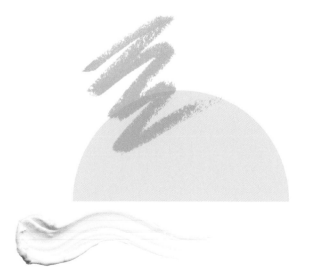

6 HOT TIPS FOR HOW TO MASK:

CLEANSE BEFORE YOU MASK.

If you put a mask on a dirty face, you'll prevent all the delicious, buttery goodness from penetrating into your skin.

DON'T MASK FOR TOO LONG.

I like to follow the instructions and add 20 minutes, if I'm being honest. Obviously, if you're doing a sleep mask you can sleep in it.

KNOW YOUR MASKS.

Everyone is different, so test out a few and find out what works for you. Also test them on your hand or a small patch of skin on your arm.

KEEP IT *THE SKINNY CONFIDENTIAL–* **STYLE.**

Mask and multitask. Mask while you're cooking, cleaning, returning emails, on a conference call. I love to mask while passively multitasking.

WASH WITH COLD WATER.

Wash off your mask with cold water. This seals the skin. I also love to ice roll with my *The Skinny Confidential* Ice Roller right after a mask. It feels oh so good.

DRY YOUR FACE WITH BABY WASHCLOTHS.

We went over this when we talked about exfoliating. They're soft and meant for a newborn, so if you think about it, it's the perfect towel for your face.

FINISH WITH A MOISTURIZER & OIL.

TA-DA.

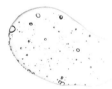

OH BOY, OH BOY,

now we're going to hear from the pros. The founder of Drunk Elephant is going to talk double cleansing, Aimee Song will tell you all about her olive oil trick, and Arielle Lorre shares her must-have products.

Tiffany
Masterson

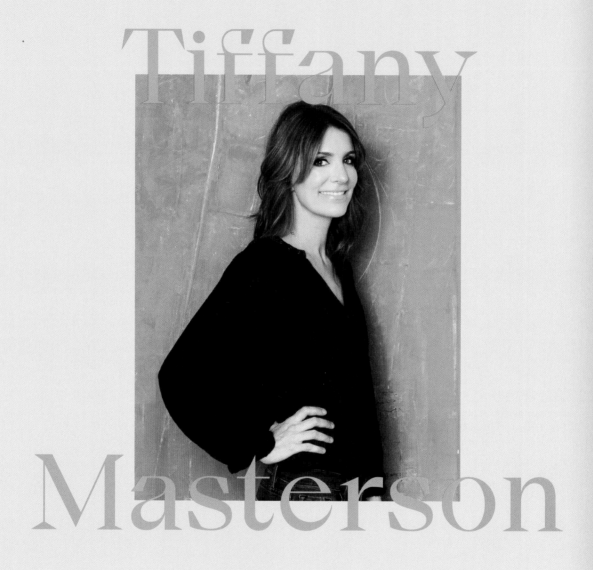

/ @drunkelephant

FOUNDER OF THE SKINCARE LINE
DRUNK ELEPHANT

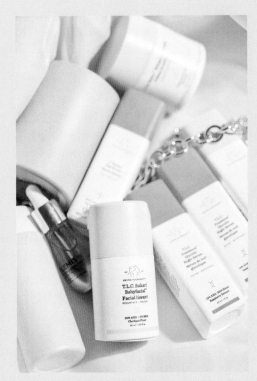

WHAT IS THE MOST PRACTICAL, RELATABLE ADVICE YOU'VE RECEIVED FOR PREVENTATIVE SKINCARE?

Just don't overdo it. If you feel like you're in a panic and you're trying everything that's out there to fix your issue, the answer is almost always *do less.* When first approaching skincare, you just need the very basics: Cleanse your skin well with a mild cleanser that is close to skin in pH; moisturize and protect it with a great physical sunscreen, which is the single most important preventative thing you can do. Then you can add actives like vitamin C and retinol, which are not only preventative, but also corrective. Great actives and lots of protection, in other words.

WHAT IS THE WORST ADVICE YOU'VE EVER HEARD WHEN IT COMES TO TAKING CARE OF YOUR SKIN?

To double cleanse twice daily and follow up with a toner. I'm a big believer that cleansing once daily is sufficient, at night. Our acid mantle is critical to the health of our skin, and removing it with cleansers and toners can be very damaging. Using biocompatible skincare, meaning only ingredients your skin can recognize, process, and absorb, allows you to do your nightly routine and wake up without having to cleanse anything off, like silicones and heavy occlusive ingredients. Start every day with perfectly balanced, happy skin.

WHAT IS A HABIT YOU'VE DEVELOPED OVER THE YEARS THAT MAKES A DIFFERENCE IN YOUR SKIN?

Not wearing foundation or mineral powder or anything like that, plus using sunscreen daily.

My philosophy is to use biocompatible ingredients that support the acid mantle, which is the protective barrier on the surface of our skin. Also, to avoid ingredients that are disruptive and confusing to skin, but ironically can be found in most products on the market. I refer to them as "the suspicious six," and they are silicones, chemical sunscreens, essential oils, fragrance, dyes, SLS, and drying alcohols. Avoiding them has totally changed the behavior of my skin, and I did not have easy skin to deal with.

WHAT STEPS DO YOU TAKE DURING YOUR DAILY SKIN ROUTINE?

So, when I wake up in the morning, the first thing I do to my skin is apply a mixture of vitamin C, retinol, and moisturizer. These are Drunk Elephant C Firma, A-Passioni Retinol Cream, and Lala Retro moisturizer. I mix all that in my hand, put it on, and then I cover it with Umbra Tinte SPF 30, which is a physical zinc oxide sunscreen.

At night, I cleanse with either Drunk Elephant Beste or Slaai depending on if I have eye makeup on or not (although they both remove my makeup) and then I pat dry. Then I use TLC Framboos, which is the pink chemical exfoliation mixed with the Virgin Marula Oil. I'll also use my C-Tango eye cream and put Lippe Balm on my lips. Most nights I top it off with my sleep mask, called F-Balm. ♥

Aimee Song

/ @aimeesong

AMERICAN FASHION DESIGNER
AND FASHION BLOGGER OF
SONG OF STYLE

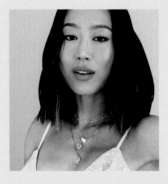

WHAT IS THE WORST ADVICE YOU'VE EVER HEARD WHEN IT COMES TO TAKING CARE OF YOUR SKIN?

I need to exfoliate more and add vitamin C immediately because your pores are opened and more susceptible to receiving the benefits of vitamin C. My skin is extremely sensitive, and a random facialist did this using an abrasive tool to exfoliate, then immediately applied vitamin C, and I broke out in hives. I was red and blotchy for 3 days.

WHAT IS YOUR "WHY" FOR TAKING CARE OF YOUR SKIN?

I feel pretty when my skin is clear and, as shallow as it sounds, I'm in a good mood when I feel pretty, but it all goes back to what I put inside my body, not just what I put on my body/skin. I feel good when I'm sleeping well, eating well, and taking care of all of my mental and body needs.

WHAT IS AN UNUSUAL OR SOMEWHAT WEIRD PRACTICE YOU DO TO KEEP YOUR SKIN YOUTHFUL?

I put on olive oil after getting out of the shower. It's super hydrating, and I love the smell of it. When I have a bad eczema flare-up and it's getting itchy, I sometimes put apple cider vinegar on it. I smell incredibly bad, so I can only do it at night or when I'm not leaving the house. ♥

Arielle Lorre

/ @ariellelorre

WELLNESS INFLUENCER AND
PODCASTER OF *THE BLONDE FILES*

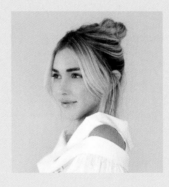

WHAT HAVE YOU FOUND TO BE THE MOST EFFECTIVE SKINCARE PRODUCT UNDER $50, AND WHAT'S YOUR BIGGEST SPLURGE?

Babor's two-step cleansing system comes in right around $50, and it has TOTALLY changed my skin! Nothing cleans it like this—it's amazing, I'm talking holy grail product here. Don't be deterred by the $50 price tag if you're looking for a steal; you only need a little bit at a time, and it'll last months. Basically, the first step, called HY-ÖL, contains natural plant oils, and in combination with the second step, the phytoactive base, it removes both oil- and water-soluble particles super thoroughly without leaving the skin feeling tight. This is from their site, but Quillaja Extract acts as a dirt magnet and enhances the cleansing effect. Your skin will feel like a baby's, I promise. On the other end of the spectrum, I've definitely spent four figures on moisturizers that did not live up to the hype. If we're talking a splurge that's worth it, Augustinus Bader is worth every penny; The Cream is absolutely amazing for fine lines and wrinkles, dryness, and suppleness. I swear, it makes your skin look younger. If it's good enough for Victoria Beckham, it's good enough for me.

WHAT IS THE WORST ADVICE YOU'VE EVER HEARD WHEN IT COMES TO TAKING CARE OF YOUR SKIN?

People used to say that a tan or sunlight (on your face) would clear up acne, and while there may be an iota of truth in there, it also leads to soo many more problems down the road! Unfortunately, I heeded this advice earlier in my life and had to deal with the ramifications (hello, lines + hyperpigmentation) years later. My face hasn't seen the light of day in at least 7 years, but now, in my 30s, all of those years sunbathing and using a tanning bed are catching up to me. I just got diagnosed with basal cell carcinoma on my face, thankyouverymuch. I think people are way more cognizant of the damaging effects of the sun nowadays, but I know there is a mindset

"I will try anything and everything when it comes to keeping my skin youthful."

among younger people that it'll never happen to them, that the day will never come when they're in their 30s experiencing these things. I'm making myself sound really old right now, but I'm here to say it'll happen and it's real! Thankfully, there are lots of advancements with lasers and treatments that address sun damage, but I wouldn't rely on those. Do as Lauryn does and wear SPF and visors!

WHAT IS A HABIT YOU'VE DEVELOPED OVER THE YEARS THAT MAKES A DIFFERENCE IN YOUR SKIN?

In addition to the foundational things I mentioned earlier (SPF, hydration, sleep, diet), I'm pretty careful about regularly washing my makeup brushes and my pillowcases (daily . . . I'm kind of a freak about it). These can just hold on to bacteria and transfer it right back onto our skin after we clean it. ALSO, this one is going to sound very LA and woo-woo, but meditation has helped a lot with breakouts. We all live very fast-paced, stressful lives, even if we don't think so. Just being bombarded with technology daily is enough to jack up our nervous system and alter our hormones. I got to a point where I was so frustrated because I felt like I was eating all the right things, using the right products, and as clean as can be but was still breaking out. I had to step back and recognize that I can be doing all the right external things, but if there's inner turmoil, constant nervous system activation, constant high cortisol (our stress hormone)—my biology is going to be altered from that. Hormonal changes and stress WILL lead to breakouts, period. So doing meditation (specifically Transcendental Meditation) has calmed that inner turbulence that we all get just from living in the world we live in, and has had a dramatic effect on my overall stress and how that shows up in my body.

WHAT IS AN UNUSUAL OR SOMEWHAT WEIRD PRACTICE YOU DO TO KEEP YOUR SKIN YOUTHFUL?

I will try anything and everything when it comes to keeping my skin youthful. I don't mean I will lift my face to the high heavens so I don't have one wrinkle and try to look eternally like I'm 25. But please give me all the stem cells and embryos and whatever is out there to maintain the nature of the tissue. I think the weirdest thing I've used productwise is the Biologique Recherche (human) placenta serum. It smells like what you would imagine placenta to smell like. My poor husband. It's one thing if it's your own, but a stranger's placenta—whose is it? How did they get it? So many questions. Aside from that, I do all the peels, laser, facials, you name it.

WHAT ARE YOUR THOUGHTS ON PLASTIC SURGERY, BOTOX, FILLERS, LASERS, AND OTHER COSMETIC MEDICAL PROCEDURES?

I do it all, and I'm very vocal about it. No shame! I've had tweaks over the years, and I couldn't be happier with all of it. Everything I've done cosmetically has been to just lighten things up on my face. Very subtle surgery, in my opinion, is way more natural and attractive than a face frozen with Botox or filled to the brim. I still do a little Botox and filler here and there, but I mean tiny amounts. Someone in the industry who is very knowledgeable told me that you never want to denature the tissue, and that's essentially what a lot of noninvasive treatments do. Of course, there is a lot of bad surgery out there, too. I think people run into problems when they try to emulate someone else's look and not just enhance their individual beauty. It's all available to us, and it's so advanced now—why NOT take advantage of that? ♥

THE
Hamlin
Sisters

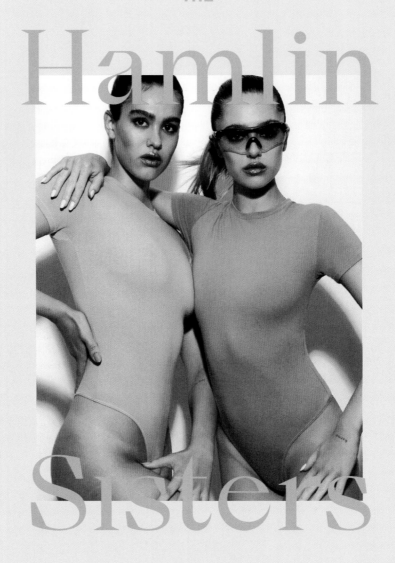

SISTERS, ACTRESSES, MODELS
WHO FREQUENTLY APPEAR
ON *THE REAL HOUSEWIVES
OF BEVERLY HILLS*

Amelia Gray Hamlin

/ @ameliagray

Delilah Belle Hamlin

/ @delilahbelle

WHAT HAVE YOU FOUND TO BE THE MOST EFFECTIVE SKINCARE PRODUCT UNDER $50, AND WHAT'S YOUR BIGGEST SPLURGE?

AG: I've found that I'm absolutely obsessed with Neutrogena makeup-removing wipes. Love them. I think my biggest splurge is definitely on sweat suits. I'm a hoarder when it comes to comfort.

DB: Mario Badescu facial spray with aloe, herbs, and rosewater.

WHAT IS THE MOST PRACTICAL, RELATABLE ADVICE YOU'VE RECEIVED FOR PREVENTATIVE SKINCARE?

AG: First of all, it is so important to know your skin type, but something that relates to everyone is making sure that your products are non-comedogenic. That means that they do not have pore-clogging properties. All skin types suffer from pores being clogged.

DB: Less is more! I used to do a full 15-minute skincare routine after washing my face, and I had awful acne. I then started using only three products and my skin cleared up a ton.

WHAT IS THE WORST ADVICE YOU'VE EVER HEARD WHEN IT COMES TO TAKING CARE OF YOUR SKIN?

AG: Popping pimples!!! I NEVER EVER EVER pop my pimples. Even if it's a huge whitehead. I've managed to stay scar-free that way.

DB: Don't use oils. I actually use oils in my skincare every day and haven't broken out in months!

WHAT HABIT HAVE YOU DEVELOPED OVER THE YEARS THAT MAKES A DIFFERENCE IN YOUR SKIN?

AG: I don't wash my face in the morning, and it has changed my skin. Not only acnewise, but I feel so much more moisturized, allowing my skins natural oils to set in.

DB: Cutting gluten out of my diet definitely helped! I also always make sure to wash my face morning and night.

WHAT STEPS DO YOU TAKE DURING YOUR DAILY SKIN ROUTINE?

AG: I try to keep it short and sweet. I've noticed that with my skin, less is more. I wash my face, then apply a toner and a moisturizer. When I was 12, I had really bad bumps on my forehead, not cystic acne, but I had these bumps also on my chest and my back until I was about 16. At that time, I went to Coachella and had the worst breakout on my chest and back. I wouldn't go on set for so long, it made me so self-conscious. And when I say bumps, I literally mean thousands of bumps on my chest and back. I was always lucky with having clear skin on my face, but it was so bad. I thought it was the end of the world, and it made me really depressed. After going back and forth to doctors, I started washing my chest and back with Nécessaire body wash, and it cleared my skin right up. I don't know what's in it, or what's not in it, but it actually changed my life. The body scrubs, the lotion, the body wash, to everything they have, is amazing.

I also use Biologique Recherche Lotion P50, and their Lait E. V, Lait VIP O2, and Lait U, which are face washes that I alternate. The Lait U is super dense and creamy. I also just feel fine without makeup so I don't really give a shit. I grew up with my mom, Lisa Rinna, never wearing makeup so I've just never felt like it was something that had to be part of my day. Although I look back at some *Real Housewives of Beverly Hills* episodes and think, shit, I should've put something on.

DB: First I use Biologique Recherche Lait E. V face wash, then I use their lotion P50 toner followed by Dr. Barbara Sturm Hyaluronic Serum.

WHAT WOULD YOU SAY TO YOUR YOUNGER SELF ABOUT SKINCARE IF YOU COULD?

AG: STOP SCRUBBING YOUR FACE AND WEAR SUNSCREEN!!!

DB: I would tell myself to start Accutane sooner. I would also stress wearing sunscreen to prevent wrinkles! ♥

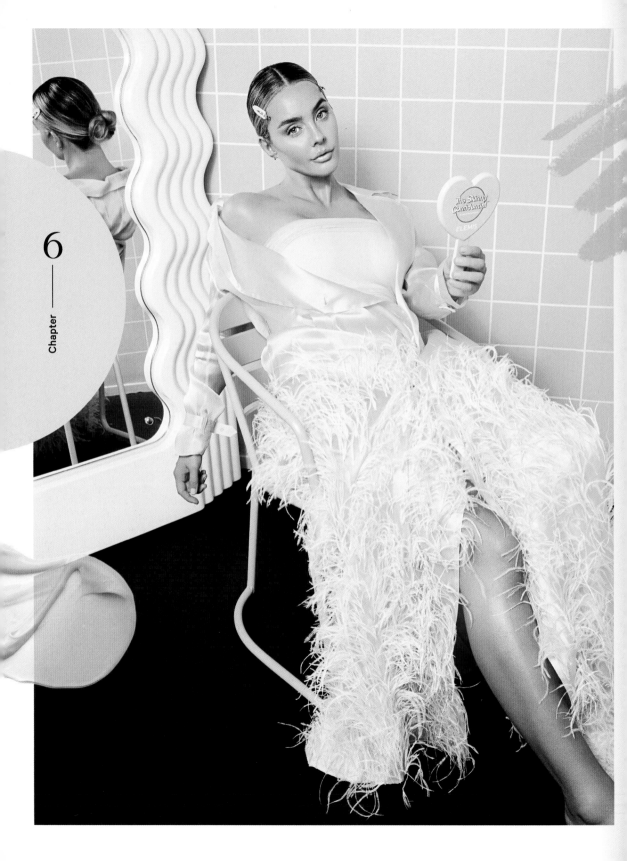

6

FILLERS, BOTOX, LASERS & ALL THAT JAZZ

O oh la la. What a FESTIVE chapter! Ready for all the preventative secrets when it comes to needles, lasers, and treatments? Fuck yes.

To recap: I've been getting Botox since I was 21, which might be young by some people's standards, but I was seeing the dreaded number 11 on my forehead.

Filler is something that's new for me, but we'll get into that. We tend to only see bad filler, so it gets a bad rep. But here we're going to cover everything you need to know about how to get good filler.

Lasers have not worked for me, but I am open to trying more. I have tried them many times for my horrific hyperpigmentation aka brown moustache—sometimes I think they made the brown spots worse. Everyday skincare and staying out of the sun have helped most with my hyperpigmentation. In the future, though, I believe lasers will evolve quickly, and in 5 to 10 years we will see some cool shit.

Millennials are more open to the idea of procedures, which are no longer as taboo as they once were. Instead of wanting to look like celebrities, young people today seem to prefer looking like an enhanced version of themselves. I don't want to look like anyone else. I just want to be the best version of ME!

I love a no-judgment zone when it comes to beauty. Nowadays it's important to DO YOU—whatever that looks like. What you do is nobody's business, especially when it comes to your body.

So why did I start getting Botox?

The scene is still as clear as day.

I was driving to my sister's graduation, all dressed up, of course—think white deep V-neck with a cute mini and pumps. I remember the whole thing like it was yesterday. My latest Dave Matthews was blasting from the car's speakers, and it was that time of day where the light shines directly in your face.

As I was driving along, I casually glanced up at the rearview mirror and there it was, a total number 11. That's right, smack between my eyebrows. I wasn't being crazy. And the light? Well, it was very much intensifying the sitch.

Almost 95 percent of girls are overly critical of themselves—including me. We could all be a little kinder to ourselves. The point is, I'm no different from you, and the deep-set 11 was annoying. As you know, I'm very detail-oriented and sometimes . . . a perfectionist. But I figured I was young and I could leave it for a while. Well, after a year, the 11 was still bugging me. A lot.

SO I DID WHAT I DO BEST: RESEARCH.

I asked everyone with credibility almost every question in the book about Botox.

Should I? Shouldn't I? What are the pros and cons? Does it hurt? Does it work? Is it preventative?

Being younger . . . and more carefree, I went for it. I got Botox.

The real reason I decided to pull the trigger was not just because of Mr. Eleven. The real reason is that it's preventative, meaning that the 11 wouldn't continue to get deeper, making the wrinkle worse. As you've heard me say, I'm all about prevention.

BOTOX BREAKDOWN

WHAT IT IS: Botulinum toxin type A, the neurotoxin that, when injected in the face, will reduce muscle movement and lessen the appearance of wrinkles.

COST: Prices vary depending on the extent of the procedure. For the area I chose, it was around $200.

WHAT I EXPECTED: Needles. A lot of scary needles. I hate needles. Honestly—I have a condition called "vasovagal syncope," which causes my body to overreact when exposed to a certain trigger: needles. Every time there's a needle, I need to eat a banana before, and lie down while the needle is administered. Plus, I have to lie there for 5 minutes after the process. The needle for this was so small and not as bad as I thought, primarily because my eyes were closed the entire time. Also, I wanted to be extremely conservative; no *Real Housewives* look-alikes for me.

WHAT IT'S ACTUALLY LIKE: I went into the doctor and she told me to lie down. Then, she whipped out a mirror and had me show her what I didn't like. She agreed that the 11 would be better off with a little Botox, and it would prevent it from getting deeper. She asked if I wanted a numbing cream; I declined because I don't mind a little pain (just the needles). After that, she got the needles ready and did four injections in what seemed like

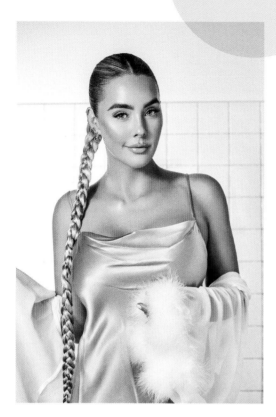

just a minute. It was quick, easy, painless, and I didn't see the needle— it felt like a more intense eyebrow pluck. Then, I was done! Every time I've had it since, it's been the same story: quick.

THE AFTERMATH: Since then, I've gotten it once a year, maybe twice, depending how long it takes to wear off.

SOME OF MY TIPS:

- I would never touch my eyes; there's something weird about getting Botox around your eyes.
- I would never recommend getting Botox by the smile lines, because you want to smile. If you get Botox there, it would paralyze the muscles.
- Supposedly it will last 3–4 months. For me, it has lasted up to 9 months.
- Avoid Botox if you're pregnant or breastfeeding.
- When it comes to bruising, there was only one time I got the tiniest bruise, but it disappeared the next day.

After Botox, it's important to not exercise, bend over, or lie down all day. Experts and doctors say to wait only 4 hours, but I always wait all day. Another friend of mine got Botox and then went to try on shoes at Nordstrom afterward. It had only been 2 hours, and well, we all know we lean down when trying on shoes. He ended up with a lazy eye for a month straight. Hence, why I'm overly careful the day I get it.

A HUGE CON: What's in Botox is just an overall con. Again, I don't recommend any-one get Botox unless they've done extensive research.

ONE BIG PRO: It's hard to explain, but it kind of opens your face in the best way, and I feel refreshed after.

FILLER

After my jaw surgery, I noticed that my lips were kind of turning in—they weren't as plump either. So I wanted a little GOOSH— you know, a little filler. So I got my lips filled on a trip to New York City awhile ago by Dr. Lara Devgan, who is a board-certified plastic surgeon, the chief medical officer of RealSelf, the CEO of medical-grade skincare line Dr. Devgan Scientific Beauty and the host of the hit podcast *Beauty Bosses*. AND I LOVE THE RESULT—soft and plump—but also youthful and not overly filled.

It hurt a little, not too bad, but I would definitely recommend going to someone who numbs the area. Make sure they numb around the lip, too. I wasn't too swollen. To be hon-est, I sort of liked the swelling. It was fun for a minute.

Here's my two cents: Go to an artist whose work you like. Don't use an online coupon ever (I have heard horror stories), go slow, do your own research and do not let anyone tell you what or what not to do with YOUR body (for my lips specifically, I wanted a little more full-ness with the "M" of the lip lifted—no duck lip).

FOR MORE JUICE ON BOTOX AND FILLERS,
HERE IS A LITTLE Q&A WITH **Dr. Lara Devgan:**

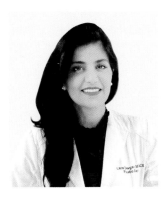

WHAT ARE THE PROS AND CONS OF BOTOX?

Botox is one of my "desert island" procedures—a quick, no downtime wrinkle-smoother that I couldn't live without. I started doing Botox on myself at age 27—before I had any visible signs of aging—as a preventative measure and a way to micro-optimize little things like the arch of my eyebrows. It's NOT about freezing your face. It's about playing up your own natural, beautiful facial features and preventing you from getting deeply etched lines.

The most beautiful and natural way to use Botox is to smooth the skin, symmetrize the face, shape the eyebrows, and preserve natural facial expression. Botox can also be used to treat migraines, reduce the gumminess of a smile, slim the lower part of the face, help relieve teeth grinding and jaw clenching, slim the shoulders, slim the calves, shrink pores, and so much more.

WHAT SHOULD SOMEONE LOOK FOR WHEN FINDING A TALENTED "INJECTOR"?

When finding someone to take care of your face, you want to think about the three Es: experience, expertise, and examples. For experience: Find someone who is well versed in these procedures and has done them over 10,000 times—that way, you are much less likely to encounter the devastatingly bad results that you've probably seen on the Internet or around town: things like droopy eyes, Spock eyebrows, asymmetries, frozen foreheads, and unnatural results. For expertise: Find a provider who is well trained and a true expert in facial anatomy. There are more than 43 muscles of facial expression and thousands of nerve and vessel branches involved in making you look the way you do. Medical aesthetics is a tricky field because there are many people who dabble in it after a weekend course, since there are very few regulations in the industry. For examples, look at real patient examples and see if your goals match your provider's sense of what is desirable and achievable. There is no one way to be beautiful, and we each have our own unique facial features, goals, and preferences for our faces, but you should be on board with your plastic surgeon's aesthetic sensibilities. The same way every painter or sculptor has a certain "look" they are known for, every plastic surgeon has a "look" they gravitate toward also. Look at someone's Instagram, before and after galleries, and patient case studies to understand whether they are a good fit for what you're looking for.

HOW CAN SOMEONE MAKE THEIR BOTOX LAST LONGER?

Botox lasts about 3–4 months in most people. It is slowly metabolized away as time passes and you move your face. One way to keep your Botox results more stable over time is to try to reduce needless scrunching of your face—use your hand gestures and vocal inflections to express emotion, and try to avoid crinkling your forehead and squinting your eyes as much as possible during regular interactions. Try to use Botox as a way to retrain your facial muscles to behave the way you want them to, even when you don't have any Botox in place. If you "fight" your Botox, it's like revving the gas pedal with the parking break on—you will run down the tank and get less value from it. Another important thing to do is make sure your skincare routine is helping you: Use a retinoid, a vitamin C, a hyaluronic serum, a great eye cream, and an SPF every day. Daily maintenance and excellent habits are what allow some 35-year-olds to look 25, whereas others look 45.

HOW OFTEN SHOULD SOMEONE GET BOTOX?

I recommend maintaining Botox every time the season changes—about four times a year. As with manicures and hair color, the challenge is to maintain a plateau in your appearance rather than having massive changes over time.

A WORD OF CAUTION TO ANYONE UNDER 21:

Georgia Louise

/ @georgialouisesk

CRITICALLY ACCLAIMED FACIALIST WITH A NOTEWORTHY CLIENT BASE AND OVER 20 YEARS' EXPERIENCE IN THE SKINCARE INDUSTRY

One piece of bad advice I hear that I would love to never see happen again is the idea of getting preventative Botox. My advice is don't start Botox to try to prevent what hasn't happened. Botox is a neurotoxin. I have people who tell me that Botox should be started when you've just finished puberty. The truth is that you were born to move the muscles in your face, and the full facial structure doesn't finish forming until the age of 21. This means that early Botox can have a profound effect on the way you look forever. Wait it out; use peptides and microneedling instead.

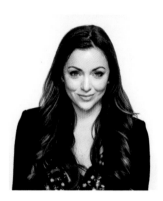

FILLERS

What are the pros and cons of fillers?

Filler has become almost a dirty word because of the sheer number of overdone, puffy, odd-looking, and dysmorphic faces all over the place. But volume loss is a real and unavoidable part of facial aging, and judicious replacement of lost volume can look very natural and beautiful. Filler can also be used to do what I think of as "facial optimization"—where many tiny millimeter-level changes all over the face can make a meaningful improvement in facial beauty. It's the principle of a Snapchat filter or Facetune: Very subtle changes can be very transformative.

We can use filler to sculpt model-esque cheekbones, improve the harmony of the jawline and chin, subtly plump and shape the lips, reduce the appearance of hollowing under the eyes, and even straighten and lift the nose. The technological advances with fillers in the past decade have truly allowed a new elegance and refinement in results.

That being said, when filler is overdone, it can diminish facial beauty. Ducky lips, puffy cheeks, and a surgical and artificial look are undesirable consequences of filler. These are judgment- and technique-related problems, so seeing an expert is important. There are many risks of filler, including benign ones like bruising and swelling, and very serious ones like tissue necrosis and blindness. This is why experience and expertise are important.

How can someone make their filler last longer?

Filler lasts months to years, depending on the amount and times used, and the locations where it is injected. The main determining factor in filler duration is your metabolic rate. It's the same way you can give ten people the exact same diet, and some of them will be very thin, some will be full, and some will be in between. To get the most out of your filler results, avoid touching and pressing the areas, and try to sleep on your back rather than your face. This will reduce movement and filler degradation.

How often should someone get filler?

Filler gradually and slowly dissipates over time, like a glass of water evaporating. My goal is to maintain the level of water in the glass without making it overflow (a puffy filler look) or making the glass run dry (too much volume loss). Typically, patients maintain filler twice a year.

LASERS

In the past, I've felt that microneedling was way more effective than lasers, mostly because the lasers I tried—IPL—brought out the hyperpigmentation on my face. But the technology has changed a lot, so for more insight, I went straight to the expert of all experts, Dr. Dennis Gross:

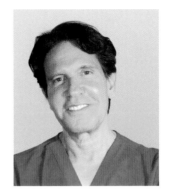

Dr. Dennis Gross ON LASERS

WHAT IS LASER?

Laser treatments are nonsurgical and noninvasive treatments that use light wavelengths to heat tissue beneath the surface. They work by directing short, concentrated pulsating beams of light at the skin. And they work in different ways: Some destroy the top, wrinkled layer of skin to expose the lower layers and encourage new growth of smoother skin (as well as the growth of new skin-firming collagen); others can target and heat up fat cells, essentially liquefying them (thereby contouring the face and/or body); some can tighten the skin, helping to make it more youthful looking; and still others can selectively target pigmentation or veins on the skin, erasing them.

It's important to remember that there is no such thing as one laser treatment that does it all. The best results come from using the one laser that specializes in that particular problem. That's how I do it in my practice—a cocktail of lasers to give you the best result. If someone is telling you that one laser can do it all—run the other way!

WHO CAN BENEFIT FROM LASER?

Nearly everyone. The results you get from lasers are better than ever before, and most have little to no downtime or pain. As I mentioned above, there are different lasers that target so many different concerns. If you have unwanted hair; discoloration; sagging skin; stubborn, unwanted areas of fat; acne scars; lines and wrinkles; there is a laser for you.

However, it is important to note that not all lasers are safe for all skin tones. Skin with more pigment is more susceptible to post-inflammatory hyperpigmentation, which can be caused by some lasers. You need to be sure to have a consultation with a dermatologist or aesthetician that regularly treats darker skin types and has a full understanding of the risks associated with certain lasers. As with most aspects of dermatology, experience, expertise, and skill are everything.

WHY ARE YOU SUCH A BELIEVER IN LASER?

Laser results are backed by science, and the results are real.

Maintaining a daily topical skincare routine is important, but lasers are able to go beneath the skin's surface to hyper-target the concern you are tackling. Lasers like Ulthera are even replacing invasive plastic surgery procedures like facelifts without the downtime, pain, or risk. That is the ultimate goal of anyone who comes into my dermatologist office—they want to see real improvements. Lasers do just that!

WHAT RESULTS HAVE YOU SEEN FROM GOOD LASER TREATMENTS?

Some of the best results I've seen for lasers are when they are used for maintenance—not just a "one and done" treatment. This is especially true for the lasers that stimulate collagen. Remember: Collagen is the key to younger-looking skin. Think of laser treatments like a steady and balanced diet—you will get the best results with consistency and a variety.

WHAT SET OF QUESTIONS SHOULD WE ASK A DOCTOR TO ENSURE WE'RE GETTING THE BEST LASER FOR OUR SKIN ISSUES?

♥ **When did this laser become available for in-office use?** Lasers are serious business. You do not want to be the guinea pig for new technology. I always do extensive, thorough research when bringing a new laser into my practice. I look at the studies and ask other people who have used it for their opinion on its effectiveness. You don't want to be trendy when it comes to lasers.

♥ **Is there any downtime, and if so, for how long?** Some lasers have downtime, and the downtime varies. If you have a big event coming up, you should give yourself plenty of time between the appointment and when you want to look your best. If you have a wedding next week, it's probably not a good idea to schedule a deep laser appointment.

♥ **Is this laser appropriate for my skin type? What are the risks?** As I mentioned earlier, some lasers cannot be used safely on darker skin types without risking hyperpigmentation. Be sure to ask your dermatologist about this.

HOT TIP ♥ **JOY KANG** *is the co-founder and CEO of Eunogo, a one-stop service where you can discover and book verified Korean beauty procedures in Seoul, Singapore, and Bangkok. She says that post-procedure, they offer clients pumpkin extracts, which are high in vitamin A & antioxidants to help reduce swelling and build the immune system.*

PLASTIC SURGERY

Since this is entirely out of my wheelhouse, I wanted to ask the best of the best for the inside scoop:

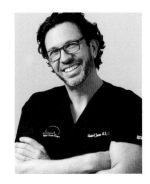

Dr. Andrew Jacono

/ @drjacono

FACIAL PLASTIC AND RECONSTRUCTIVE SURGEON AND AUTHOR OF *THE PARK AVENUE FACE*

WHAT'S A PLASTIC SURGERY PROCEDURE THAT PEOPLE ARE GETTING RIGHT NOW BUT THAT NO ONE IS NECESSARILY TALKING ABOUT?

In 2020, we have seen more permanent and customized solutions to facial aging, including bespoke implants—specifically cheek, chin, and jawline. Through the combination of CT scanning and computer aided design (CAD), custom facial implants can be created using precise measurements based on the patient's own physical model. Oftentimes, people rely on fillers to gain higher cheekbones, stronger chins, and more prominent jawlines, but with new custom implant technology, the implants fit like a glove and give the permanent results that so many seek without the upkeep of fillers.

TELL US ABOUT BUCCAL FAT REMOVAL.

Buccal fat removal procedures can help to reduce full, rounded cheeks, leaving patients with a slightly more chiseled look.

Excess fat pads located in the lower portion of the cheeks can give off the appearance of being overweight. Unfortunately, the hereditary condition of excess fat in the lower cheeks, which is called buccal fat pads, cannot be reduced by exercise or diet. For patients that are dealing with this unflattering condition, a buccal fat removal surgery may be the answer.

CAN YOU BREAK DOWN "THE GOLDEN RATIO" AND EXPLAIN IT?

I touch on the concept of the Golden Ratio in my latest book, *The Park Avenue Face*. While beauty trends come and go, the Golden Ratio has stood the test of time.

It is a term for the mathematical ratio of 1:1.618, and describes the relationship of one length to another. It is often called Phi (named for the acclaimed Greek sculptor Phidias, who regularly used the ratio). The Golden Ratio is found in people, animals, flowers, trees, geometry, art, and architecture. It's found in the wings of a butterfly, the curves of a nautilus shell, the size and shape of the Parthenon. Even the double-helix structure of a DNA molecule follows these proportions, perhaps explaining why we are so drawn to this ratio; it's literally in our genes.

Plastic surgeons learn about the Golden Ratio early in their training, as it's a very helpful way to teach them how to assess the correct relationship of length and proportion within individual facial features (such as the lips) or the relationship of different features to each other (such as the eyes to the eyebrows). In fact, a California-based maxillofacial surgeon named Stephen Marquardt derived a perfect—or rather, a perfectly *proportioned*—face from this Golden Ratio. He refers to it as the Golden Mask, and by superimposing this mask onto an image of a face that isn't quite balanced, it allows surgeons to better pinpoint areas or features that are deficient or excessive, then illustrate their findings and their suggestions for correction or improvement to their patients.

YOU'RE KNOWN FOR "THE PARK AVENUE FACE." WHAT ARE FIVE FEATURES OF THE FACE THAT ARE UNKNOWINGLY PLEASING TO THE HUMAN EYE?

Five features that are unknowingly pleasing to the human eye are brow shape—specifically arched; almond-shaped eyes; a heart-shaped face; a short distance from the bottom of the nose to the upper lip; and a defined gonial angle, which is the angle formed by the back of the jawline under the ears.

WHEN IT COMES TO THE FACE, WHAT'S THE BIGGEST PLASTIC SURGERY MISTAKE YOU SEE PEOPLE MAKING?

The biggest plastic surgery mistake in my opinion is overdoing it. Whether it's surgery or injectables, too much can actually make you look older. It's also a lot about technique. You can get a facelift that pulls and distorts the face and our eye reads that as old. The same goes with overfilling the face, or what we call "filler fatigue."

IS THERE ANYTHING OUT THERE THAT CAN GIVE YOU SIMILAR RESULTS TO PLASTIC SURGERY (THAT ISN'T SURGERY)?

Surgery is the only permanent solution to facial aging, but for those in their early 40s or younger, Botox and filler can work wonders. The trick is to go to a skilled injector that knows where to add filler and when to stop.

WHAT ARE THE DOS AND DON'TS OF NOSE JOBS?

Seek a specialist who has done thousands of noses and can produce not only before and after shots, but also patients that you can talk to.

Oftentimes I see patients that are looking for a certain celebrity's nose. This is not the correct approach in that not every nose is made for every face.

HOW CAN SOMEONE ACHIEVE THE PERFECT FACELIFT, AND WHAT'S THE RIGHT AGE TO HAVE ONE?

Aging is a very personal journey. There is no perfect age or time to undergo a facelift, as it depends on how much improvement you are looking for given the downtime and costs associated, but more than ever I've seen patients in their late 40s with the desire to look 10 years their junior for personal or professional reasons. You can't knock more than 4 years off your appearance with filler—a lot of people will try to make you believe you can.

Technique is very important when considering a facelift. A skilled surgeon will be able to deliver a superior result.

WHAT ARE SOME QUESTIONS THAT PEOPLE SHOULD BE ASKING THEIR FACIAL PLASTIC SURGEON?

It's important to know how long they have been in practice, the number of procedures they have completed, and what they specialize in, as you want to avoid those that are the jack-of-all-trades, but master of none. Also, ask for their credentials. Those with more experience in their specific speciality are often more well versed and have better outcomes.

ANOTHER POINT OF VIEW—
AND GENIUS NONSURGICAL
LIFTING HACK:

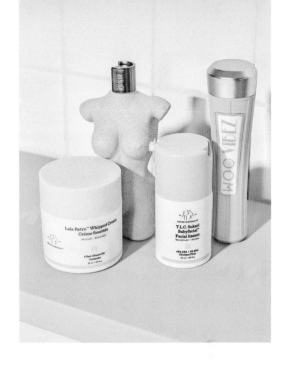

Hrush Achemyan

/ @styledbyhrush

CELEBRITY MAKEUP ARTIST
WHOSE CLIENTS INCLUDE
THE KARDASHIANS

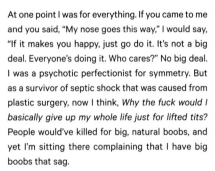

At one point I was for everything. If you came to me and you said, "My nose goes this way," I would say, "If it makes you happy, just go do it. It's not a big deal. Everyone's doing it. Who cares?" No big deal. I was a psychotic perfectionist for symmetry. But as a survivor of septic shock that was caused from plastic surgery, now I think, *Why the fuck would I basically give up my whole life just for lifted tits?* People would've killed for big, natural boobs, and yet I'm sitting there complaining that I have big boobs that sag.

Now I think I'm somewhere in the middle. Would I have plastic surgery? No. Would I do it again? No. It was just too traumatic. I was supposed to have reconstructive surgery to fix all the scarring, and I just couldn't do it. Just the idea of being put under, I might stop my own heart from the anxiety, because my life was perfect, went to sleep, woke up, and then my life was a shit show. That is what really scarred me. Maybe one day I'll get over it. Who knows? Life is so beautiful, and it's so short. Basically anytime you get plastic surgery, you're laying your life on the line to look prettier. There are other ways to look prettier.

Here are some of my hottest tips on how to tape your neck for a lifted, snatched look.

HRUSH'S TIPS FOR TAPING YOUR SKIN

Taping your skin is a great option if you can't afford or don't want filler or Botox. You can buy face tape from almost any beauty store—it's such a good option to hide wrinkles or facial bloating. Just note that if you're wearing your hair up, you shouldn't use this method.

- Put the tape higher on the forehead for more of an eyebrow arch.
- Put the tape closer to your temples for straighter, more-even brows.
- Pull up the top half of your hair evenly with clips.
- Use toners to clean the area around the temples or forehead so there's no slipping and sliding.
- Place the string behind your head and place the tape on each of your temples.
- Don't do it to the very tightest option, but you do you!
- Put your hair down to hide the string, then blend foundation on the tape on your temples.
- It's great if a friend can help you!

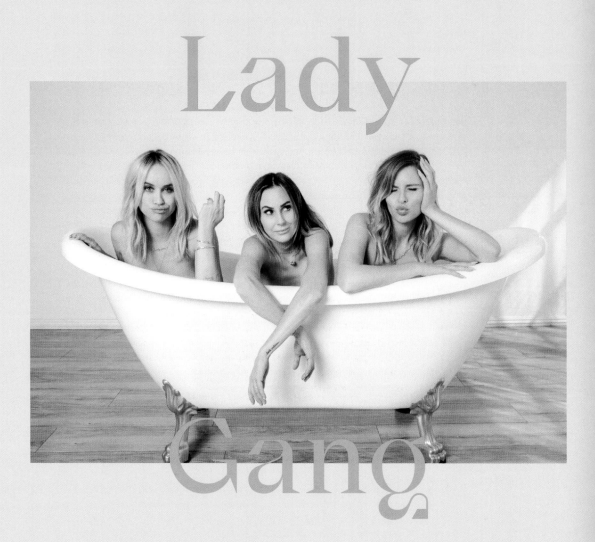

THE

Lady

Gang

PODCAST HOSTS AND AUTHORS
OF THE *NY TIMES BESTSELLER*
ACT LIKE A LADY

Keltie Knight

/ @keltie

EMMY-WINNING TV HOST

Becca Tobin

/ @becca

ACTRESS, SINGER, AND DANCER

Jac Vanek

/ @jacvanek

FASHION DESIGNER AND
ENTREPRENEUR

WHAT IS THE WORST ADVICE YOU'VE EVER HEARD WHEN IT COMES TO TAKING CARE OF YOUR SKIN?

BT: The worst advice I've personally received was that at 30, you have to start using Retin-A. It's not a universal miracle potion for everyone, and if you have sensitive skin . . . STAY AWAY!

JV: I went to an esthetician when I first started developed BAD adult acne. It was cystic, nasty, painful acne, and I needed HELP. First, she swindled me into buying all of her overpriced bull-shit products (and I got them, 'cause I'm a sucker), and then she told me the magic cure for acne was to splash your face with water six times after washing. No more, no less! Well, I tried that for months (because again, I'm a sucker), and sadly (and SO shockingly), the magic didn't work for me.

WHAT HAVE YOU FOUND TO BE THE MOST EFFECTIVE SKINCARE PRODUCT UNDER $50, AND WHAT'S YOUR BIGGEST SPLURGE?

KK: I love Weleda Skin Food, it's about $13, and I found out about it when I was on a flight next to the Victoria's Secret makeup artist for the supermodels; she told me it is what they all use! My biggest splurge is getting chin filler twice a year.

BT: The most effective product I have found for under $50 is anything by Rhonda Allison. My favorite product from the line is the sensitive skin complex. My biggest splurge is the La Mer Treatment Lotion Hydrating Mask. It's absolute heaven.

JV: Whenever my skin FREAKS OUT, my esthetician always recommends CeraVe moisturizer. It's like $15 for a freakin' TUB, and it helps calm irritated skin, and it's great for eczema. Biggest splurge was La Mer Crème de la Mer moisturizer. I mean look, it was thick and luxurious and probably made of angels and rainbows, but I won't be spending $200 for it ever again.

WHAT HABIT HAVE YOU DEVELOPED OVER THE YEARS THAT MAKES A DIFFERENCE IN YOUR SKIN?

KK: I'm a major exfoliator queen. I use all types—chemical, scrubs, masks, microdermabrasion, enzymes—but my number 1 favorite is shaving my face with a men's razor. It takes off all the old skin cells and dirt and allows your product to really get in!

BT: I have started doing microneedling a couple times a year, and it has changed my skin. My dark spots and acne scarring have minimized, and the texture of my skin feels like I'm in my 20s again.

JV: I have been getting clinical acne facials every month for the past 8 years. I'm talking chemical peel, painful extractions, the whole shebang. I could use every overpriced skincare product in the world, but nothing sucks the gunk out of my pores quite like extractions.

WHAT IS AN UNUSUAL OR SOMEWHAT WEIRD PRACTICE YOU DO TO KEEP YOUR SKIN YOUTHFUL?

KK: I love SNAIL. I learned about it at a K-beauty pop-up, and I love the way it makes my skin shine. Allegedly, the snails secrete a serum that rejuvenates skin. I swear it works!

BT: I shave my entire face once every couple weeks with a DermaFlash. Game-changer!

JV: If I'm out of spot treatment, I do find myself using toothpaste on pimples overnight. It really does the trick.

WHAT IS THE MOST PRACTICAL, RELATABLE ADVICE YOU'VE RECEIVED FOR PREVENTATIVE SKINCARE?

KK: 100% to just stay out of the sun. People always ask me about my skin, and I've def done stuff, but mostly I haven't spent any time in the sun trying to tan since I was 22 years old.

BT: I do anything that Dr. Diamond suggests! (I know it's not relatable, but it's really mostly Botox and regular facials.)

JV: The greatest duo of all time is prescription Retinol and SPF! I'm still struggling to find the balance of frequency of retinol because I have naturally dry and sensitive skin to begin with, but it's a never-ending journey right? ♥

Patrick

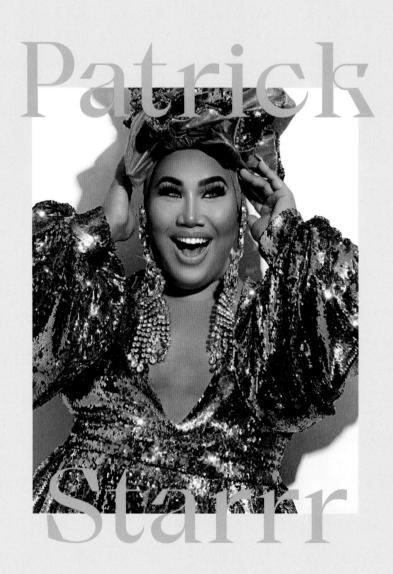

Starr

/ @patrickstarr

MAKEUP ARTIST, YOUTUBER,
AND INFLUENCER

WHAT IS THE WORST ADVICE YOU'VE EVER HEARD WHEN IT COMES TO TAKING CARE OF YOUR SKIN?

Worst advice when it comes to skincare is, "Don't moisturize because you have such oily skin." I thought as a teenager that I didn't need to wear any moisturizer because I was already "moisturized." There are many types of moisturizer suited for many different skin types! I love a less-dense moisturizer like Tatcha Water Cream for my skin.

WHAT HAVE YOU FOUND TO BE THE MOST EFFECTIVE SKINCARE PRODUCT UNDER $50, AND WHAT'S YOUR BIGGEST SPLURGE?

The best skincare product that I have come across under $50 is the Paula's Choice 2% BHA Liquid Exfoliant! It has literally transformed my skin into baby skin. I have very textured skin, and the BHAs have helped my skin feel bouncy and bright! My biggest splurge would have to be the Tatcha Silk Peony Eye Cream for $60! It is so smooth and it fills in my fine lines and wrinkles.

"A combination of exfoliating products and chemical exfoliants makes a huge difference!"

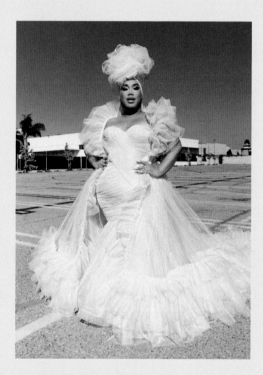

WHAT HABIT HAVE YOU DEVELOPED OVER THE YEARS THAT MAKES A DIFFERENCE IN YOUR SKIN?

A habit that I have been doing religiously for years is exfoliating! I was always insecure about my texture. Especially since I am a man in makeup and I have prominent facial hair and stubble. A combination of exfoliating products and chemical exfoliants makes a huge difference!

WHAT STEPS DO YOU TAKE DURING YOUR DAILY SKIN ROUTINE?

My daily steps for my skin routine are from my acronym "Cows Eat More Than Squirrels Eat, Mood" aka Cleanse, Exfoliate, Mask, Tone, Serum, Eye Cream, then Moisturize." I may skip masks here and there, but for the rest of the steps—DAILY! 💜

Jade Chapman

/ @jadeywadey180

CELEBRITY AESTHETICIAN, MAKEUP ARTIST, DIGITAL CREATOR, AND EDUCATOR

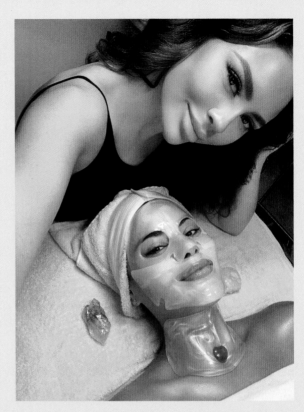

WHAT IS THE MOST PRACTICAL, RELATABLE ADVICE YOU'VE RECEIVED FOR PREVENTATIVE SKINCARE?

Start investing in a balanced skincare routine *now*. Planning for the future is always a good idea, and I've felt that way about my skin since a young age. My mom always taught me to hydrate with serums and of course protect with sunscreens. She is actually the reason I became an aesthetician at 19. Our skin begins losing firmness and elasticity in our early 20s, so preventative skincare is highly suggested for all ages.

WHAT IS THE WORST ADVICE YOU'VE EVER HEARD WHEN IT COMES TO TAKING CARE OF YOUR SKIN?

I once had a client tell me they were suggested lemon juice to get rid of their acne. Being in the beauty industry, I always hear new tips or tricks on how to take care of the skin; most of it is very helpful, but there is a lot that is false. My best advice is to seek a professional aesthetician that can help curate a custom skincare regimen for you personally. Just remember, everyone's skin is different. If a product works for someone else, great, but it does not mean that it would work the same for you.

WHAT HABIT HAVE YOU DEVELOPED OVER THE YEARS THAT MAKES A DIFFERENCE IN YOUR SKIN?

Proper exfoliation. I have always had a strong belief that to achieve clear, smooth skin, consistent exfoliation is key. Many people get intimidated by this step in their routine, but for me its been the golden rule in my regime. I like to mix between chemical, mechanical, and physical exfoliants. One of my favorite treatments to get is the HydraFacial. It uncovers a new layer of skin with gentle exfoliation and relaxing resurfacing.

WHAT IS AN UNUSUAL OR SOMEWHAT WEIRD PRACTICE YOU DO TO KEEP YOUR SKIN YOUTHFUL?

I like to create my own aloe vera products. I actually grow my own plants and create pastes and elixirs from them. They are high in antioxidants, vitamin A, and enzymes that can help heal the skin. Whenever my skin is feeling congested or I have a few stubborn blemishes, I like to topically apply this magical botanical! ♥

Shea Marie

/ @sheamarie

FOUNDER AND CREATIVE DIRECTOR OF SAME AND CEO OF THE FEELIST

FILLERS, BOTOX, LASERS, & ALL THAT JAZZ

WHAT HAVE YOU FOUND TO BE THE MOST EFFECTIVE SKINCARE PRODUCT UNDER $50, AND WHAT'S YOUR BIGGEST SPLURGE?

Tea tree oil is one of my all-time favorite affordable beauty buys. I'll add a few drops to my facial cleanser if I am breaking out. You don't need to find a fancy brand; you can pick it up at Whole Foods.

My biggest splurge was starting my own skincare company, The Feelist, so I could create the products I've always truly wanted! We focus on clean, plant-based formulas with superpowered botanic ingredients.

WHAT IS THE MOST PRACTICAL, RELATABLE ADVICE YOU'VE RECEIVED FOR PREVENTATIVE SKINCARE?

Stay out of the sun. I wish I had listened to that advice when I was younger! Of course, as a teenager growing up in California, I spent a lot of time at the beach and (as much as I hate to admit it) in tanning salons. My mom was always trying to stop me, but of course, at that age you don't listen and you think you'll never get older. Now I slather on the highest SPF I can find on my whole body, especially my face, neck, and hands. For my swimwear brand Same, I even went as far as to design suits with high necklines and long sleeves for ultimate sun protection.

WHAT IS THE WORST ADVICE YOU'VE EVER HEARD WHEN IT COMES TO TAKING CARE OF YOUR SKIN?

My position in the industry has allowed me to try nearly every product, treatment, and beauty/health offering under the sun. There was a time I had a morning beauty routine of probably 30+ products. I used to think the more expensive a product was, and the more intimidating-sounding ingredients it had—the better it was. The more I started to research and learn about skincare, the more I realized how far off that thinking was. I've always been extremely conscious of what I put in my body, what I eat and drink, so why was I not the same with what I put on my body? Especially since the skin is the body's largest organ. What I learned throughout this whole process, and what it took to get my skin back to a good place is that (1) sometimes less is more, and (2) nature is powerful.

"Your body is your home. It's the only one you've got! Treat it with love and respect."

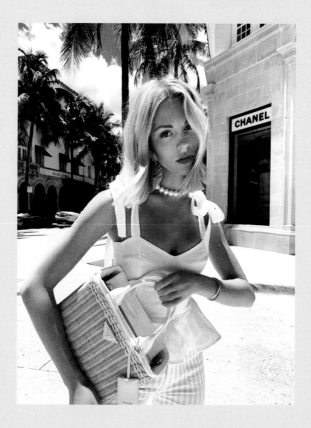

WHAT IS A HABIT YOU'VE DEVELOPED OVER THE YEARS THAT MAKES A DIFFERENCE IN YOUR SKIN?

Becoming more conscious about clean skincare and reading, learning, and truly understanding ingredients and their purpose in products I'm using. I really became interested in the world of clean beauty over 5 years ago when I started developing sensitivities to many products I was using. Over time, I realized that my skin reacted much better to clean and plant-powered ingredients.

HOW DOES YOUR NUTRITION AND WELLNESS PLAN AFFECT YOUR SKIN?

I've always been conscious of my health and eating well, and as clean as possible. Learning that your skin is your biggest organ made me realize that what you put on your body is just as important as what you put inside of it. I think gut health plays a huge role in wellness. I usually eat super clean, but after a few days of eating unhealthy, I immediately notice a change in my skin. For clear and beautiful skin, you need to be conscious of both what you put *in* your body and what you put *on* your body. It's all about the synergy between the two.

WHAT STEPS DO YOU TAKE DURING YOUR DAILY SKIN ROUTINE?

You don't need to overwhelm your skin with too much product. I learned that the hard way. Finding clean essentials that work for you is key. For me, that's a cleanser, a face oil, and a hydrating body lotion (I believe that skincare doesn't stop at your face). I created our face oil, Most Wanted, because I was looking for a product that could double as a serum and a moisturizer. I run two companies, as well as my personal brand, and am planning a wedding, so I need products that work well and are effective and to the point.

WHAT IS YOUR WHY FOR TAKING CARE OF YOUR SKIN?

Your body is your home. It's the only one you've got! Treat it with love and respect.

WHAT WOULD YOU SAY TO YOUR YOUNGER SELF ABOUT SKINCARE IF YOU COULD?

Stay out of the sun. Eat healthy. Drink more water. Drink less alcohol. Get enough sleep.

WHAT IS AN UNUSUAL OR SOMEWHAT WEIRD PRACTICE YOU DO TO KEEP YOUR SKIN YOUTHFUL?

Trying to sleep on my back—it's SO impossible to get used to. I've even gone so far as to buy ridiculous pillows to keep me in the right position! But it really does prevent fine lines and wrinkles.

WHAT ARE YOUR FAVORITE BOOKS, WEBSITES, PODCASTS, OR OTHER RESOURCES YOU REFER TO FOR PREVENTATIVE SKINCARE ADVICE?

Through my work in the industry, I've become friends with a lot of dermatologists and estheticians; I am constantly picking their brains for new and innovative skincare treatments and products.

WHAT ARE YOUR THOUGHTS ON PLASTIC SURGERY, BOTOX, FILLERS, LASERS, AND OTHER COSMETIC MEDICAL PROCEDURES?

I'm all about people doing what makes them happy and feel their best, as long as they aren't comparing themselves to others or to unrealistic beauty standards. I think what makes us different makes us sexy, so we shouldn't try to be anyone else. ♥

GET THE F♥CK OUT OF THE SUN

Emily
Schuman

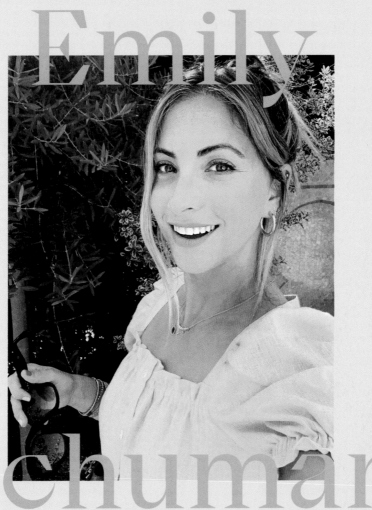

/ @emilyschuman

BLOGGER, DESIGNER, AND
AUTHOR BEHIND THE BRAND
CUPCAKES AND CASHMERE

WHAT IS THE MOST PRACTICAL, RELATABLE ADVICE YOU'VE RECEIVED FOR PREVENTATIVE SKINCARE?

I'm 37 years old and started my blog at 24, which is when I started having more photos taken of me than ever before. I have never done any sort of cosmetic procedure to my skin, but when I compare my skin now to 13 years prior, it looks better now than it ever did—and that's because I finally started a consistent routine: I was well into my 30s before I started wearing sunscreen and taking makeup off before bed, and while I splurge on skincare products I believe are worth every penny, great skin is so much more about consistency and finding a routine no matter your budget. Find what works for your skin and stick to that and invest in routines specific to you. For example, if you're someone who has acne-prone skin, spend a bit more on a really good salicylic acid product; if you have dry skin, consider splurging on a serum. Understand your skin so you can best manage it and invest in it.

WHAT IS THE WORST ADVICE YOU'VE EVER HEARD WHEN IT COMES TO TAKING CARE OF YOUR SKIN?

Back when I first started caring about beauty products in college, I was recommended the St. Ives exfoliating wash—which I think was pretty much everyone's gateway product into skincare at the time. I would dollop a huge amount onto my dry skin and go to town. It was the product equivalent of just taking a rough loofah to my face. I thought I was doing the right thing by sloughing off that layer of skin, but it was pretty much the last thing I should have been doing. I have really sensitive, prone-to-redness skin, and when I exfoliated it so roughly, my skin would flare up. Now I use primarily chemical-based, more gentle exfoliants that are right for my skin.

This goes back to knowing what works for your skin: If a magazine (or blogger!) recommends a product, just be sure to make an informed decision based on your skin type. What works for someone else may not be the best product for you.

WHAT IS A HABIT YOU'VE DEVELOPED OVER THE YEARS THAT MAKES A DIFFERENCE IN YOUR SKIN?

I first learned about dermaplaning when I was getting a facial and the esthetician asked if I would be open to it—and I was mortified. At the time, I thought it was her way of telling me I had a five o'clock shadow, but then she explained that the process (essentially shaving your entire face a few times a week with a superfine razor) gets rid of practically invisible peach fuzz and is a great way to get your skin smooth. I got over my initial embarrassment about having facial hair and now use Tinkle Eyebrow Razors across my entire face once or twice a week—my forehead, where a mustache and sideburns would be, and cheeks. I find that it not only makes my skin feel incredibly soft, but helps my skincare products sink in that much better, from mists to serums to lotion. Makeup also applies more smoothly—but it doesn't work for everyone. My best friend tried it and broke out in a full face rash, so begin with a small area of skin before you commit to dermaplaning your entire face!

WHAT STEPS DO YOU TAKE DURING YOUR DAILY SKIN ROUTINE?

In the morning, I put my hair back in a scrunchie and splash cold water on my face (no soap). Then I dab my skin dry with a towel so it isn't bone-dry, and spritz it with Caudalie Beauty Elixir. I will put on a couple of drops of Vintner's Daughter and press it into my skin. I wait a couple of minutes for it to sink in—I'll sometimes brush my teeth during this time—then apply lotion. In the middle of winter, I use Caudalie Premier Cru, but if it's not too dry out, I use their S.O.S Cream. I follow that up with Eve Lom Eye Cream, and finally Supergoop! Glowscreen.

My nighttime routine looks nearly identical: I wash my face with Caudalie Foaming Cleanser and twice a week I will use the Vita Liberata Self-Tanning Lotion, just because it gives my skin a nice touch of color. Because one of my skincare issues is discoloration and redness, I find that I need far less makeup when I apply the tanner—which I appreciate! Otherwise, I apply the same products as in the morning, with the exception of sunscreen. Before bed, I add Lanolips 101 Ointment.

GET THE F●CK OUT OF THE SUN

> "If a magazine (or blogger!) recommends a product, make an informed decision based on your skin type. What works for someone else may not be the best product for you."

WHAT ARE YOUR THOUGHTS ON PLASTIC SURGERY, BOTOX, FILLERS, LASERS, AND OTHER COSMETIC MEDICAL PROCEDURES?

It's not for me—at least right now. I take a lot of pride in taking good care of my skin, and I think the vast majority of women look best in their natural state, with undone hair, smile lines that show they've lived a full, happy life, and I try to remind myself that "no wrinkles" does not necessarily equate to looking younger. But the most important thing, which I try to use as my guiding principle, is just that everyone should do whatever makes them feel their best. For me, that's aging gracefully and leading by example with my daughter, so that when she's older and begins getting wrinkles, she doesn't feel like "What's wrong with me?" ♥

Rocky Barnes

/ @rocky_barnes

TOP MODEL, INFLUENCER, AND ENTREPRENEUR

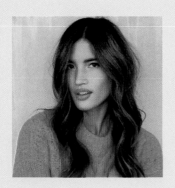

WHAT IS THE MOST PRACTICAL, RELATABLE ADVICE YOU'VE RECEIVED FOR PREVENTATIVE SKINCARE?

The rule of thumb that I use is the trifecta: retinol at night, vitamin C in the morning, and sunscreen throughout the day. I've heard this advice from multiple beauty gurus. I'm never tied to one brand in particular, always willing to try new products, but I do stick to this routine. Before I heard about the trifecta, I found beauty to be somewhat daunting.

There are so many options out there, and having this structure to go by has made my skincare routine less overwhelming.

WHAT IS THE WORST ADVICE YOU'VE EVER HEARD WHEN IT COMES TO TAKING CARE OF YOUR SKIN?

The worst advice I've ever received was that lasers will do wonders for your skin. I think for many people, it might! However, for someone who has skin that is pigmented like mine, it is one of the worst things you can do. Taking other people's advice on skincare can be dangerous. You have to do your own research and look into what's best for you.

We all have different skin types, and there isn't a magic treatment that works for everyone. If I had taken the advice of the person who told me to get lasers, my entire face would be riddled with issues.

WHAT IS A HABIT YOU'VE DEVELOPED OVER THE YEARS THAT MAKES A DIFFERENCE IN YOUR SKIN?

No matter where I am or what I'm doing, I always wash my face before bed. Even in college, on my drunkest nights, I'd always wake up with a clean face. I was never that girl with the raccoon eyes in the morning. Over the past few years, I've made a conscious effort to drink more water as well which, as we all know, is a no-brainer for maintaining clear skin.

WHAT STEPS DO YOU TAKE DURING YOUR DAILY SKIN ROUTINE?

/ **A.M.** /

1 Wake up, rinse face. Just water, that's it!

2 Apply vitamin C serum: Beautycounter Vitamin C Serum

3 Apply moisturizer and SPF: Dr. Barbara Sturm Face Cream, Nars Tinted Moisturizer SPF

/ **P.M.** /

1 MARA Beauty Algae Enzyme Cleansing Oil

2 Charlotte Tilbury Magic Night Cream

3 Tata Harper Restorative Anti-Aging Eye Crème

4 Murad Retinol Youth Renewal Night Cream

When I was pregnant, I lathered MUTHA Body Butter all over my body. ♥

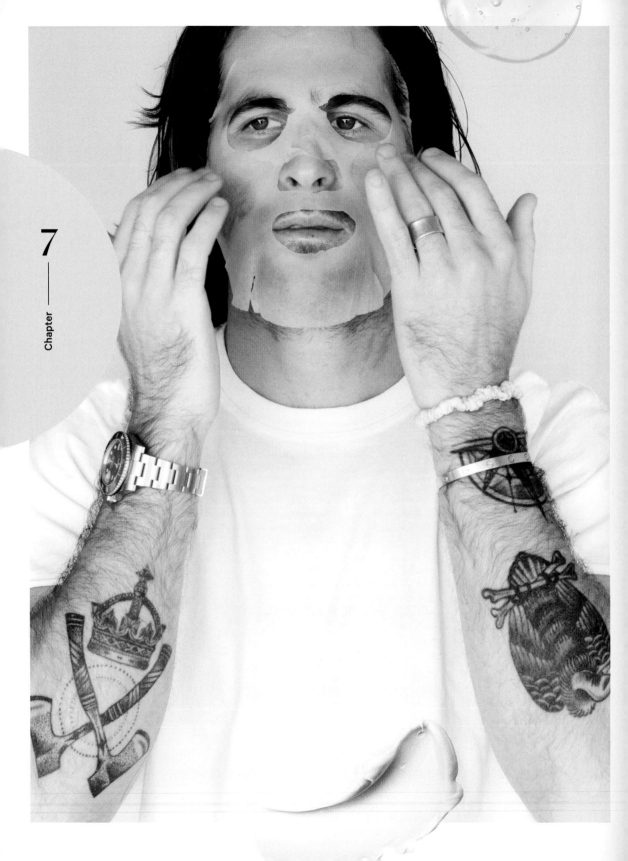

HOW TO MANI-PULATE YOUR MAN INTO SKINCARE

This, my friends, is one of my favorite topics, and THAT is because I feel like if I'm good at one thing, it's manipulating men into skincare. When I first started dating my husband, he had absolutely NO skincare routine. Like he'd maybe slap some Herbal Essence shampoo on his face and then some Coppertone sunscreen if we were lucky? Yikes.

I knew if he kept up this routine his skin would be weathered by the time he was 40. So I needed a plan of action and had to think fast . . .

My plan was simple, efficient, and, most importantly, EFFECTIVE.

Anyway, we're going to hear from my husband soon so we are both going to give you all the secrets to get your S/O into skincare.

The first step is having your own skincare completely under control.

You want to have your routine locked and ready. Have all the products laying out on your vanity with the labels turned out. Now, if you don't share a bathroom with your significant other, you want to take your products to HIS bathroom and make your routine seem SO delicious.

For each step of your routine, you want to really turn on the "ooooohhhhh" & "aaaahh-hhhh." Extra credit for a deep sigh. Pretend you're eating the best ice cream you've ever had in your life.

Obnoxious comments also work wonders.

For instance, when using your toner, say things like, "Wow, this is so refreshing. I've never felt so refreshed in my life." When you finish applying your buttery moisturizer and hop into bed, make a remark about how plump and dewy your skin feels and how you can't wait to wake up with no fine lines or wrinkles. Things like, "Oh my god, my skin has never felt so good," go a long way.

And right before you lie down on your silk pillowcase, with your silk eye mask & your red light therapy hue all over the room, maybe say, "I can't wait to wake up with flawless skin."

So, as your significant other sits there with his God-knows-what on his face that's actually meant for your elbows, he'll start to feel guilty. That's what you're going to lead with here: FEAR. You want him nice & fearful that he'se not taking preventative measures for his skin. And shit . . . that's what this whole book is about . . . preventative measures.

The next thing you're going to want to do is play a podcast on skincare while you guys are getting ready. A little shout out to Dr. Dennis Gross, Dr. Barbara Sturm, Georgia Louise & Dr. Jason Diamond on *The Skinny Confidential HIM & HER Podcast.* You can play these while your man is putting gel in his hair (and probably on his blackheads, too, because he has no idea what the fuck else to use).

This is going to subliminally signal to your man that he needs to take skincare seriously.

Just a heads-up, this isn't a "one and done" type of situation. You're probably going to have to do this Broadway presentation at least 10 times before they MIGHT ask for a moisturizer. That's the thing with men—they're going to ask you for things to try a little bit at a time. He might ask for a little spritz of your mist or a dime of your moisturizer, maybe even a little bit of oil on his wrinkled forehead. The main thing here is to go slow. Like, just the tip to start.

My husband said what really worked for him was when I'd give him one product to try at a time & didn't overwhelm him with everything at once.

First, I had him start with a really buttery cleansing balm. I made sure the bottle had masculine colors & told him to just use it in the shower. Sometimes I even got in the shower with him and did facial massage with it for him. He seemed to like it.

A few months later, I gave him a nice moisturizer with SPF in it.

THEN, you guys, positive reinforcements along the way really made him pop a boner.

I'm telling you, praise them. Tell them their skin looks so good and that you can really see a difference since they've started their new routine. Before I knew it, my husband had a six-step skincare routine with all masculine-colored products, occasionally even stealing my pink, white & teal–colored products. One time he even stuck his dirty fingers into my La Mer jar and rubbed it all over his knees and elbows thinking it was body cream. He came to bed smelling like a Bergdorf's department store, thinking I had no idea that he had gotten into my stash. But that's how obsessed he has gotten with skincare.

Now, he asks me to order him products by Dr. Lancer, Dr. Dennis Gross & Elemis. His routine rivals mine, and sometimes he even looks dewier than me in the morning. His fine lines are disappearing & his confidence is up.

THAT is how you manipulate your man into skincare.

SO JUST TO RECAP, HERE ARE ALL THE STEPS FOR WHEN YOU'RE MAKING YOUR PLAN OF ATTACK . . .

- ♥ Have your own skincare routine completely under control, locked & loaded.
- ♥ Do your skincare routine in front of them with lots of obnoxious sounds like "ooooohhhhh" & "aaaahhhh." Don't forget comments like, "I can't wait to wake up with flawless skin."
- ♥ Remember to lead with FEAR. Fear that they aren't taking care of their skin.
- ♥ Play podcasts about skincare in front of them so someone else is subliminally suggesting they get into skincare.
- ♥ Introduce one product/step at a time. Starting with a cleanser or toner is ideal. You know, like sex . . . "just the tip."
- ♥ Positive reinforcements after a few days. Compliment their skin whenever you can.
- ♥ Before you know it, they'll be thinking it was their idea. Ta-da!

PRODUCTS FOR MEN & HOW TO APPLY THEM:

Cleanser

Put a dime-size amount of cleanser onto your fingertips, then gently apply to your face in small, upward circular motions. I prefer cold or lukewarm water (hot makes redness appear sometimes).

Rinse with warm water, then gently pat your face dry (with a baby washcloth, preferably).

Toner

Soak a cotton pad with toner, then lightly swipe it over face, neck, and chest.

Serum

The standard application is 2 pumps or a dime-size amount.

Eye cream

Always apply your eye cream with your ring finger. Use weakest finger always!

Mosturizer

Gently pat on skin in an upward motion.

Oil

Gently press on skin.

Masks

Masks for men are SO underrated. My husband likes to do a sheet mask in bed—he just lies there like Michael Myers from *Halloween*. He thinks he's so bougie, and by the time he's done showing it off on Instagram Stories, he's sleeping like a baby with plump skin.

Tip of the year: Get him to start with a sheet mask, because they're the coolest.

Speaking of the coolest, let's chat with my husband on all things skin—this section is an ideal read for anyone who's looking to give their S/O a "little nudge-nudge, wink—get your fucking skincare game in check or else."

I got you. ♥

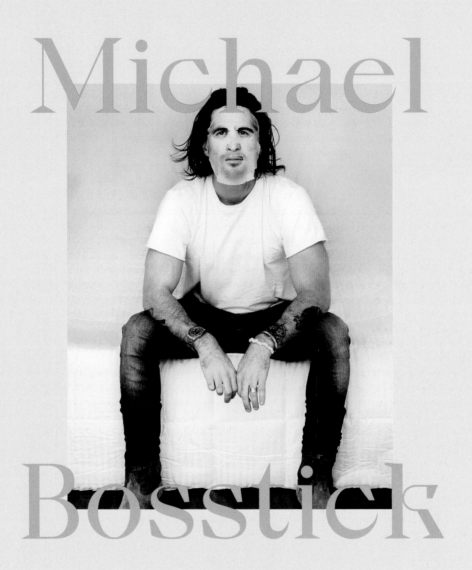

Michael
Bosstick

/ @michaelbosstick

CEO OF DEAR MEDIA, CO-HOST OF
THE SKINNY CONFIDENTIAL HIM & HER
PODCAST, HUSBAND TO LAURYN, AND
FATHER TO ZAZA AND TWO CHIHUAHUAS

WHAT HAVE YOU FOUND TO BE THE MOST EFFECTIVE SKINCARE PRODUCT UNDER $50, AND WHAT'S YOUR BIGGEST SPLURGE?

Under $50, I would say razors. Now, that might sound weird, but I think shaving really renews the skin & helps exfoliate. You don't even need to shave the whole face to get some solid exfoliation. The problem, though, is that Lauryn always steals my razors for herself and uses them . . . on God knows where. Note to self, don't shave with the stolen ones . . .

Dr. Dennis Gross Vitamin C + Collagen Serum is my biggest splurge. My entire life I've had dark undereyes, maybe from a lack of sleep, maybe because my eyes are deep-set, or maybe bad nutrition (working on this), but this serum really works for my skin. When I started using it, my skin became firmer, I could see the fine lines disappear, and my skin was brighter. This is the first product I used where I could really see results. It's also the first product I learned about for skin besides face wash and moisturizer. It opened my eyes to a whole new world of products. Literally, LOL.

We started having all these skincare experts come on *The Skinny Confidential HIM & HER Podcast* who I would've never had access to if we weren't sitting directly across from them for an hour. Dr. Dennis was one of the first guests we had on the show, and listening to him speak about skin really gave me an understanding of skincare at a cellular level. He showed me that there is a huge benefit to taking good care of your skin and even gave me Botox live on the show (it's no big deal, stop being scared!). He was the first person to explain the biology of the skin & why we need to take care

of it, so it became very apparent to me that I needed to start doing something, and the Vitamin C + Collagen Serum really showed me that good skincare products work.

WHAT IS THE MOST PRACTICAL, RELATABLE ADVICE YOU'VE RECEIVED FOR PREVENTATIVE SKINCARE?

That taking care of your skin will make you look and feel better. Sounds like a no-brainer, but for some reason men think they don't need to take care of their skin. People are living longer & longer. I don't want to live the last 30 years of my life looking like I'm already in the grave when I don't have to. For whatever reason, guys have a hard time getting into this stuff, but just washing your face, even in the shower, takes no time at all. I used to just splash my face with water in the shower and thought it was enough, but using a cleanser or face wash takes 2 seconds. Same with putting on a moisturizer. Just washing your face & putting on some moisturizer can make a big difference.

And if you can't do that, at least throw on a little bit of sunscreen. It just makes sense because the sun is really powerful & can do a lot of damage to the skin. I don't tend to lie out & bake, but I also don't hide from it like my wife. If I know I'm going to be in the sun, I like to throw on a little SPF for some protection.

WHAT IS THE WORST ADVICE YOU'VE EVER HEARD WHEN IT COMES TO TAKING CARE OF YOUR SKIN?

Using a ton of different products & mixing them all. It can be really

overwhelming for guys when you're told to start using all these different products & mixing different lines, all at different times of day. The majority of us can't keep up, and if we feel overwhelmed we are going to lose interest. Keep it simple.

Personally, I like to use one product line at a time. For example, I'll use Dr. Dennis Gross's products for a couple months, then when I can see that I've gotten results, I'll start using another line, like Dr. Lancer's men's products, Dr. Barbara Sturm or Drunk Elephant or Elemis (some of Lauryn's favorite brands, too).

Mixing & matching is a bit difficult. Your skin doesn't know what to do & it'll eventually freak out. As a man, it's overwhelming when your wife or girlfriend hands you a bunch of stuff. It was so easy when Lauryn came to me with three products, three steps, and told me what to do. Now it's become a routine & I don't even think about it, like brushing my teeth. So, I suggest picking one brand & sticking to it to really see results.

WHAT IS A HABIT YOU'VE DEVELOPED OVER THE YEARS THAT MAKES A DIFFERENCE IN YOUR SKIN?

Lauryn always jokes that I have a six-step routine now, but it's not quite that long. But I do have an A.M. & P.M. routine now that has become a habit. Maybe it's been drilled in me a bit more than the average man because of the podcast & interviewing so many skin experts, not to mention living with my wife. So having that routine of washing my face, applying a serum & a cream have really made a difference. It takes an extra 6 minutes out of my day. If you don't have 6 minutes to look and feel better, you don't have a life.

HOW DOES YOUR NUTRITION AND WELLNESS PLAN AFFECT YOUR SKIN?

I don't have the best diet, but I don't have the worst, either. My wife would say my problem is I don't eat, but I typically practice intermittent fasting. I like to do 16 hours of fasting & I drink a lot of water. Hydration is number one for skin. I also noticed that when I added more greens to diet my dark undereye circles cleared up. I also take a lot of supplements. To name a few: glutathione, a men's daily (A.M./P.M.), B vitamins, zinc, vitamin D, colostrum, magnesium, amino acids & more. I think making sure you get the right vitamins in your diet is important.

As soon as I wake up, I drink a huge bottle of water, probably 1 liter. Then I'll have a coffee or some kind of caffeine after I've had water. Caffeine & alcohol both really dry out your skin, so I always follow up with another liter of water so my skin doesn't dry out. Some of us only drink caffeine all day long & it really dries out the skin.

WHAT STEPS DO YOU TAKE DURING YOUR DAILY SKIN ROUTINE?

I'll wash my face in the shower usually. Most days I only wash my face once because I don't want to strip it or over-cleanse. Then I'll get out & use a toner, depending on what brand I'm using at the time. Next, I apply a serum & moisturizer and then finish with an eye cream. Like I said, I don't always wear sunscreen, but if I know I'm going to be out in the sun I will put some on. Lauryn would scold me because she'll say I'm getting incidental sun exposure, but if I know I'll just be driving & in the office all day, I don't put any on. Sorry!

I think this might sound like a lot to some people, especially men, but this whole thing doesn't take more than 3 minutes. If I think I need a good exfoliation, I'll use Dr. Dennis's peel pads. At night I'll do a night cream or night serum depending what my skin needs. If I'm a bit dry or need some extra help, that determines what I'll use. Once you start taking care of your skin, you learn to know what it needs when it's not looking its best.

WHAT IS YOUR WHY FOR TAKING CARE OF YOUR SKIN?

For me, straight vanity. When I started using products, I saw the difference right away. Before I got into skincare, I was looking like an old, weathered saddle & my wife & a lot of experts showed me how easy it can be. My wife, my friends & people sitting across from me on the podcast were telling me that my skin was looking better. It made me feel good.

Then I obviously just want healthier, better skin that's going to look better for longer. I'm the kind of guy who likes to weigh the positives & negatives, and I just couldn't find a negative when it came to looking after my skin, so why wouldn't I? A lot of guys say that they don't care & that's fine, you don't have to care, but to me, there's a much bigger downside to NOT doing it than doing it. It's easy, it's fast, and the results are noticeable.

WHAT WOULD YOU SAY TO YOUR YOUNGER SELF ABOUT SKINCARE IF YOU COULD?

I wish someone told me to start taking care of my skin when I was younger. I wish I was able to speak with someone to explain what was happening with my skin at a cellular level as it aged. The most I knew was to throw on some Cetaphil or Dove soap, and they used to run Proactiv commercials for people with acne. That's all I knew.

I think if I had gotten into it, I would have prevented a lot of the fine lines that I have now. We live in a society where we try to fix everything, but really, this stuff is preventable. We can prevent a lot of aging & skin issues instead of correcting them later in life.

WHAT IS AN UNUSUAL OR SOMEWHAT WEIRD PRACTICE YOU DO TO KEEP YOUR SKIN YOUTHFUL?

Not sure if this is that weird, but whenever I see my skin getting bad I'll shave or trim my facial hair. I like to keep a bit of facial hair, but when I shave or trim it renews & refreshes the skin. So if my skin isn't looking too great I'll do that, then steal one of Lauryn's face masks that says HYDRATION & do that.

WHAT ARE YOUR FAVORITE BOOKS, WEBSITES, PODCASTS, OR OTHER RESOURCES YOU REFER TO FOR PREVENTATIVE SKINCARE ADVICE?

Obviously, I have to shout out my own podcast. Really, that's the only place I go to. Second would be my wife & her blog. We have all these built-in resources & the best part is we get to invite these people to our platforms for a one-on-one conversation where we get to ask the exact questions we want answers to. I haven't found a better resource than that.

WHAT ARE YOUR THOUGHTS ON PLASTIC SURGERY, BOTOX, FILLERS, LASERS, AND OTHER COSMETIC MEDICAL PROCEDURES?

From an aesthetic standpoint, less is better is my opinion. But I'm all about people doing whatever makes them happy. I've done Botox because the lines on my forehead were really deep. After talking to Dr. Dennis, he explained to me they would only get worse, so I went for it to paralyze the lines.

People should do it because it makes themselves happy, though, not anyone else. Don't go get a bunch of filler or lip injections because your friends are doing it, or because you think that's what guys/girls like. Don't make decisions on how you look from how other people want you to look. Do it for you and be honest about what you really want.

WHAT WAS YOUR SKINCARE ROUTINE LIKE BEFORE YOU MET LAURYN?

I didn't have one. I literally would just get in the shower and rub shampoo on my face while I washed my hair. As I said, I looked like an old weathered saddle and really didn't realize what I was doing to myself. I also think a lot of young people think they will look that way forever. It wasn't until I hit my 30s that I started to see how wrong I was. Listen up, young people! Enjoy it now, because it goes quick if you don't take care of yourself.

HOW DO YOU THINK LAURYN MANIPULATED YOU INTO A SKINCARE ROUTINE? WHAT TACTICS DID SHE USE THAT WORKED?

The best thing Lauryn did was introduce only one or two products at a time. Also, she'd get me things like a "gentleman's facial"—never anything too crazy or intimidating. Then, of course, I had the benefit of sitting in podcasts with her and these doctors and experts telling me exactly how to take care of my skin. So it really rubbed off.

Positive reinforcements didn't hurt, either. Getting compliments (Lauryn really knows how and when to lay it on thick) let me know that what I was doing was working, and over time, she introduced more products in a way that was easy to understand. Seeing the benefits while having it become part of my everyday routine made it an easy habit.

IF YOU HAD TO GIVE SOMEONE ONE TIP TO GET A MAN INTO SKINCARE, WHAT WOULD IT BE?

As I said, what worked best for me was only being introduced to one or two products at a time and positive reinforcements. The biggest mistake is to overwhelm us men. Slowly introduce things and use them together. Do your skin routines together and show your partner how to use each product.

Once in a while, Lauryn would get forceful and just put something on my face, but then it would feel good so I wanted to use that product more. She would also say that she could tell I wasn't using certain things from the way my skin looked, so I'd get all self-conscious. But that actually worked, because it told me that when I do take care of my skin the difference is noticeable.

WHAT'S YOUR FAVORITE THING YOU'VE LEARNED ABOUT SKINCARE THROUGH LAURYN?

That if you keep up with the maintenance you'll constantly see benefits. But if you stop, you'll see the consequences, too. As soon as you start taking care of your skin, you can see all the good it's doing. It helps you become aware of the state of your skin and know what it needs. If you take care of your skin you can slow aging, but the most important thing I learned from Lauryn is knowing your skin and knowing what it needs. The downside of this for me personally is that I now analyze the skin of literally everyone I meet. Things I didn't notice before I can now see right away. I can tell if someone has good skin or not. I can tell if they take care of it or not. It's hard to unsee once you see the light! Next, we'll hear from a few more men who are true experts in their beautifying fields (plus one totally batshit outlier, so hold on to your seats for that one). ♥

Justin

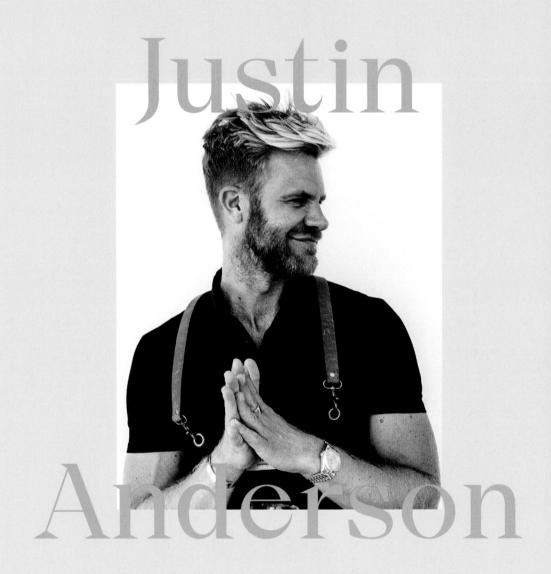

Anderson

/ @justinanderson and @justinandersoncolor

CELEBRITY HAIRSTYLIST AND
FOUNDER OF DPHUE

WHAT HAVE YOU FOUND TO BE THE MOST EFFECTIVE SKINCARE PRODUCT UNDER $50, AND WHAT'S YOUR BIGGEST SPLURGE?

Best skincare product under $50 is an ice pack for my face I purchased from Amazon that I wear in the morning after a night of eating too much salt or drinking. The pack helps reduce swollen, puffy skin. My biggest splurge is the 3Lab WW Day SPF 40. I love that it's a clear sunscreen and goes on matte. Other sunscreens always make me greasy.

WHAT IS THE WORST ADVICE YOU'VE EVER HEARD WHEN IT COMES TO TAKING CARE OF YOUR SKIN?

I remember when I was younger I was told the sun would help dry out acne. In actuality, a sunburn over an acne scar will leave a lasting mark.

WHAT HABIT HAVE YOU DEVELOPED OVER THE YEARS THAT MAKES A DIFFERENCE IN YOUR SKIN?

When I am consistent with taking a shot of apple cider vinegar every morning, I notice my skin is the clearest.

> **"...I use TAZORAC Cream, which I find to be the best thing to shrink my pores. It's much more expensive than a retinol cream, but I truly believe it works the best!"**

WHAT STEPS DO YOU TAKE DURING YOUR DAILY SKIN ROUTINE?

Since I wash my face following my early morning workout, when I get home, I just rinse in the shower then immediately apply a toner. Every other day, I use Dr. Dennis Gross Alpha Beta Extra Strength Daily Peel. I am also a huge fan of vitamin C, so I apply it after the toner. However, I have to be very strategic about how I apply vitamin C because of my blond hairline and beard. No matter which brand I use, it always tints the hair in those areas orange. On days I can't risk an orange hairline, I use the MARA Beauty Universal Face Oil, followed by the 3Lab SPF. I only use the SPF if I know I will be in direct sun, because I find that daily use of SPF makes my pores larger, and I prefer to wear a hat when needed.

At night, I wash, tone, use Universal Oil and every other night, I use TAZORAC Cream, which I find to be the best thing to shrink my pores. It's much more expensive than a retinol cream, but I truly believe it works the best!

WHAT IS AN UNUSUAL OR SOMEWHAT WEIRD PRACTICE YOU DO TO KEEP YOUR SKIN YOUTHFUL?

I convinced my aesthetician to buy me a professional-strength microderma roller that I use at home once a week or every other week before applying my serum. Also, a few times a week, I fill my sink with cold water and ice then stick my face in it before bed and always before an at-home selfie!

WHAT ARE YOUR THOUGHTS ON PLASTIC SURGERY, BOTOX, FILLERS, LASERS, AND OTHER COSMETIC MEDICAL PROCEDURES?

Huge fan! I believe starting Botox early helps with wrinkles and is very preventative. I also love a Clear & Brilliant two to three times a year. I'm all about cosmetic procedures as long as you aren't changing the shape of your face. ♥

Hyram Yarbro / @skincarebyhyram

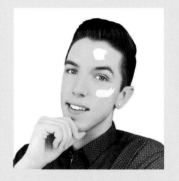

WHAT HAVE YOU FOUND TO BE THE MOST EFFECTIVE SKINCARE PRODUCT UNDER $50, AND WHAT'S YOUR BIGGEST SPLURGE?

Youth To The People Kale Superfood Cleanser. It's one of those cleansers that just works so well, and anytime I remove it from my routine, my skin is noticeably different. It's more textured, more clogged. I've recommended it to everyone, and so many people say that it's life-changing.

My biggest splurge has probably been the Foreo UFO LED heating and cooling mask. It's a really cool device that has just three different types of LED lights using a warming and cooling processor to basically help you better apply your skincare products and your face masks.

WHAT IS THE MOST PRACTICAL, RELATABLE ADVICE YOU'VE RECEIVED FOR PREVENTATIVE SKINCARE?

Sunscreen, definitely. Just sunscreen. Very simple, but in reality, that's what will just prevent the majority of skincare problems. And it's something that I and so many others pushed back against initially, but in reality, it's the most practical advice I've been given. My favorite is probably the Purito Unscented Centella SPF50. It's a Korean sunscreen that performs so beautifully. It feels like a light moisturizer, no white cast. The ingredients are incredible, and it utilizes innovative Korean UV filters that have performed so much better than what we have in the USA.

WHAT STEPS DO YOU TAKE DURING YOUR DAILY SKIN ROUTINE?

I'll usually start my nighttime routine as soon as the sun goes down so that I'm getting the full benefits of the nighttime routine, as opposed to only right before I go to sleep. So I will usually use a cleansing balm or a cleansing oil. I don't use makeup wipes, and I don't solely go in with a cleanser because that'll be most effective for removing sunscreen. And then I rinse off, using a water-based cleanser to get all the cleansing oil or balm out, and then sometimes I'll go in with a treatment. I like to use the treatment first so that it's not interrupted by any moisturizing agents or ingredients on top. Right now I've been using the Versed Gentle Retinol serum for nights that I do retinol. On the nights I'm exfoliating I've been doing the KraveBeauty Kale-lalu-yAHA treatments, glycolic acid treatments. I'll offset my retinol and exfoliating treatment. I'll exfoliate about two times a week and use the retinol about two times a week.

And then in between those I'll just do a night solely focused on restoring the moisture barrier to make sure it's protected. And afterward, I usually go in with a product called KraveBeauty Great Barrier Relief. That one is pretty much my ride or die for protecting the moisture barrier. And it has all of my favorite ingredients in it. And then, depending on how dry my skin is and what time of the year it is, I go in with a really hydrating moisturizer. Right now I'm using a lightweight gel cream from Rovectin, Clean Lotus Water Cream; it's a Korean brand. Then I use the Milk Makeup Melatonin lip mask. I think the routine is relatively simple, because I offset some of those. I don't do all of this every single night, but I like to have at least 4–5 steps. 🖤

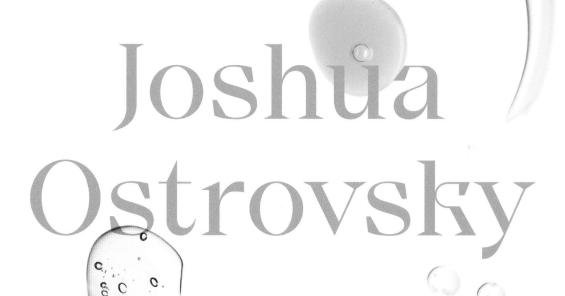

Joshua Ostrovsky

/ @thefatjewish

AMERICAN CELEBRITY AND
ENTREPRENEUR KNOWN AS
THE FAT JEW

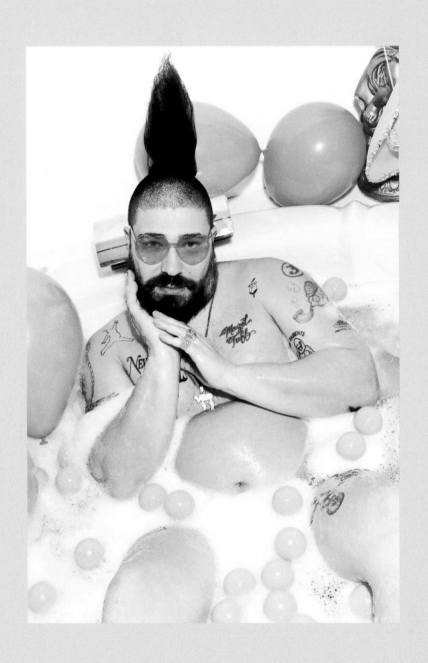

WHAT HAVE YOU FOUND TO BE THE MOST EFFECTIVE SKINCARE PRODUCT UNDER $50, AND WHAT'S YOUR BIGGEST SPLURGE?

My skincare routine is as follows: I'll start the day with a Nicaraguan Manuka honey. I'll get a dollop of that (usually from Moon Juice) & I'll smear it all over my face. Then I'll take a Reishi powder and dump it all over my pores & into my mouth. Then I spit it back into my hand, so it's like a paste, then rub that all over my body. Jk jk jk, I literally use Noxzema cream like a teen from the '80s. For my biggest splurge, I guess it would be Badescu. I bought some Badescu, didn't really care much about it, but then I was like—THIS IS FUCKING GREAT. My skin was glowing. I looked like I was pregnant.

WHAT IS THE MOST PRACTICAL, RELATABLE ADVICE YOU'VE RECEIVED FOR PREVENTATIVE SKINCARE?

Someone told me to use a fucking Bioré strip once. And to be honest, I have giant Russian pores on my face & things are just getting in there. All kinds of wild shit gets in there. We have a whole group chat where we send pics of our used Bioré strips. It's so gnarly. Guys are so disgusting, honestly. Our dicks smell & our Bioré strips are heinous.

WHAT HABIT HAVE YOU DEVELOPED OVER THE YEARS THAT MAKES A DIFFERENCE IN YOUR SKIN?

A good plan is to grow a beard up to your fucking eyeballs so no one can see your face, then everyone will be like, "Oh, his forehead looks good." People think my skin is flawless because they can only see 10 percent of it.

HOW DOES YOUR NUTRITION AND WELLNESS PLAN AFFECT YOUR SKIN?

My nutrition has never affected my skin. It made me really fat until I literally looked like fucking Shrek and started sweating when I pooped, but my skin has always been flawless. I have never had any body acne (or body hair)—I actually look like a giant smooth infant when nude. It's a blessing, and also kind of creepy.

WHAT IS YOUR "WHY" FOR TAKING CARE OF YOUR SKIN?

Because I'm a narcissistic monster who looks at a group photo and only focuses on how *I* look!

WHAT IS AN UNUSUAL OR SOMEWHAT WEIRD PRACTICE YOU DO TO KEEP YOUR SKIN YOUTHFUL?

When I was in the Dominican Republic, there were these guys who do this thing where they manually masturbate whales. They jerk off these whales & procure the semen, and it's basically a super exfoliant. So I bought some. I think it worked?

WHAT ARE YOUR FAVORITE BOOKS, WEBSITES, PODCASTS, OR OTHER RESOURCES FOR PREVENTATIVE SKINCARE ADVICE?

The Skinny Confidential. You're the only one I'll watch a 397-step skincare routine for. You also do really nice charcuterie boards. Like, I've gotten weird erections from your charcuterie boards—I guess I'm attracted to them?

WHAT ARE YOUR THOUGHTS ON PLASTIC SURGERY, BOTOX, FILLERS, LASERS, AND OTHER COSMETIC MEDICAL PROCEDURES?

YES YES YES YES YES. I was with a group of people at dinner the other night (five men, five women) and one of the guys was like, "None of you ladies need any work, you're all beautiful," and I was just like STOP. We all need work.

I do think we're starting a little young. Kylie Jenner used to look like an unloaded baked potato, so for her, that was probably a good move. She looks great now. You don't really need to do much in your 20s, but once you hit your 30s . . . go the fuck off. Get your whole face redone, get a new face welded onto your face.

Very recently I met J.Lo, and she is actually Benjamin Button, completely aging in reverse. Honestly, she looks so fucking good. I would literally pick corn out of her feces. She looks amazing. Who is her Persian plastic surgeon? GIVE ME HIS FUCKING NUMBER, JENNIFER. ♥

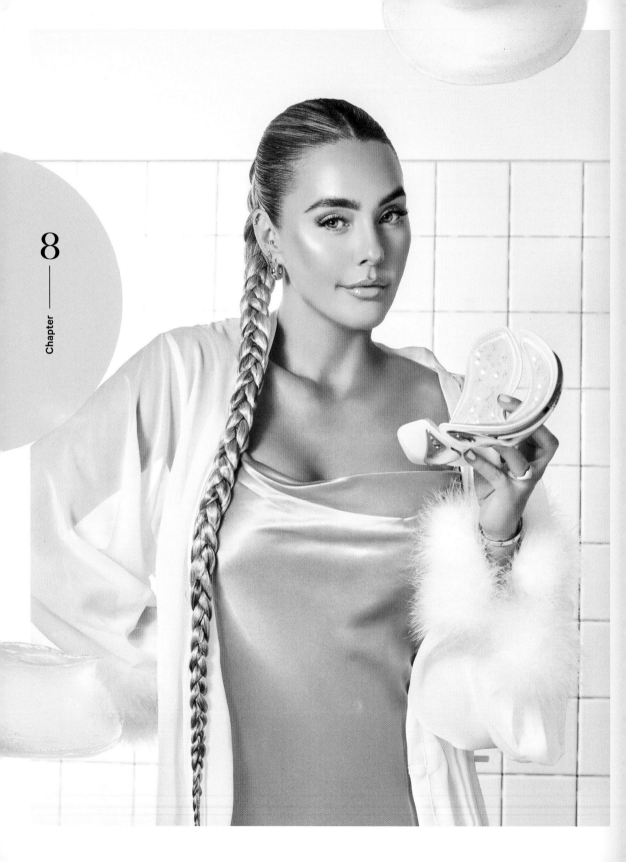

BUT LIKE, WHAT DO THE DERMATOLOGISTS, AESTHETICIANS & PLASTIC SURGEONS SAY?

A huge part of my platform is sharing what the everyday girl is doing, my journey, and which supermodels love a certain eye cream. But we also need the nitty-gritty, scientific 411 from the experts. Having the podcast and the blog has allowed me to sit down and pick the brains of these experts—like people who really know their shit.

Keep reading for all the nerdy details we all want to know. Many people in this chapter have not only gone to college for a billion years to really study their craft, they've also started huge businesses and empires (As if you need another reason to respect them!). Additonally, they've all made standout products that I love and use every day, and maybe you guys do, too.

THE EXPERTS

Without further ado, allow me to introduce you to the gurus:

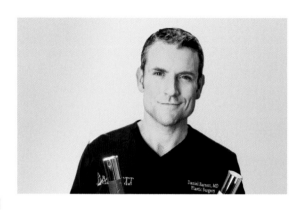

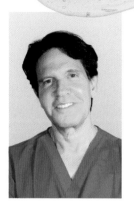

DR. DANIEL BARRETT
BOARD-CERTIFIED PLASTIC SURGEON

DR. DENNIS GROSS
DERMATOGIST AND CO-FOUNDER OF DR. DENNIS GROSS SKINCARE

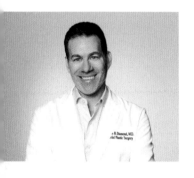

DR. JASON DIAMOND
DOUBLE BOARD-CERTIFIED CELEBRITY DERMATOLOGIST KNOWN FOR HIS MODERN FACE-LIFT

GEORGIA LOUISE
CRITICALLY ACCLAIMED CELEBRITY FACIALIST OFTEN REFERRED TO AS .THE "FACE SCIENTIST"

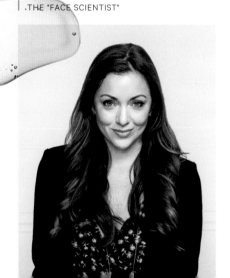

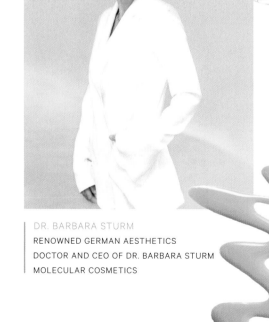

DR. BARBARA STURM
RENOWNED GERMAN AESTHETICS DOCTOR AND CEO OF DR. BARBARA STURM MOLECULAR COSMETICS

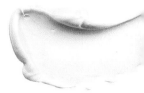

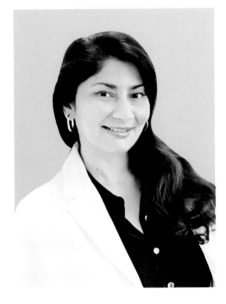

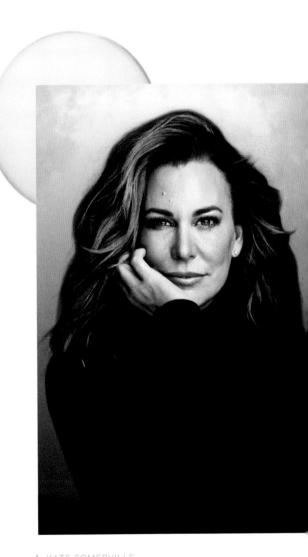

DR. KAY DURAIRAJ
CELEBRITY FACIAL AND NECK PLASTIC
SURGEON AND VOTED ONE OF THE TOP 100
INJECTORS IN THE US

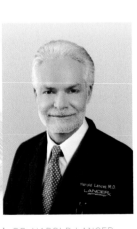

DR. HAROLD LANCER
BOARD-CERTIFIED CELEBRITY
DERMATOLOGIST AND FOUNDER OF
THE LANCER METHOD

KATE SOMERVILLE
FOUNDER AND CREATOR OF KATE SOMERVILLE
SKINCARE AND KATE SOMERVILLE SKIN HEALTH
EXPERTS

Dr. Daniel Barrett

/ @drdanielbarrett

BOARD-CERTIFIED PLASTIC SURGEON

WHAT'S THE MOST EFFECTIVE TREATMENT OR PROCEDURE, AND WHY?

I get asked all the time for quick fixes: Should I laser this or dermaplane that? Skin procedures and treatments such as these are only a small piece of the beautiful skin puzzle. In many ways, they're a lot like a get-rich-quick scheme: They sound good on paper, generate a lot of enthusiasm, and ultimately don't work.

One example of this is the IPL (intense pulsed light) laser. Many companies make these and sell them to providers as a fix-it-quick option for pigmentation concerns, like melasma (sometimes called "pregnancy mask"). The problem is that melasma and many pigment disorders are multifactorial in origin. Yes, an IPL treatment gives instant initial improvement but ultimately creates worse hyperpigmentation in nonconditioned skin. This is because the heat from the laser blasts away pigment while heat trauma actually increases pigment production in the skin's melanocytes. This is brilliant for the laser company and the service provider as it keeps people coming back for more frequent fixes, but is not in the best interest of the individual.

The most effective skincare treatment is a carefully-crafted skincare routine and a healthy lifestyle. Once this is obtained, ancillary treatments such as lasers, peels, dermaplaning, facials, and microneedling can augment your skin's appearance. They are never good as stand-alone treatments, and each one has its unique advantages and disadvantages.

WHAT'S THE BIGGEST MISTAKE YOU SEE PEOPLE STILL MAKING WHEN IT COMES TO THEIR SKIN?

Trying to figure out on their own what is best for their skin. Our skin is one of the largest organs in/on our body, and it protects us from the environment. With skin being so important, and with so many different skin conditions out there, why do people try to figure out what's best for them online or by asking a salesperson in the cosmetics aisle at Whole Foods? Go to a qualified skin professional and you will save time & money and keep your skin looking fresh & youthful.

WHAT IS YOUR ABSOLUTE FAVORITE SKINCARE PRODUCT IF YOU HAD TO CHOOSE, AND WHY?

ZO Exfoliating Polish Face Scrub. I use it every morning. It is the most refreshing thing I do and feels amazing! It was named one of the top exfoliating face scrubs by Good Housekeeping Institute Beauty Lab, and for good reason. It has ultrafine magnesium crystals that don't destroy your skin like apricot scrubs, as well as vitamins A, C, C-ester, and E, which deliver a powerful antioxidant boost during the exfoliation. My favorite part is the tea tree oil because it smells amazing and reduces inflammation.

Mechanical exfoliation is the fastest way to smooth and refresh skin. I often have my patients who are skeptical of skincare products try the ZO Exfoliating Polish first. They are back within a week, ready to hear more of what I have to say because it works that fast! Not only does exfoliation get rid of inflammatory sebum, dead skin cells, and other dirt & debris on your face, allowing other products to penetrate deeper, it increases dermal turnover and repair. This is a crucial mechanism that decreases how old your skin looks by thickening it, reducing pigment, and reducing wrinkles. If you want strong and youthful skin, don't forget to exfoliate.

WHAT'S A HEALTH OR WELLNESS TIP THAT MAKES A BIG DIFFERENCE IN PEOPLE'S SKIN?

The foundation of beautiful skin begins with lifestyle. Sleep, diet, and environmental protection are more important than anything you can do or apply to your skin. I have many 20-something patients who come to my office asking for undereye filler for dark circles. When I ask them about their lifestyle, they tell me they are staying up late at night, drinking excessively, getting bad sunburns at pool parties, and eating horrible food. I charge over $1,000 to inject one syringe of filler under the eyes, but addressing these lifestyle factors is completely free and beneficial in so many other ways.

Be sure to carve out time to a exercise every day. Mostly, this is to help you sleep better at night. Go to bed and wake up at the same time every day—including the weekend. Get 7–8 hours of sleep. Yes, moms, this can be achieved for you as well. I have two young daughters, and my amazing wife and I still are able to make sleep a priority. Be disciplined about this and your skin will reward you tenfold more than what I can do for you in my office.

A more recent revelation in wellness that can help your total body inflammation is earthing or grounding. That is, connecting your body to the earth in some meaningful manner every day similar to how humans evolved with daily earth connection. Some people walk barefoot on the grass or beach, others connect grounding patches to their body. The early research behind this is promising. One review study suggested that grounding improves the living matrix, which is the central connector between living cells. Tiny electrical signals course through our body, and it's suspected that if the charge is left to build up, it damages our immune system and increases inflammation. I bought into this and use grounding patches and shoe straps when I exercise, walk barefoot when I can, and sleep on a grounding mat at night. My first morning after trying this I woke up more refreshed than I've felt in a long time! I like the products from Ultimate Longevity and Erthe grounding shoe straps.

WHAT SHOULD WE BE EATING FOR OUR SKIN?

Diet is not one size fits all, so be flexible. I'm no diet expert, but I've found some common factors that help with skin health. They all revolve around lowering the inflammation in your body, and hence your skin. Here are three areas you should start with:

Address food sensitivities. There are several studies on our own body's intuition when it comes to what we eat. Children naturally select food that contains nutrients they are deficient in. So it's important to listen to your body, but also to supplement that with a food sensitivity test such as a Cyrex Food Sensitivity Test. Recently I discovered I had a strong

sensitivity to peanuts—and had no idea. I was eating two or three peanut-containing products every day, and when I stopped, my skin, sleep & bowel habits dramatically improved.

Another tip is to start taking digestive enzymes with every meal to lower the immune response of the foods you eat. I like a product called Masszymes. I immediately felt less bloated when I started taking it. Restore is another great product that helps with leaky gut syndrome and combats glyphosate bombardment.

Practice intermittent fasting. Humans did not evolve over millions of years to eat three meals a day. In fact, doing so is detrimental to our health in so many ways. Most humans evolved to eat once, maybe twice a day. Dr. John Kellogg coined the phrase "breakfast is the most important meal of the day" in a 1917 publication and single-handedly invented breakfast. Prior to this, many cultures would not eat until afternoon. It may sound crazy, but when you stop eating for at least 12 hours, you give your gut a break and dramatically switch the hormone levels in your body. This switches your body from being carbohydrate dependent to a ketone or fat-burning mode.

This is important for many reasons, like improving insulin sensitivity (reducing diabetes), helping with weight loss, preventing dementia, improving mental clarity & heart health, and lowering the overall oxidative stress in your body and skin. Intermittent fasting is also one of the best ways to naturally reduce acne and many other skin problems. Again, there are entire books on this subject, but my recommendation is to start intermittent fasting today with a 12-hour eating window and a 12-hour fasting window. For example, finish eating dinner at 6 P.M. and don't eat again until 6 A.M.

For more benefits, increase your fasting window to up to 16 hours (and lower your eating window to 8 hours). Every month you can do a 24-hour water fast, and every quarter you can try a fasting-mimicking diet for 3 days or go all in with a 3-day water fast. This will have a dramatic cleansing effect on your body.

Be careful at first, and supplement your fast with activated charcoal and bentonite clay to absorb the toxins that are released the first few times you try this. When your body finally taps into your fat cells, it releases many environmental, fat-soluble toxins that you've absorbed over the years. This is one reason why many people get headaches when first trying intermittent fasting. Power through the first week and don't give up—beyond that it gets easier!

Avoid inflammatory foods and oils. As a general rule, don't eat anything in a package or box that isn't fresh. Stay far away from fast food, since the oils in fast food are extremely inflammatory to the skin, and will cause breakouts and premature aging. The preservatives may not kill you or cause cancer (at first), but they can torment your skin.

Stick with raw or fresh foods, shop the perimeter at the grocery store—don't buy anything in the aisles! Furthermore, eat more foods that reduce inflammation and are high in omega fatty acids, like fish. Stay away from non-organic produce and factory-farmed meats. A factory-farmed cow will impart its GMO-grain-fed-inflammation straight to your skin, whereas pasture-raised bison will do wonders for it. Being vegetarian or vegan is OK, but realize that many choose to be vegan based on skewed meat studies showing the toxic implication of eating factory-farmed meat, not organic pasture-raised meat. There is a big difference. If you are avoiding meat, make sure to supplement your protein, collagen, minerals, and omegas appropriately.

WHAT VITAMINS & MINERALS ARE BEST FOR THE SKIN?

By now, everyone should know the basics. Vitamins C, D, E, K, biotin, and zinc all do wonders and can be found in a good multivitamin like Thorne Research Multi-Vitamin Elite A.M. & P.M. But beyond the basics are some more powerful and recently-discovered antioxidants—like the carotenoid astaxanthin and polyphenols like resveratrol—and its newer cousin pterostilbene that are better absorbed. Astaxanthin is produced by algae—and shrimp and salmon contain a lot of it. That's what gives them a pink glow. Farm-raised salmon has to be dyed pink because it is naturally gray. FYI, farm-raised salmon is toxic, and I don't recommend consuming it. If you take astaxanthin every day, it gives your skin a gentle glow. According to some studies, it is 1,000 times more potent than vitamin C and serves as a natural built-in sunblock. I recommend taking 12 mg daily, and my favorite version of this product is Hawaiian BioAstin.

There are many more beneficial supplements to ward off aging and benefit your skin. I recommend downloading the Kaufmann protocol app and plugging in all of your details to see what supplements you might benefit from. Again, just like diet, it's not one size fits all.

HOW CAN WE ALL GET SUPERSTAR SKIN?

Superstar or rock star skin is probably not the best skin. Can you imagine the stress experienced by celebrities and performers and how it impacts their skin? Being on the road traveling, poor diet choices, late performances, tons of makeup and sweat? For superstars, the fundamentals are even more important. Any semblance of normalcy they can incorporate into their skincare routines and lifestyle will be very beneficial. However, the biggest challenge for my high-profile and celebrity clients is to tackle stress. If this is you, or you have a high-performance job or work environment, listen up. Stress levels have a tremendous impact on our skin health and quality. Hormones, like cortisol, that are induced by chronic stress, are beauty and skin destroyers. The good news is that they can be mitigated by several daily habits, including my favorite, meditation.

Imagine you have 57 different apps running on your phone at one time. That load is eventually going to bog down your phone and consume all your battery power. The same is true for your brain! If you have a million thoughts running at once in your brain, you won't be able to focus well on any task and your brain will tire out. More important, stress hormones will increase. Meditation is like hitting the reset button on your brain and body. It filters down meaningless thoughts, anxieties, and emotions just like closing the apps on your phone and restarting it.

The benefits of a regular meditation practice are well studied. It's been shown to improve mental clarity &

focus, and to decrease blood pressure and incidence of heart disease, cancer, depression, irritable bowel syndrome, chronic pain & inflammation. It also has a tremendous positive impact on your beauty and skin.

The root causes of many skin problems such as psoriasis, eczema, acne, and vitiligo are stress, anxiety, fear, and worry. In one study of psoriasis patients, the group that listened to meditation tapes while under a UV light healed four times faster than the group that did not listen to the meditation tapes. Meditation reduces negative emotions, which not only lowers your stress levels, but also decreases how often you frown—something that can cause wrinkles over time.

Have you ever seen the face of a Zen master? They look totally relaxed & at peace and have far fewer wrinkles than most folks their age. Want to save money on Botox? Try meditation.

Meditation also slows the aging process from the inside out by allowing increased delivery of oxygen to your internal organs and skin. It boosts your mood, overall confidence, and willpower so you can make smart diet choices and lifestyle changes that impact your skin.

Meditation may seem nutty or intimidating to some. Others wonder where to start. A single breath can be a meditation. It's that easy. A great option for beginners is the guided meditation apps that are available. I started with those and eventually took a 4-day course in Transcendental Meditation that consisted of two 20-minute meditations daily. I liked that I had access to meditation instructors who could answer my questions as I was incorporating the practice into my life. I liked it so much I asked my wife to join me! Daily practice has done wonders for my health and our marriage.

TALK TO US ABOUT THE DIFFERENT SKIN TYPES, I.E., COMBINATION, SENSITIVE, OILY, ETC.

Many of our patients complain that they have sensitive or dry skin. We hear it all the time, and many of them use it as an excuse to justify a bizarre skincare regimen. There is no clear consensus on skin types, but there is a lot of evidence that combination skin (oily in the T-zone and dry everywhere else) doesn't really exist. Some studies suggest that only 15 percent of the population actually has dry skin and the majority simply have regular oily skin.

What people most often have is SICK skin! Skin that is lacking appropriate barrier function or skin that is weakened by aggressive moisturizing regimens. Aggressive moisturization can signal the dermis to stop producing its own natural moisturizer. Appropriate skin conditioning can heal sick skin and get you back on track. Consult with a skincare expert to diagnose your skin type, and more important, develop a routine that will work for you.

WHAT SHOULD WE BE LOOKING FOR ON SKINCARE LABELS?

When I'm looking at the labels of skin products, the ingredient list is what I turn to first. Ingredients are listed in order of how much is in the product. For example, if alcohol is listed as one of the top three ingredients, that product might not be the best thing to put on your face.

Next, check the open jar symbol and expiration date. The open jar symbol is how good the product is once it's opened: for example, 3M, 6M, 12M. The M stands for months. Be sure to use the product in that time frame and avoid expired products. Expiration dates *do* matter for skincare, especially with combination formulations. Most products that are vegan will have this on their label. Products that are cruelty-free will have a bunny symbol on them.

When it comes to the actual ingredients, this takes a little more research. There are some ingredients that I have to look up because I've never heard of them and sometimes can't pronounce. I used to think this was a negative, but some ingredients that sound ridiculous are actually good for you.

Example:
TOCOPHEROL: vitamin E
PALMITOYL TETRAPEPTIDE-7:
   a beneficial growth peptide
TETRAHEXYLDECYL ASCORBATE:
vitamin C

All sound intimidating at first but are actually beneficial. Bottom line, labels are important to understand, but do your research on ingredients.

WHAT'S YOUR ADVICE FOR ANYONE CONSIDERING BOTOX & FILLERS?

Do your research when selecting a professional to inject neurotoxin or dermal fillers into your face. Even the best injectors experience complications, so don't trust your face to someone you haven't fully vetted. I call it the "beauty expert selection pyramid."

The foundation begins with the credentials of your provider. Make sure they are a board-certified physician in the specialty they are practicing. If you are getting lip injections in someone's garage, you've definitely made a mistake. Next up, check out their before and after photos. Do they exist? If so, do you like the results you're seeing? Do the results look like what you are trying to achieve?

Next, check out their reviews. Yelp is my go-to here in Los Angeles because its reviews can't be bought, and it heavily favors the consumer. Don't just believe the testimonials on the provider's website. Then, call the office. Is there a person answering the phone? If so, are they nice? Can they explain the process to you?

Lastly, schedule a consult and make sure it's a good fit. If it doesn't feel right, don't feel bad, it's not always meant to be. Find someone who is passionate about what they do and not just trying to make a buck. You are trusting this person with your health and beauty. Keep looking if it doesn't feel right. Filler or Botox gone wrong can cause permanent injury and even blindness in very rare circumstances. Invest time in the selection process.

HOW BAD ARE SMOKING & TANNING FOR THE SKIN & WHY?

Smoking and excessive tanning or sun exposure are *perhaps the worst things* you can do to your skin.

Let's start with smoking. This one is personal, as my father passed away from lung cancer when I was 15 years old after smoking his entire life. The ingredients in cigarettes harm every major organ in your body, including your skin. Looking back at old photos of my father, I can see the skin damage the smoking caused. The main mechanism of smoking works by constricting blood vessels that deliver oxygen and nutrients to your skin. The result is damaged elastin, which causes sagging everywhere,

and damaged collagen, which leads to premature aging and increased wrinkles. Including the worst wrinkles to treat—smoker's lines.

Tanning and excessive sun exposure are almost equally bad. Although I recommend a small amount of daily sun exposure to at least 25 percent of your body for 15 minutes, you don't have to expose your face. There are actually photoreceptors on many parts of your body, including the back of your knees. The reason why a little bit of sunlight is good for your body is that it helps maintain your circadian rhythm and produce essential vitamins like vitamin D and certain hormones. It improves your mood, sleep, and stress levels. There is a reason why people get seasonal depression when they are kept in the dark during winter months.

A little bit of UV light is OK for the above reasons, but too much causes some of the most difficult-to-treat skin damage. UV light penetrates deeply into your skin and breaks the DNA strands in your skin cells. This causes them to mutate and increases your risk of skin cancer. Not only this, but there is an increase in the production of free radicals that damage the beauty factors in your skin, like collagen and elastin.

Be smart about your sun exposure. You can always protect your face with sunblock and allow your body to soak up a few minutes every day. If out for more than a few minutes, be sure to wear protective clothing to minimize damage. If you have even the slightest sunburn, you've failed your skin and will probably be seeing me sooner rather than later.

In regard to tanning beds, there is a better solution—red light therapy. Red light therapy exposes your face and body to high-energy-specific wavelength light in the red light

and infrared spectrums. These light waves do not damage your skin but rather boost skin quality by increasing mitochondria function, collagen levels, and circulation. They also help muscle recovery, lower blood pressure, decrease inflammation, and help repair skin damage like stretch marks, scars, and wrinkles. Red light therapy also makes you feel good, just like a tanning bed.

There are numerous devices on the market—from handheld options to double-sided bed options. Two companies that I like are LightStim and Joovv. I have a large four-panel Joovv in my living room. I stand in front of it for about 20 minutes every morning, and I love the way it helps me get my day started. If you can't afford to purchase one, there are several spas and offices like mine that have these panels available for patient use.

HOW CAN WE CONTACT YOU FOR MORE INFO?

I'll leave my number right here: (310) 859-9816. When you look your best, you feel your best, and when you feel your best, you do your best.

Dr. Dennis Gross
ON PREVENTATIVE
BEAUTY & SPF

You have a window of opportunity to prevent problems. It's absolutely possible nowadays to prevent instead of treat & correct. Aging just creeps up on us, but it's totally predictable. Younger people are getting involved in taking care of their skin, and that is a good thing. This generation can look young forever because we know the technology & concepts you need to exercise when you're younger. This means starting with devices or or certain ingredients, doing little treatments, doing baby Botox. We'll talk about this later in this chapter. Preventative beauty is key.

I cannot emphasize enough how super important prompt intervention & treatment is. When you start to see a line or a wrinkle, or you start to see a little bit of looseness in skin, that's all about collagen. It's all about how your skin has lost those fibers that make skin firm, that give it thickness, and that starts to happen in your early 20s. You may not see it, but it's actually inside your skin and then, boom, a wrinkle is born.

If you were outside for 10 or 20 minutes a day, just running into the store, to the car, back and forth saying hi to somebody for a few minutes, or whatever, at the end of the year, that equals sitting in the sun or lying on the beach for five full days straight, if you do the math. That's just totally unacceptable. So the sun is really a hazard.

Driving is a huge factor in incidental sun exposure. You can literally see more crow's feet & more sagging & even larger pores with the loss of collagen as the skin thins out.

You should be wearing sunscreen even if you're not actually actively sunbathing. And I'm telling you, this is how you're going to look younger in years to come.

Dr. Kay Durairaj
ON NEW, POPULAR
PROCEDURES

Liquid Rhinoplasty

Liquid rhinoplasty is a filler injection & runs around $1,000 or so per visit. It's used very creatively, and you have to be a good artist with it. I use it to fill the hump area. If you want to disguise the hump, you're going to put some filler above and slightly below. I also use it to mold and shape the tip of the nose to give the illusion of the light hitting a certain way, so paradoxically you're adding volume but you're adding it in a way that you have the right shadows and light reflecting and contouring, so it looks straight and lifted.

It lasts about a year, or up to 18 months, because the nose is very stationary—so it lasts. The lips move a lot so the filler goes away pretty fast in comparison.

Kybella

This is kind of amazing, like a little miracle in a bottle. It's a fat-melting enzyme, and never have we ever had a shot that dissolves fat that is known and proven to work. There have been a lot of products injected in Europe like Mesotherapy, but they don't really work. This actually dissolves fat, and it's made from a natural enzyme that's in your digestive tract (in your gallbladder) called deoxycholic acid. Some genius had the idea to harvest that and then use it to dissolve distinct deposits of fat. And chin fat is very resistant to exercise and weight loss. It's kind of hereditary fat.

Lipo & chin lipo work. So a lot of people say, "Well why not get lipo, why do you want to do shots there?" It just boils down to money. Chin lipo is around $4,500, so if you don't have a lot of fat it may be cheaper to melt it with Kybella, which is about $600 per vial. I tell patients, "If you can pinch an inch, plan on doing three vials."

You can do two vials the first time, and then one vial for follow-up if you want really fast results. Otherwise, just once a month, or whenever you have the time is good for maintenance. Another really interesting thing: Sometimes women feel a little bit of chubbiness right over their pubic bone, and they just don't like it because yoga pants don't feel right, they feel awkward. So that's something that two treatments of Kybella can melt away.

The biggest downside of Kybella is that you swell for about 4–5 days.

THE EXPERTS
ON LED LIGHTS

KATE SOMERVILLE

I do everything that I can to keep my clients off drugs because this is going to have an effect later on in their life. We've had people that have severe, severe acne, and we put them on the lights. Love the lights! We've been using LED lights for about 15 years in my clinic & it's really changed my clinic. I used to see somebody with cystic acne & I'd be able to get them 70–80 percent clear with facials and products. Now, with the lights, I can literally get them clear.

What's so awesome about the lights is you do a blue and red light for acne. The blue eradicates the bacteria, and then the red stimulates the collagen and it helps with healing.

You need to make sure you're getting the one that's strong. There are a lot of at-home ones out there that I don't feel are effective enough because they don't have the power that we do in the clinic. But LED lights changed my clinic and changed the acne experience.

DR. DENNIS GROSS

You wear my LED mask for 3 minutes a day. You just have to just push the button & it releases LED light, and LED lights are used to stimulate collagen. So vitamin C serum, retinol serum, the SpectraLite mask, the eye device—all these things are ideal for millennials because it's so easy, but you can really prevent aging.

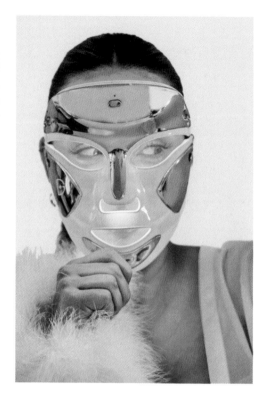

THE EXPERTS
ON PROCEDURE SAFETY

DR. HAROLD LANCER

I think education is first in terms of finding out what the problem is you're trying to fix. Once you know what it is you're trying to fix, you need a menu, you need a program, you need an approach. Haphazard use of products or procedures will lead to a problem.

DR. DENNIS GROSS

I love hyaluronic acid fillers. The Restylanes and Juvéderms of the world, all good. But the biggest danger I think your audience should know about is getting the wrong filler. Even if it's safe, even if it's approved, the wrong filler in the wrong place is a problem. I have patients who come to me because they want me to undo the problems.

Silicone in a bottle that you put in a needle and shoot it into someone's skin, that's being done out there. It's illegal & completely unpredictable and it leads to lumps—and then you're stuck with it forever.

You always need to stick to the stuff that we know is safe and approved. Temporary stuff is good because if you don't like it, it wears away. If you don't like it, there's an enzyme that can get rid of it.

One thing you can safely tell people is to do their research and look for a high-volume injector. You don't want to go to someplace where the person's doing their 10th lip injection. You need to see me, because I'm doing my 10,000th lip injection! But you need to go to a place where you can see consistent, reliable results.

Word of mouth is always great if your girlfriends have tried something and they've come out looking pretty good. But if you're doing a dangerous area like around your eyes, there's risk of blindness and you just can't mess around with that. It's just not worth it.

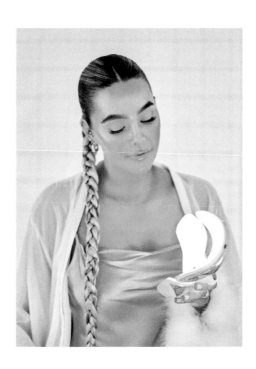

Don't pay all this money and then come out with round chipmunk cheeks that just don't look good. It saddens me, because it's the placement of the filler, not the filler itself. It's the technique, it's the art, it's the skill behind knowing where to put it in someone's anatomy.

DR. KAY DURAIRAJ

Take the time and have things done correctly the first time. If you have someone who really screws it up, please don't go back to them. Give them a chance, have them look at it, and have them assess what they would do. But if you don't get a good feeling from a person or you can just tell when you don't feel confident or they're not injecting you in a confident way, feel brave enough to stop and say, "This isn't working for me, I'm going to get another opinion."

THE EXPERTS
ON STARTING PROCEDURES

DR. HAROLD LANCER

People always come in with some problem that came from a procedure. They are trying to fix something with some bizarre med spa IPL treatment or they get some chemical peel and the problem is compounded. So I think when you're trying to repair something, you first want to evaluate what caused it. For something like blotchiness or color mismatch, you always want to treat it topically first, medically first. And that's why the Lancer skincare part of it is usually the first treatment before we even think about procedures. Before you get to the lasers and the radio frequency and the chemical peels, it's always about medical rehab first.

The number-one tip is to cut back in terms of the amount of stuff you do. I think that if you're doing neuromodulator, whether it's

Botox or Dysport or Xeomin or a Jeuveau, whatever brand that is, do less of it. If you're doing volume correction, known as fillers, do less volume correction. So I think the more subtle, under-the-radar maintenance correction is a good, current beauty tip. It's a composite of repetitive treatment so you get a bigger cumulative end result.

DR. DENNIS GROSS

I think if it's something you really want, go slow. I really feel strongly about going slow, and if we need to do more, we add it. You can't take it back once it's in. And so, you can always think you're going to get it perfect, but you just never know. So never overdo it.

You can fix bad Botox if the fix involves giving more Botox. You can't fix bad Botox by taking it out.

DR. KAY DURAIRAJ

When you start doing filler at a very young age, it's important to start very light-handed. You can always come back. It's always good to start with just a touch, let it settle in, make sure you love it.

I see patients in their 20s routinely now who are doing preventative Botox, and there's a lot of controversy about that, but I'm a big believer. There's no reason to make your skin wrinkle over and over. Skin is like a piece of paper. The more you fold it, the more it creases. Even when you unfold that paper, it has maintained those creases after years of crinkling.

If you see something that is eroding away at your self-confidence and your self-esteem, you need to fix it, and you need to fix it early. It's like letting a poor adolescent suffer with acne to the point that they have really scarred, damaged skin, and their psyche is scarred. As long as we have technology that is safe and effective and affordable, why not do it?

If you're getting your lips done or there's some feature you want to enhance, it really helps the surgeon to bring in a picture. Then we get your vibe and your aesthetic and what you like and what you want to project. And then I can add those features to your face in a way that matches your face.

DR. JASON DIAMOND

People now know that they don't need to wait until they're 60 to address something that bothers them. If something bothers them when they're in their 20s, 30s, then it's OK to have that addressed. I make the analogy to everybody: people often ask, "Isn't it vain, or shouldn't you accept what God gave you?" Well, my answer to that is, right now as we speak, what would be our guess as to how many people are in a gym worldwide, a billion?

Right now, there are probably a billion people exercising somewhere, minimum, maybe more. And why are they exercising? They're exercising to reduce the fat, to get a six pack, to slim out their thighs, to improve their biceps, and that's because people want to improve their self-esteem or want to feel better about themselves.

The face you can't exercise away. You can't exercise to make certain types of changes. So what's the difference between exercising to get a six pack or doing a little filler to your chin to create a better chin shape and improve the weakness that you have? To me, it's the same exact principle and the same concept.

DR. BARBARA STURM

Don't start too early because you weaken your muscles. From my experience, I started at 30. Now, if I don't use Botox, my eyebrows are so low because they're so weak. I would just wait. Don't get crazy on this stuff too early.

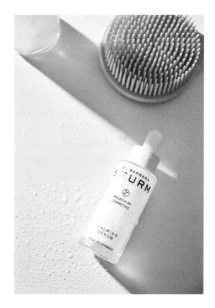

THE EXPERTS
ON SKIN ROUTINE

DR. BARBARA STURM

Don't go too crazy. I know people love it because there's so much temptation out there: Here's something, and the packaging is so cute, and this mask has so much glitter. Just don't do it.

A skincare routine needs to be simple but effective, especially when you're young. I think the key is to stay away from what you think the grown-ups do and all these aggressive treatments. Totally stay away.

If you suffer from acne (which young and old people do), don't try to destroy your skin because of it. Be nice to your skin. If your skin acts out with acne, don't put it in

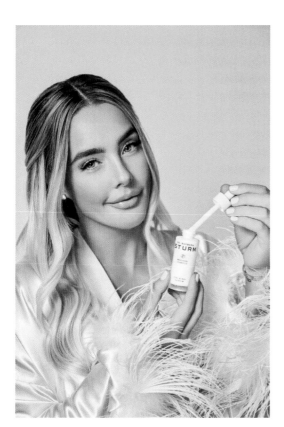

a time-out—just love it & then love it even more. Love it means give it enough hydration, don't overpower it, don't use too much oily stuff, but don't dry it out. Don't be aggressive and dry it out, because when you dry it out all your physiology is disturbed, and when it's dry there are little ruptures in your skin and bacteria can come in and make it even worse.

If you want to treat your acne, treat the areas, don't treat your whole skin. What's actually really working is white toothpaste overnight or even some Neosporin (you can put on during the day). We, for example, just came out with a spot treatment that is tea tree oil, which is even a little tinted. You can just put it on the spots and then hydrate your skin; make sure you clean your skin, don't touch your skin with your dirty hands (they're dirty all the time). That's also because you transport bacteria into your skin. Have your skin cleaned once a month and that's it.

GEORGIA LOUISE

Use your water-based things first. Then you put an oil on. Lay them in order of thickness. So lightest to heaviest. You don't want to put an oil on and then use a serum, because it's not going to push through the skin. For example, Dr. Barbara Sturm's hyaluronic serum is amazing. You could put that on first because it's super hydrating. It really penetrates quickly & is more water-based.

Once you get that down, then you can start to use a thicker base serum. For example, I may use a retinol A. I think retinol A is the best thing for breakouts & for fine lines. It's really the most proven antiaging product out there still. But in my opinion, from a skincare point of view, don't use one that's prescribed. Go for one that's a skincare product with a vitamin A, because it doesn't irritate the skin, and irritation is the worst thing you can do.

As far as my own routine: It's a whole thing. I close the door from the kids. I light the candle and it's like a whole ritual. I start with La Mer micellar water and take off my eye makeup. To be honest, I don't wear a lot of makeup. It's usually just mascara and a La Mer compact powder. That's it.

So, after the micellar water & removal of makeup, I then use the balm, because the balm is like the first oil cleanse. I ceremoniously massage it into my skin. Then I remove that with a warm towel so all the oil and all the debris are pulled out.

Then I'll cleanse again. If your skin is dry, go with a milky hydrating cleanser. If your skin is oily, go for the cleansing wash and foam it all out.

So once I've done my two-step cleanse, which is the oil and then the cleanser, I go ahead and dry the skin with Kleenex tissue. Next, I tone my skin. Toning means introducing hydration back into the skin, preventing the skin from feeling stripped and dry. You're basically hydrating the layers of skin. So toning is an important step in this process. Once I've rose-misted my skin, then we get down to layering the hydration like I said above.

THE EXPERTS
ON PRODUCTS

DR. DENNIS GROSS

Here's the bottom line: I think that there are incredible things you can do with science, and I take ingredients that are proven to work and then we figure out how to make them work better by combining them with other ingredients, how to make them have better delivery to the area we want, and how to combine them with other ingredients so they're multitasking. I love products that do more than one thing.

No matter what you do, you have to get the skin to love what you're applying. That means never overdoing it and yet introducing things that all work together. My skincare line is all designed to work together. The moisturizer, the peel, the mask, the eye creams, the retinol, all these things are integrated & designed to work. All you have to do is follow instructions.

I am convinced people are buying more products & using more products and that people are more concerned than ever to look good. And I think it's backfiring. There are products containing ingredients that are actually causing breakouts and acne.

DR. BARBARA STURM

You think we live so organic, but the truth is, if you do real studies on it, it's a very polluted place. Yeah, we have to make sure that you keep your skin hydrated, because hydration is important for skin barrier functions. If your skin barrier doesn't function right, pollutants can come, and also sunlight can penetrate your skin easily and can cause premature aging, cancer & hyperpigmentation issues. So we need to hydrate our skin all the time to strengthen our skin barrier function.

That's where the anti-pollution drops come in. We need to create a shield for particulate matter to be held out of the skin but also our anti-pollution drops contain polyphenols, which help with the digital light. It's basically a thinner version of the hyaluronic acid or hyaluronic serum. It's a thinner version but has all these hero ingredients. I mix the hyaluronic acid in the morning with the anti-pollution drops and put it on as a first step.

I think we all have to do it, and it's a great product for kids and teenagers. Our kids are in front of the screens all the time, and they're also in the polluted world. Yeah, we think let's not overpower the skin, but it's herbal, very natural ingredients; otherwise, I wouldn't put my skincare on my kids.

If you think our skincare needs to be aggressive, harsh, and full of very active ingredients, then I wouldn't put it on my child's skin, but that's another big thing that is wrong in the skincare industry. People seem to think they need to quickly fix something and go for very aggressive treatments or skincare routines. Pouring acid on your skin basically causes inflammation and destroys your skin barrier function and makes your skin super vulnerable. Hello sun, hello pollution, just come in.

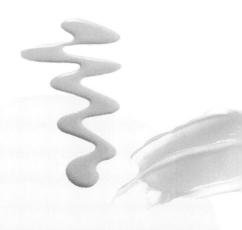

Motivational speaker and author **Gabrielle Bernstein** is a huge fan of Biologique Recherche Lotion P50 and Weleda Skin Food. She used to have acne but it totally went away when she cut sugar and dairy. Her secret tip is using petroleum jelly under her eyes to keep them super soft. Gabby also loves getting facials—it's like lying there and meditating.

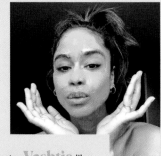

Teddi Mellencamp of *The Real Housewives of Beverly Hills* uses the Nurse Jamie UpLift Roller before she applies her makeup. The little massaging stones feel so good and make your skin look youthful and your makeup apply much better. She loves going to FACEGYM, too, because the face has muscle just like any other body part and they work them out! One of Teddi's fave products is Kate Somerville DermalQuench Liquid Lift. She says it's a miracle worker that instantly plumps up any line or wrinkle like a dream.

DJ and music video director **Vashtie** likes to massage her face with her knuckles when applying moisturizer and serums—she uses quite a bit of pressure to do this. She also loves The Ordinary's hyaluronic acid serum because it's super affordable and always gives her skin a moist and dewy feeling. She's a big fan of the Celluma Pro LED light therapy device, too. You can find Vashtie wearing sunscreen and in the shade these days. She said that 15 years ago "a Black aesthetician suggested I wear sunscreen. I laughed and said, 'Our skin doesn't have to worry about that.' She quickly schooled me about how damaging the sun is on *all* complexions."

Model and founder of Babe Body, **Hunter McGrady** splurges on Clé de Peau Intensive Fortifying Cream. It's so expensive, but she says it's such a great lightweight formula to wear at night. Her other favorite products are Weleda Skin Food and Supergoop! Unseen Sunscreen. Hunter is also obsessed with facial acupuncture for boosting collagen and increasing circulation. Plus, check out her daily skin routine:

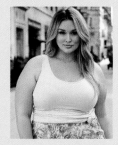

The first thing I do when I wake up is wash my face with Biologique Recherche Lait VIP O2. Then I will take a cotton pad and load it up with Biologique Recherche Lotion P50V toner, which has been a godsend! It is a bit pricey, but this has truly transformed my skin. After that I will do a thin layer of Biologique Recherche Creme Placenta and top it off with Weleda Skin Food, and if I am going out in the sun I always put the Supergoop! Unseen Sunscreen on! I repeat this process at night with the addition of the Clé de Peau Intensive Fortifying Night Cream.

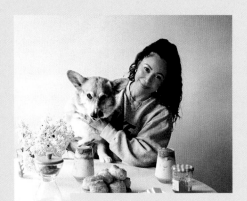

Adrianna Guevara Adarme of *A Cozy Kitchen* loves The Ordinary Niacinamide. For $6, it's her favorite workhorse. "The texture is amazing, my skin loves it, and it's super effective at brightening an evening out my skin tone." Adrianna is also a big fan of the "double cleanse"—using a cleansing balm before a water-based cleanser.

Jacey Duprie of *Damsel in Dior* is obsessed with Dr. Dennis Gross's facial steamer. She uses it four times a week and sets it up while she blow-dries her hair. Jacey swears it helps her skin absorb the key ingredients in her products. Jacey notices a huge improvement in her skin when she starts her day with a Fab Four Smoothie by *Be Well By Kelly*'s Kelly LeVeque.

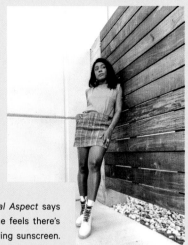

DeAnna Rivers of *The Visual Aspect* says that since she's African American, she feels there's this huge misconception around wearing sunscreen. When she was younger she thought she didn't have to wear sunscreen because of higher levels of melanin in her skin. At about 10 years old, she went to a pool party and only put on sunscreen once and was in the pool for hours, like 5 hours! Afterward, she went home and was 10 shades darker. Her dad was so mad. DeAnna didn't know at that time that her family had a history of health problems and that she couldn't be out in the sun like that for hours and not reapply sunscreen. It was a great lesson learned, and she also learned about the plethora of health issues that run rampant in her family lineage. So, DeAnna says, "no matter how much melanin you have in your skin, you need to wear sunscreen every day and reapply often!"

Rumi Neely of *Are You Am I* loves a pre-shower mask in the morning—something either brightening or hydrating. Right out of the shower she applies a vitamin C serum, moisturizer, and sunscreen. At night she likes to use a cleansing balm to melt away makeup and a gentle face wash before applying U Beauty serum and either Augustinus Bader's Rich Cream or Vintner's Daughter Serum, which just feels like heaven. Extra steps she's introduced now and then are microneedling (before the serum application) or following up with a few minutes of gua sha.

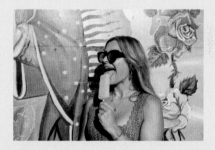

Stephanie Simbari of *That's So Retrograde* goes for Osea Malibu Sea Vitamin Boost as her under-$50 mist. As she says, "If I could drink it I would; I'm obsessed."

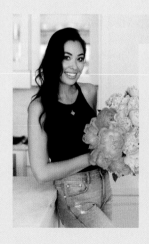

Kat Tanita of *With Love From Kat* wakes up by splashing her face with cold water. After lightly tapping her face dry (never rubbing!), she applies Dr. Barbara Sturm's face cream and eye cream, then tops off with her anti-pollution drops. Once that dries she adds a layer of Supergoop! Unseen Sunscreen and, if she's not wearing makeup, a bit of face oil for some facial massage. At night, Kat uses Elemis Pro-Collagen Cleansing Balm or Holifrog gel wash to remove her makeup. Finally, she'll use RVL skincare toner pads by Dr. Rita Linkner, then applies Vintner's Daughter Serum.

Lisa Allen of *Salty Lashes* swears by alternating her prodcuts. Once you build up a tolerance to your retinol, the best thing to do would be to alternate every other night, between retinol and glycolic. She does it religiously and swears it makes the biggest difference in your skin because it never fully acclimates to either product. At the same time, you don't have a reverse reaction to either one if you're alternating every other night. Her other hot tip is to *not* wipe off your hands after you apply your serums and your creams. Instead, rub them into the back of your hands because your hands are the first place to show aging.

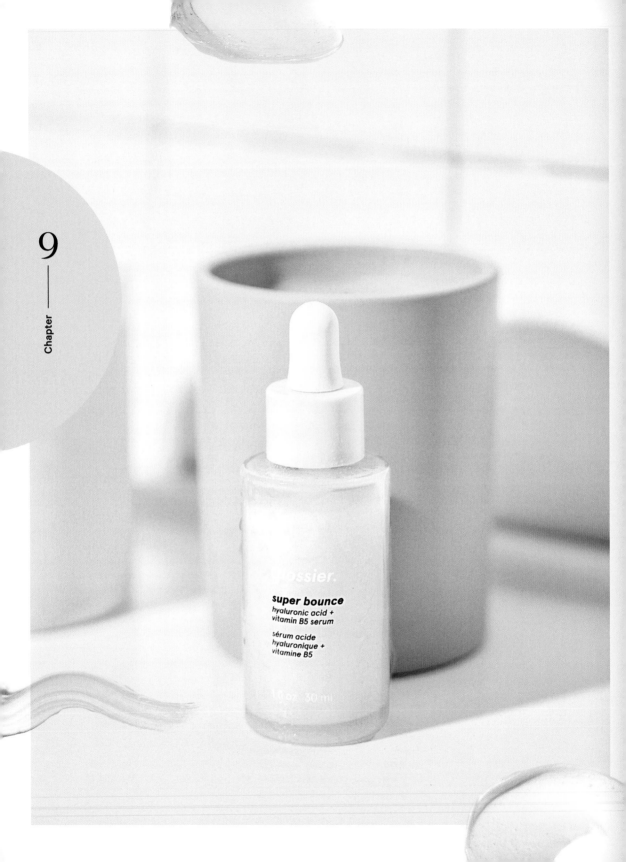

9

HUNGOVER SKIN, TRAVELING SKIN, HUMID SKIN, DRY WEATHER SKIN, PERIOD SKIN & KOREAN SKINCARE

ALL the hacks for all the different kinds of situations that can fuck with your skin. We're going to go over the best ways to de-puff when you're hungover, how to take care of your skin when you travel & tips for bombass skin in humid or dry weather.

HOW TO BE PROACTIVE WITH YOUR HANGOVER

NIP THAT SHIT IN THE BUD

There is nothing worse than swollen wine face. Especially when you're trying to look snatched for an event or date. Luckily for you, I have compiled a list of magical tricks—you ready?

In the spirit of keeping things hydrated, I'm going to share with you one of my favorite hangover cures/elixirs. I got this tip from Ms. Suzanne Somers. She always delivers when it comes to the best beauty tips and tricks.

This is one of those elixirs I keep going back to that I think not only makes you feel better, but also hydrates the skin.

THE HANGOVER ELIXIR

♥ spoonful of ascorbic acid powder

♥ 3 ALA antioxidant capsules (alpha-lipoic acid)

♥ *Directions*: Mix the ascorbic acid powder with water & ice, STIR, STIR, STIR. After sipping on that, swallow three ALA capsules. I like to do this routine after I've eaten something small!

Benefits of the mixture? Ascorbic acid benefits include: prevents the common cold, boosts the immune system, AND the best: maintains elasticity of the skin.

ALA, also known as alpha-lipoic acid, is an antioxidant, and the benefits are absolute magic. Lucky us, the antioxidant is also known to fight off pesky hangover.

Ultimately I'm just not one of those "drink coffee" to cure a hangover type of person. In fact, I feel like the coffee makes it worse? Is it just me?

Peppermint tea & ginger tea are ALWAYS fantastic the day after a bender, too. And of course, WATER, WATER, WATER.

A little eye mask tip for ya: drumroll, please . . . keep your eye masks in the fridge. This will tighten the skin and cool you down in the best way. In fact, I even have a special skin fridge. When your eye pads are cool, they feel so much better. Plus, when they are chilled, it does a better job at tightening your undereye bags. I was getting very annoyed that I had to walk to the kitchen every single time I wanted to get a chilled skincare product, like my eye masks. It was annoying to do in the morning, and it was seriously messing with my efficiency. Now with my special skin fridge, I can keep all my products in one place. I just wake up, grab, and go.

Speaking of the cold, I use my *The Skinny Confidential* Ice Roller every single fucking day, whether I'm hungover or not. It especially helps de-puff wine face and bloat. Rolly roll!

HOT TIP ♥ **DR. DENNIS GROSS:** *When you're hungover, hydrate. And I would definitely take a vitamin B pill & vitamin C. But vitamin B complex gets rid of a lot of the water you retain that leads to puffiness the day after drinking. Plan on doing aerobic exercises the next day, too. So, you wake up and you're hungover, right? Well, what you want to do is the Alpha Beta peel pads. Peeling is the fastest way to overhaul your skin. That's what people come into my practice for. They just plop down and say, "I look tired. I look horrible. Fix me quick." I always do a peel.*

HOW TO TRAVEL BUT KEEP YOUR SKIN ALL DEWY

Traveling is such a bitch on your skin. I'll never forget when I was in New York City and started to realize that the bags under my eyes were getting darker and thicker. I started talking to women about it, and most of them thought it was from lack of sleep because NYC is such a hustling city.

After researching it, I realized it's actually because of the pollution and excess fluid under our eyes that needs to be drained. (Hello lymphatic drainage—see chapter 3).

Anyway, each city comes with its own shit. For instance, in LA my skin is glowy and shiny, but I worry about the sun (hyperpigmentation, brown spots & wrinkles). The point is, no matter where you are in the world, it can be hard on your skin. You want to have the tools to combat whatever is necessary.

VERY THE SKINNY CONFIDENTIAL-ESQUE PACKING TIPS FOR ALL YOUR BEAUTY NEEDS:

FACE RAZOR: When you're on vacation, you simply need a facial shaver. You really don't want a situation where you're in the sun and your boyfriend is staring at the long black hair on your upper lip. Trust me, I've been there.

Having a face shaver on hand is best for everyone involved. Plus, I like to shave my face in general. I go all over my cheeks with this.

TAN TOWELS: If you're not going to do the sun or are unable to spray tan, use a tan towel. In just 5 seconds, they very much get the job done. Plus, some of them are infused with a clear self-tanning formula that works with the proteins/amino acids of skin to give you a nice, healthy tan within hours.

SHEET MASKS ALWAYS: I am that person who is wearing a sheet mask for 3 hours, mid-flight. But it makes all the difference in your skin's hydration; there are even times when the flight attendants ask if I have an extra mask. When you're done with the mask, rub the rest of the serum into the skin for extra goodness; there's no need to rinse after.

HOW TO BE IN DRY CLIMATES

You need moisture in the air, so if you can get a humidifier going, do it. This will help counteract the dryness from the plane, hotel AC, or heat, and/or the climate where you're staying. My sister, Mimi, recently spent a few months in South Korea and said they're all the rage with Korean women. In fact, they can't live without one. So much so that Mimi eventually ended up purchasing a small humidifier that . . . wait for it . . . goes on YOUR DESK. At work! How clever. So while you work you're working on your skin—if that's not fucking multitasking at its finest, I don't know what is.

BENEFITS OF A HUMIDIFIER FOR THE SKIN

- ♥ Helps with itchy, cracked skin.
- ♥ Promotes healing when it comes to skin rashes.
- ♥ Can help with acne.
- ♥ Keeps your skin feel hydrated & soft.

It has made SUCH a big difference in my skin and really helps with allergies, sinuses, and cracked, chapped lips. Make sure you're switching out the water in your humidifier every week. Otherwise, it can grow mold & bacteria.

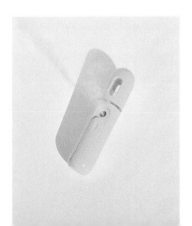

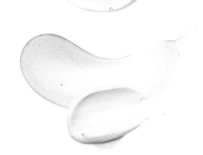

HOT TIP ♥ *One of my best tips for traveling in dry weather is slathering your feet in lotion or oil, then sleeping with socks on. It keeps your feet nice and smooth, because there's nothing worse than cracked, old calluses on the bottom of your feet in dry weather.*

Opt for gentler products.

In dry weather, you want a lot of oil. Instead of a cleansing balm, you should cleanse with an oil. Just pour some oil on a cotton pad to remove your makeup, then apply more to moisturize.

If you don't have oil, just call room service and ask for a side of olive oil—works like a charm. Oil also works great as an eye cream in dry weather & Aquaphor is a great drugstore find to apply under your eyes, on your lips, or on your elbows.

Speaking of lips, I'm a huge fan of a lip mask in dry weather, too.

Everyone is always worried about wrinkles on their face, chest & hands, but not their *lips*. Your lips are so important. I feel like I'm always drinking out of a straw, so this is very much necessary for me.

The cool thing about a lip mask is you put it on before you go to sleep, and when you wake up, it's still on. And I mean it REALLY stays on, guys. You seriously wake up with these plump, soft, pillowy lips. I don't wipe it off when I wake up, I just keep it on—but that's just me. We're a little extra over here. I also use it as a lip gloss during the day—it makes a great primer under your lipstick.

I always go for a freezing cold shower in dry weather.

But if you can't do freezing cold, go for luke-warm. Just be sure to not go too hot in the shower in dry weather; it dries your skin out like a prune. Especially on the face—if water is touching my face, I always make sure it's cold. I also recommend dry brushing more in dry weather. It removes all the dead skin and promotes circulation & lymphatic drainage.

While we're on the subject of showers, want to know how to turn yours into a eucalyptus spa-like experience?

This hack is so easy & so therapeutic that you're going to want to run to your local farmer's market asap.

All you need for this project is eucalyptus leaves & a black hair tie. Yup, that's it. What you do is take the eucalyptus leaves—I get mine from the farmer's market because the fresher the better—and run them under water to get rid of any bugs, dust, or debris, because you definitely don't want that shit trickling down on you in the shower. (Again, this is why I like the farmer's market: no pesticides on my eucalyptus leaves, PLZ. Also, they're like $4.39.) I run them under the water for about a minute, then shake the water off. Next, grab a rolling pin or something similar (an empty wine bottle works, too!) and roll it over the leaves to release the aroma.

Then, take a hair tie & wrap it around the bottom of the leaves, hang it upside down, and wrap the hair tie around your shower-head so it hangs down under it.

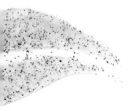

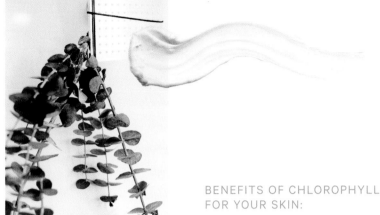

If you don't want to hang it on your showerhead, you could also just fill a vase with water & the eucalyptus leaves & keep it in your shower.

Every time you shower, the water will trickle through the leaves & it will create this beautiful, soothing, decongesting aromatherapy throughout your whole bathroom. It's going to stimulate & detoxify your skin & totally decongest you, and it will smell like the most amazing garden. This combined with a salt lamp night-light in your bathroom at night makes your bathroom feel like a bougie spa.

If you're more of a bath person, you could always put a few drops of eucalyptus oil into the water with Epsom salt. Epsom salt is fab if you've worked out hard and have sore muscles, and it's so good for the skin. It softens really rough and dry skin and exfoliates dead skin cells. Note: DON'T EAT IT! It's only for baths.

HOT TIP 🤍 *If you're at a high altitude (aka skiing in Aspen), drink chlorophyll. It's an energy/ immunity booster, hormonal balancer & FABULOUS detoxifier. It's filled with vitamins, minerals & essential fatty acids, too. It promotes digestive health, so if you have any gut issues—DRINK UP! It'll also make your skin glow and help with altitude sickness.You can take chlorophyll in liquid or capsule form, but I prefer the liquid because it's like instant green juice. You can easily throw chlorophyll drops in your morning smoothie or take it with other vitamins.*

BENEFITS OF CHLOROPHYLL FOR YOUR SKIN:

- 🤍 A wound healer.
- 🤍 Helps clear acne & breakouts.
- 🤍 Nourishes the skin.
- 🤍 Helps your skin look younger.
- 🤍 Reduces wrinkles.

Exfoliate less. Moisturizer, serum, and mist more.

In dry weather, you're going to want to skip the exfoliating because it can strip the skin. Instead, use an oil cleanser and a hydrating moisturizer. Lather yourself in oils, put on a calming mask, and don't forget to ask for a side of olive oil with your room service salad.

HOW TO BE IN HUMID CLIMATES

1 Wash your face.

You always want to wash your face because you'll be sweating a bit more in humid climates. Sweat breeds bacteria, so upper lip sweat begone! I also love to get a facial in humid weather. If you're staying at a hotel, you can get a great one. Since I travel a lot, I've learned how to micromanage a facial, but like, in a nice way, of course. Here are a couple things to ask for when getting a facial while traveling:

- 🤍 Lots of facial massage, like 75 percent.
- 🤍 Brightening & tightening products, please.
- 🤍 Use anything cold to de-puff like an ice roller or ice globe.
- 🤍 Gua sha tools are always welcome.

2 Keep toner with you—it helps keep you hydrated.

Toner is amazing because it's like a refreshing mist that will wake you the fuck up. I look for toners with all natural ingredients because I'm typically spraying it directly on my face. I love ones that have witch hazel as the main base.

3 Apply oil-free moisturizer to avoid oily-looking skin.

Oil-free moisturizer is your best friend here. You can use a little less oil in humid weather because your skin is producing more. Also, try some foods that will keep you hydrated & your skin balanced. Black plums (vitamin C), mangoes (known to eliminate pimples), watermelon (super hydrating), cucumber (also hydrating).

4 Exfoliate your skin . . . it helps a ton with not looking oily.

Exfoliate more in humid weather. Be sure to do a gentle exfoliation in small upward circles to bring the face up. I also like a good peel. In the summer, the humidity makes your skin less sensitive, so when you incorporate an exfoliant, it really helps minimize pores and leaves your skin all glowy.

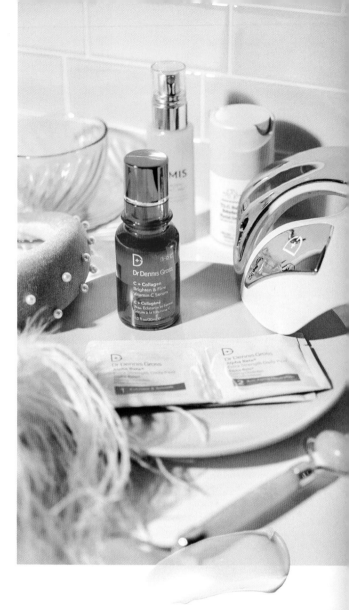

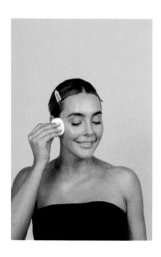

5 Apply light makeup.

You don't want to go too heavy on makeup after you've made your skin glow. You don't want it melting off your face like the Wicked Witch of the West. I opt for a damp Beautyblender with a light foundation & minimal powder (only powder your T-zone).

HOW TO GET RID OF PIMPLES, ESPECIALLY ON YOUR PERIOD.

A few years ago, I got married. And well, 2 days before the wedding, I got a huge zit. FML. Luckily for me, I packed the only three things you need to get rid of pimples or blackheads in the most efficient & quickest way: a pimple clay, a blackhead remover & some tea tree oil.

Here's the thing: If you pop a zit, the juice of the zit is what spreads the pimple. That's right, guys, bacteria spreads. And it doesn't give a shit. In fact, it's relentless—it goes everywhere—which is why when you get a zit & pop it, more zits pop up. Whenever I pop anything, I make sure not to get any of the residue on my skin.

Anyway, here's my actual zit cure.

I take this very seriously because I've very much perfected this over the years. In fact, it's kind of a magical cure.

FIRST OFF: A good zit clay. Zit clay is essential. It's nothing avant-garde. Quite simple, really. It's this clay that's infused with minerals that decrease oil production and increase healing time, so it heals pimples fast. I've been using clay forever, and I've never seen anything so magical.

Here's the main secret, though: The directions say to leave it on for 10 minutes . . . I leave it on the zit overnight. So I sleep with the clay on the pimple. Works like a charm.

OK, on to the blackhead remover, aka the little $3.99 drugstore tool.

HERE'S WHAT IT DOES:

- ♥ One end is a loop tip for pressing & extracting, the other sharp end is for piercing or poking.
- ♥ To minimize damage to your skin, the needle is an effective way to remove blackheads, acne, or pimples.
- ♥ Using the remover is a safer way to clear your pores than squeezing blackheads using your fingernails.
- ♥ With the help of these needles, you will lessen trauma to the surrounding skin.

It's nothing special, but BOY OH BOY does it get the job done. So much better than popping anything with your dirty fingernails. I like to use this after I get out of the shower because my skin is soft.

If you don't have a blackhead remover, you can try to CAREFULLY pop the zit. When you get out of the shower, wipe your face with a clean, never-been-used, freshly washed towel. Cover your fingers with a tissue. Even after showering, your hands and nails have bacteria that can infect your about-to-be-popped pimple. To do this, fold a tissue in half and wrap it around your index finger. Repeat with your other hand. Consider yourself prepped for zit surgery.

OK, SO TO SPOT TREAT DURING THE DAY, USE TEA TREE OIL. BECAUSE IT:

HEALS CUTS AND BURNS: It's a natural antiseptic, meaning it can be used to help treat wounds & burns. Tea tree oil has also been known to treat bacterial infections—love it! Use a dime-size amount of tea tree oil to heal razor burns, small cuts & even sunburns (although I'm hoping everyone avoids the sun like the plague). If you want, you can add some water to the oil, too.

KILLS BLEMISHES: This oil is known for getting rid of pimples. Recently, a study found that the oil offers similar results to a 5 percent benzoyl peroxide. Next time you're on Aunt Flow & have a zit, throw some tea tree oil on it! I use it before I apply makeup because you can't see it. It's just like a light oil that coats the skin before primer. It's kind of the ideal zit healer, no?

TA-DA. Keep it easy. There's nothing worse than someone trying to overcomplicate a zit. A zit is easy to solve. I use these three tips every time & they've never steered me in the wrong direction. The clay spot treatment mask is a real lifesaver. Just bear with me, because the directions may be in Swedish— but it's worth it. The blackhead remover is SO efficient. Really to the point & something to use when you're out of the shower. Lastly, if you're treating a pimple during the day: TEA TREE OIL. I use it whenever I feel a zit coming & post zit-picking.

PIMPLE PATCHES WORK WONDERS, FOR AUNT FLOW, TOO:

Craters, zits, pimples, whiteheads, whatever the fuck you want to call them, there's nothing worse. Especially when you wake up with one that looks like a third eye. My trusty clay treatment & a pimple popper work wonders, but since then I've found out about pimple patches.

They're like Band-Aids for your pimples that protect them from your dirt or extra gunk overnight, ALL WHILE reducing the size of the pimple by morning. It makes sense why everyone in Korea is obsessed with them: They reduce inflammation BIG TIME & really flatten the bump.

You can wear them whenever that third eye pops up. They're very incognito, so if you wear it to the grocery store & run into your ex, it's no big deal! They'll just be sad they missed out on your flawless face.

WAIT! DIAPER CREAM WORKS AS A PIMPLE ZAPPER! IT'S TRUE.

DIAPER RASH OINTMENT FOR GETTING RID OF PIMPLES IS ALL THE RAGE. Well, maybe it's not, but for me right now it is!

Having a baby really makes you run around, man. Sometimes you gotta get creative. Not too long ago, I made a wild discovery that blew my mind.

Basically, it all started when I had a small rash around my nose. No idea what it was from, but regardless, I had a little rash.

So there I was changing my daughter's organic diaper, I picked up her diaper cream & started to slap it on. As I was putting this on her I thought, *Why couldn't I use this on my face????? Like, why not????*

So there I was, in 6-day-old sweats with breast milk pouring out my boobs, putting diaper cream on the rash around my nose.

A day later, the rash had already gone down a crazy amount. I couldn't believe how

HOT
TIP

Baby your skin. That's right. Baby wipes can be used as amazing makeup removers—they're super delicate (I personally do not like to use wipes on my face, but if you're going to do it, use a baby wipe). Baby moisturizers are great for all skin types, especially if you have some kind of rash, and they all smell amazing. And sunscreen for babies has a very high SPF with fewer chemicals than normal sunscreens, and baby shampoos won't strip your color. So next time you're at the drugstore, check the baby section for products.

much redness it had taken away from the rash, so I started to think, *What if I put diaper cream on a pimple?*

We'll get to the pimple part, but first, I want to talk about the actual diaper cream I used (and still love).

The one I have is called Pinxav, pronounced "pink-salve." Its whole thing is to soothe & protect, and let me tell ya, it got the job done for my rash.

The good thing about this is that it's super inexpensive. You could really use anything all-natural here, so don't feel like you have to get attached to any brand. But you should know that the ingredients in this diaper cream are very much *The Skinny Confidential*-approved.

When it comes to pimples, I'm a huge fan of the clay that we talked about earlier. It's my number-one go-to for pimples. If you don't know about this, it's literally magic. I've been using it FOREVER. The stuff works immediately. I've never seen anything so magical.

But, if you're in a pinch, this diaper cream does work. I know this because I've tried it many times. It's super fun because it's pink and it truly coats the pimple (I actually walked to Pilates with it on my face). I don't mind how it smells.

Next time you get a pimple or a rash in any area, remember diaper cream. Boy oh boy, does it work.

Korean skincare IS QUEEN. Since I am most certainly not the expert on Korean skincare, I went to the best of the best to showcase all the juicy secrets. You'll hear from some major players in this chapter—women who have founded companies and spent their lives dedicated to making Korean skincare accessible to everyone.

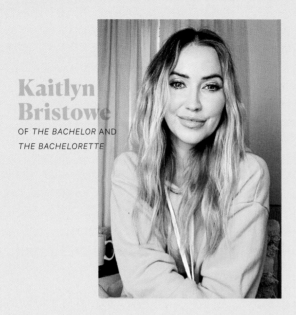

Kaitlyn Bristowe

OF *THE BACHELOR* AND *THE BACHELORETTE*

Check out her fave products and her A.M./P.M. routine:

/ **A.M.** /

♥ Wash my face with SkinCeuticals gentle cleanser
♥ SkinCeuticals C E Ferulic Serum
♥ SkinMedica HA5 Rejuvenating Hydrator
♥ ZO daily moisturizer
♥ Colorescience sunscreen

/ **P.M.** /

♥ Wash my face with SkinCeuticals gentle cleanser
♥ SkinCeuticals H.A. Intensifier
♥ SkinMedica HA5 Rejuvenating Hydrator
♥ SkinCeuticals Triple Lipid Restore 2:4:2
♥ SkinCeuticals A.G.E. Eye Complex

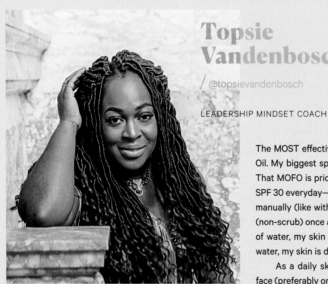

Topsie Vandenbosch

@topsievandenbosch

LEADERSHIP MINDSET COACH

The MOST effective product is by far Biossance 100% Squalane Oil. My biggest splurge is TATCHA LUMINOUS Dewy Skin Mist! That MOFO is pricey but so, SO worth it for the dewiness. I wear SPF 30 everyday—it's a must. I always exfoliate my skin 1x a week manually (like with a scrub), then I use an AHA exfoliating mask (non-scrub) once a week. Game changer. When I drink 48 ounces of water, my skin glows from the inside out. When I don't drink water, my skin is dull and boring, and I swear it randomly peels?

As a daily skincare practice, I pat an essence all over my face (preferably one from Peach & Lily), then I use a serum (either from Biossance, Glow Recipe, or Peach & Lily) then a facial oil (Biossance). I always make sure to use a cleansing balm to take off my makeup, and then I give myself a lymphatic massage. One thing I always do is sleep on a satin pillowcase, for the love of Christ. Never cotton. Psychopathic vibes if you do the latter.

I think when it comes to procedures, people should mind their business. Stop judging other people's choices if they don't affect you. And mind the business that pays you. Always. If you want to enhance your beauty, GO FOR IT. If you like it, I LOVE IT.

GET THE F♥CK OUT OF THE SUN

Actress and blogger Alyssa Lynch thinks the best advice that goes along with taking care of skin is diet and hydration. "Eating nutrient-dense foods and superfoods, and drinking enough water, is such a simple task that is so incredibly effective when it comes to glowing from the inside out. The more the body is glowing, the more the skin will be, too. Adding certain supplements can be beneficial as well, depending on your body and diet. I know people see such amazing results, as do I, from taking certain collagen products. Collagen can really help with keeping the skin looking healthy and prevent aging." Alyssa says that when she became plant-based and truly started practicing self-care—meditating, yoga, working out, diet, supplementing—is when she really noticed her skin GLOW.

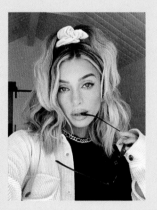

The Styled Seed blogger Delaney Childs wakes herself up by rubbing an ice cube on her face. She goes over areas that feel swollen or are looking tired and dull. The shock of the ice cube makes your skin bright and wakes it up. Some other accessible things that Delaney recommends are drinking lots of water, taking your makeup off before bed, and wearing sunscreen on your face every day. You don't have to do anything super expensive or invasive—just those things are simple and actually work. Her super hot tip is putting on a tea tree oil concentrate after she washes her face every morning. Delaney says it's really helped calm down the oiliness of her skin.

Lifestyle influencer Camille Styles never splurges on cleanser. According to her, you just wash it off, so she opts for gentle drugstore cleansers like Cetaphil, Purpose, Olay—they get the job done. She saves her splurges for serums, antiaging products, and the one that she shells the most out for on a regular basis: Vintner's Daughter Active Botanical Serum. She uses it morning and night, after toning but before moisturizer.

Camille also says that consistency is key. As a blogger, she is sent A TON of products to try. Even though it's so tempting to experiment with new products, she learned the hard way that switching things up too frequently makes her break out. "When I've got lots of fun new products in my lineup, it's impossible to know which ingredients are causing the sensitivity." Now she sticks to what she knows works and follows her regimen every morning and every night, no matter how busy or tired she is. "If I do want to try out a new product, I introduce it for a few weeks without making any other tweaks, so I can objectively see how my skin reacts."

Naomie Olindo, founder of clothing company L'ABEYE and star of the hit show *Southern Charm*, says intermittent fasting changed her life. It makes her feel better, sleep better, and improves her mood. It goes hand in hand with having good skin because she's healthier as a person. "If you eat like shit, your skin is going to look bad." If Naomie didn't use Blender Bombs in her smoothies, she wouldn't eat nearly as many nutrients. Naomie used to have little bumps all over her face, and someone once told her, "You look good on the outside, but your insides are rotting. You need to treat the inside first and then your skin will get better." Now, if she even has a soda, within a week the bumps come back. She also thinks what matters is the quality of ingredients, and sometimes the price of products can go hand in hand with that. But there are also lots of good products that aren't insanely expensive. "You don't have to use all La Mer."

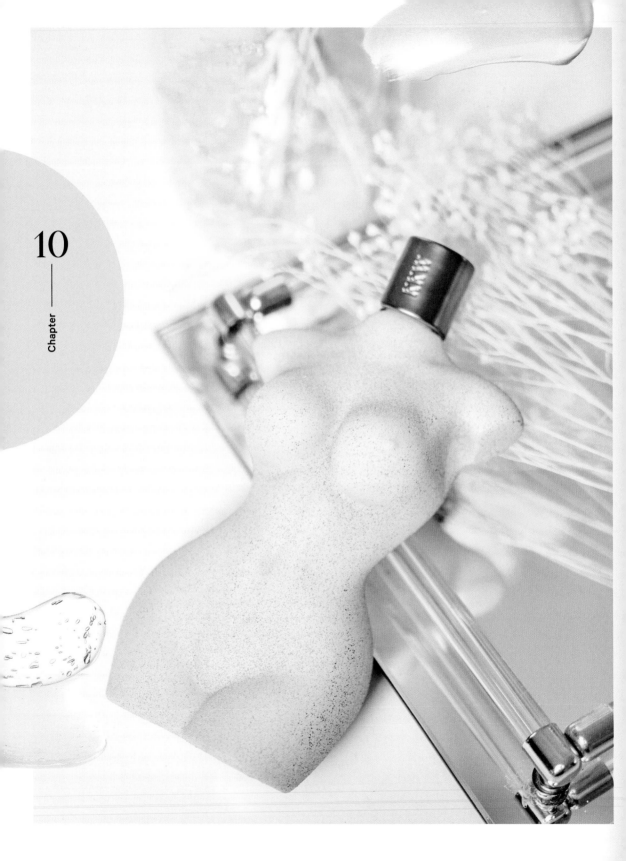

DON'T FORGET THE NECK, CHEST, HANDS, LIPS, BOOBS— YOU GET IT

H OLD UP.
This is one of the things that most people forget about & in turn, your face is all glowy, but then you have these aged neck & hands, which makes someone appear older than they are.

Don't get stuck only piling serums & moisturizers on the face & forget to take it down to at least your neck and chest. But also, give those areas a little extra TLC.

TURKEY NECK EXERCISES

I don't know about you, but I certainly had the phone switch around on me and saw turkey rolls on my neck on the camera. Since this happens, I want to talk about how to fight excess chin skin. All I know is, I never want the camera to turn on me while I'm staring at it again without doing neck exercises. Interested? Thought so. I've talked about the importance of face yoga, so why not add exercises to improve the face/neck, too? I literally stretch my face and neck every day. This exercise also helps with tech neck . . . Never heard of it? Well, it's real. And the struggle is REAL real.

So many women forget that one of the first places we age is the neck. And guess what? The cellphone sitch is REALLY not helping.

Here's the deal: If you don't stretch your neck, it may turn into a turkey neck: You know, that saggy folding skin under the chin. But by using my 5-Second Facelift exercises, you can avoid that whole gobble-gobble situation.

HOW TO COMBAT EXCESS CHIN-SKIN:

- Stay hydrated: You skin's less likely to wrinkle.
- Maintain an overall healthy body fat percentage.
- Do daily, 5-second face/neck stretches.
- As you know, I'm all for prevention, prevention, prevention. So every day I give myself a mini facelift. How? It's so easy it's kind of ridiculous.

THE SKINNY CONFIDENTIAL 5-SECOND FACELIFT:

- Lift your head toward the ceiling and lift up and down 10 times. This works really well while practicing yoga, too.
- While still sitting or standing up straight, roll your lips over your teeth and open your mouth as wide as possible, then tilt your head back. Hold here for 30 seconds, then rest for 10 seconds. Repeat two times.
- Lie on your bed with your head hanging off the edge. Slowly lift your head up until your neck is in line with your torso. Hold for 10 seconds, then lower slowly back toward the floor. Rest for 10 seconds and repeat two times.

I do these practices every day—if you see me driving and practicing them, I apologize in advance.

NECK & CHEST

Did you know the neck and chest are one of the first things that can give away age? I spotted this when I started watching *The Real Housewives*. Some of them would have these tight, snatched faces, but would neglect to take care of their chest and neck. If you're looking for a quick fix right away for your neck, there's something I recently discovered called neck tape. This is obviously not preventative, but it's good in a pinch. AND HELLO: This very much can tighten the shit out of the jowls, extra loose skin & possibly even a double chin (I know this well thanks to gaining 55 pounds when I was pregnant) quickly. You should know that most neck tape is waterproof and made of hypoallergenic, surgical-grade adhesive—however, you should check before you buy, as always. I read through those Amazon reviews like a beast before purchasing—this is *muy importante*.

We all know that the skin on the décolleté is extremely thin and delicate, so it's also important to be careful about the products you use. Basically, many doctors have told me that the neck and chest contain fewer glands than other parts of the body, so damage is easily done. The collagen and elastin also begin to break down and cause the skin to sag, resulting in those vertical creases.

The way you sleep matters for your neck and chest, too. If you sleep on your side a lot, then that's going to cause more wrinkles on your chest.

DÉCOLLETÉ (AKA NECK) SKINCARE TIPS:

This area is so important. It needs a lot of attention & some major TLC.

MOISTURIZE. Find a moisturizer that you love and take it all the way down to your tits. I personally love to mix a moisturizer with oil. I look for moisturizers that have vitamin C in them. Look for nourishing ingredients like shea butter, collagen, hyaluronic acid, etc. If you're looking for an oil for the neck and chest, look for a product with raspberry oil in it because it protects from free radical damage and locks in moisture.

APPLY SUNSCREEN. Since you've been reading this book, I feel like I don't need to tell you about applying sunscreen. Just be sure to take it to your tits & hands.

WEAR HIGH-NECK SHIRTS WHENEVER POSSIBLE. I always love to wear a high-neck shirt, especially when I'm going on a long car ride or if I know I'm going to be in the sun. If I can't wear a high-neck shirt for some reason, I try to wear a hat or visor with a huge brim.

WATCH YOUR POSTURE. It's really important & something that a lot of people forget about. I even invested in one of those dorsal vests that hold your shoulders back while you're working.

EXFOLIATE ONCE A WEEK. Don't forget to exfoliate your chest. Don't go crazy because the skin is so thin, but make sure you're paying attention to it. I like to use a coffee scrub on my neck and chest because I feel like it wakes you up. It's also great to dry brush before taking a shower. If you don't remember, the benefits of dry brushing are that it gets the lymphatic system going, improves circulation, can reduce appearance of cellulite & gets rid of dead skin cells.

AVOID SMOKING. You guys don't need me to sit here and tell you why you shouldn't smoke. But just to recap, smoking will wrinkle your face, neck, chest & lips VERY FAST.

How I like to combat that is with sunscreen, but here are Dr. Barbara Sturm's tips:

- Limit screen time (the average for people is 5–8 hours!!).
- Wear blue-light-blocking glasses (more on this in a sec).
- Move your phone away from your bed (this will help decrease your cortisol).
- Use skincare products that have blue light filters in them (like the Glowscreen or anti-pollution drops).
- Use hyaluronic acid regularly to further protect your skin's barrier function (plus, it'll keep you super hydrated).

So ya, blue-light-blocking glasses are definitely worth mentioning. Constant use of electronics used to really make me feel stressed out. I was ALWAYS on them. Like always . . . even in bed (but I'm waaaaay better now). In fact, I'm so specific about unwinding that I hardly ever go on my computer in bed anymore.

Anyway, what the glasses do is block out all the blue light from computer screens, phone screens, or any screen. Blocking out the blue light kind of tells your eyes & brain that it's time to shut down for the night. There are so many to choose from—just scope Amazon or see if your favorite sunglass company makes some, too!

You can also sit farther away from your screen. We're all hunched over our computers & phones. Personally, I try to practice a lot of mindfulness & Pilates to engage my core while I'm sitting so I'm not so hunched over.

You can also get chairs that help straighten your posture & help minimize that HEV exposure. And for all you researchers wondering, HEV is understood as the blue, artificial light that comes off all screens. It means HIGH-ENERGY VISIBLE LIGHT.

Sarah Gibson Tuttle

/ @oliveandjune

FOUNDER AND CEO OF OLIVE & JUNE

HOW DO YOU GET A SALON-PERFECT MANICURE AT HOME?

I created the Olive & June Mani System because I wanted to find a way to achieve a salon-perfect mani in one box. I found that the key is all in the preparation, which helps you avoid early chipping. Giving yourself regular manicures is the best way to show your hands some love. Weekly shaping, buffing, and painting will keep your nails looking and feeling their best.

Start by shaping your nails with our clipper and file. The best shape for your nails is the one you like the best! Then use your thumb to push back your cuticles and gently buff away any dead skin—no cutting allowed! Use the buffer to smooth away any ridges or peels on your nail plate. Dip each nail in the nail remover pot to strip your nail plate of debris, dust, and oil. Do not wash your hands! Water is the enemy of a long-lasting mani because it makes your nail plate expand and your polish chip. We also recommend avoiding any moisture or oil in your mani process until your polish is dry. This is the biggest mistake we see when people experience chipping. So don't touch anything—especially your hair or face—to avoid reintroducing any oils onto your nail plate.

Now, paint! Ideally with a long-lasting, cruelty-free, and vegan polish. In addition to our polish line, we also developed the Poppy, which is our patented universal polish brush handle, which makes painting with your non-dominant hand a breeze. Remember to always paint thin coats—the first one should look streaky! And let each coat dry as much as possible in between to avoid bubbles. Then apply a top coat (like our Super Glossy Top Coat) to add shine and make your mani last as long as possible.

KEEP YOUR HANDS LOOKING YOUTHFUL

Your hands. One of the things most people forget when taking care of their face, neck, and chest are their hands. Hands are used all day, every day, and we use a lot of soap and water that can be harsh—we do dishes, we take care of kids, we're just constantly using them. I really wanted to do a section on keeping your hands looking youthful because it really does make a difference as you age. All I want for Christmas is driving gloves. LOL.

- Wear your gloves when driving, yes, but also make sure you pay attention to when you're doing the dishes. Doing the dishes can mess up your hands, too—you will see wear and tear if you're not investing in some good ole dish gloves. They come in pink at the supermarket so you can have some fun with them.
- Moisturize, moisturize, moisturize, especially glob it on at night.
- Choose an orange/red-based polish because blue tones can bring out the veins. This may sound odd, but I have noticed that my veins don't pop as much when I opt for reddish tones.
- Exfoliate your hands.
- Spray tan instead of lying in the sun.
- & duh, don't forget the SPF.

LIPS, LIPS, LIPS! LIPS ARE SKIN, TOO.

As we all know the weather and the sun can make your lips cracked and chapped, so having a specific lip balm in your bag is always very important. I personally like an all-natural lip balm, because duh, it's by your mouth. I once heard on *Keeping Up with the Kardashians* that in a lifetime, women can swallow up to 9 pounds of lip balm! That's just so nasty. Obviously, I want something natural if I'm going to be ingesting it, ya know what I mean?

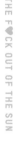

Another hot tip is a toothbrush. THAT'S RIGHT, BRUSH YOUR LIPS!

I've been doing this since sixth grade. Weird? Bear with me, because it's super easy, economical & quick.

Here's what you do: Grab a drugstore toothbrush & some cinnamon oil (it'll seriously plump your lips—trust me). Then dab the oil on the toothbrush & brush in a circular motion to gently exfoliate your lips. Afterward, I like to put on some lip balm to seal the deal. Stimulating the lips makes them bigger/poutier & I mean, ultimately no one wants white, sickie crust flaking off their lips.

WAIT! DON'T FORGET THE REST OF YOUR BOD:

These are my tips for taking care of the body parts we forget. Just because you aren't directly in the sun doesn't mean you can sleep on sunscreen. Be smart & preventative here. The more you get into the habit, the more it becomes like brushing your teeth. It'll be like second nature.

When it comes to sunscreen for the full body, I prefer a mist. It's the easiest, the quickest & not too overwhelming.

Most derms recommend SPF 30 and up no matter where you're going, so make sure your body is getting the best protection.

Most SPF can withstand water and sweat, so you shouldn't need to reapply body sunscreen unless you're lying out in the sun or swimming a ton. Obviously, I always have some nearby, though.

MAKE SURE to get your whole body, but especially: don't forget the knees! The knees sag easily, so maybe give some extra TLC to your knees and even elbows. I'm a fan of doubling up on both of those areas. This may sound aggressive, but I feel like it's one of those things you'll be glad you did when you're older.

BOOBS/TITS/TITTIES/FUNBAGS/ BREASTS/JUGS:

I have a dirty little secret . . . I'm obsessed with rubbing all-natural boob lotion (it's actually for pregnant women) or oil on my tits. I started doing it in high school using avocado. Why? Because I seriously believe it prevents stretch marks. Here's the deal: When I heard about this all-natural product for pregnant women, I did my research, added it to my shopping cart, and patiently waited for it to arrive. Now, I've been using it for some time and I'm obsessed. So obsessed it is a nightly ritual, just like brushing my teeth.

The one I like is called Boob Tube by Mama Mio.

YOU WANT YOUR TEETS TO AIM NORTH, NOT SOUTH. The goal is to prevent sagging, stretching, and dark spots.

I'm very much for that policy, thanks. But here's how to make that happen:

- ♥ Simply grab some cold-pressed, raw oil (think avocado oil, coconut oil, or olive oil) and get to rubbing.
- ♥ Or, if you find an all-natural boob lotion, look for ones that have these ingredients:
  - **CoQ10:** Nature's wonderfully powerful antioxidant that helps prevent collagen degradation to stop sagging.
  - **Milk thistle extract:** A natural antioxidant to help prevent free radical damage to delicate skin to keep it strong.
  - **Organic evening primrose, organic sweet almond, organic olive, and avocado oils:** Every single one is packed with omegas, vitamin D, and vitamin E. Superbly moisturizing, keeping skin firm and elastic.
  - **Organic shea:** The most potent healing butter. It's an omega-rich natural elasticizer that helps stave off sagging.

If that list doesn't make your nipples hard, I don't know what does.

They even have sheet masks for your boobs (and butt). They're the latest in beauty treatments and something that we're going to see more and more of.

Sarah Nicole Landry of *The Bird's Papaya* podcast swears by vitamin C serum morning and night. She swears that since implementing it in her rotation it's like she's aging in reverse.

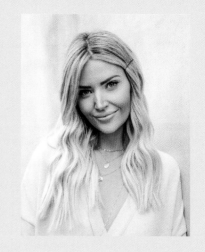

Certified health coach **Neda Varbanova** holds a master's degree in food studies from NYU and is the creator of Healthy With Nedi, a lifestyle brand. Neda says berries are one of the best fruits you can eat for beautiful skin. They're packed with antioxidants and vitamin C, which may help reduce wrinkles. She says avocados are another great skin food because of the high content of healthy fats that keep the skin moisturized. Neda's secret for clear skin is mixing baking soda into her mask. She loves Biologique Recherche's Masque Vivant and uses it twice a week with one-half teaspoon of baking soda. The deep-cleansing mask purifies while shrinking pores. Even her facialist swears by it. Another hot tip from Neda is to use Greek yogurt on your skin if you get a sunburn.

Pharmacist-turned-wellness-influencer **Dr. Mona Vand** has two simple-but-effective rituals: She does her best to change her pillowcases every night so that her faced is pressed up against something clean all night—a solid breakout preventor. And she always throws on a face mask 15 minutes before she showers. That way she can bring it down to her neck & chest and have an easy way to wash it off. She also likes to let the mask sit on her skin for about 5 minutes in the shower so the steam can help it absorb more.

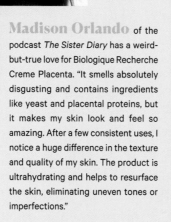

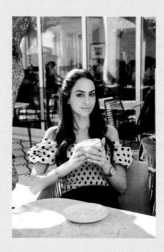

Madison Orlando of the podcast *The Sister Diary* has a weird-but-true love for Biologique Recherche Creme Placenta. "It smells absolutely disgusting and contains ingredients like yeast and placental proteins, but it makes my skin look and feel so amazing. After a few consistent uses, I notice a huge difference in the texture and quality of my skin. The product is ultrahydrating and helps to resurface the skin, eliminating uneven tones or imperfections."

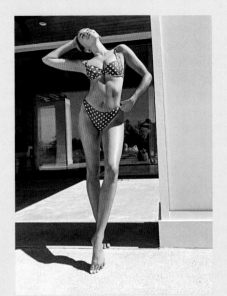

Jordan Younger, aka *The Balanced Blonde*, is never without her cocokind rosewater facial toner. At $17, it boosts hydration and has only one ingredient: rosewater. The founder also happens to be a dear friend of hers who got into the business because of her own battle with skin issues. Jordan always has a bottle in her purse so she can get a hydrating spritz any time of day.

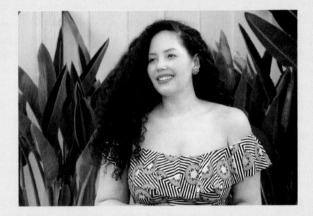

Model and influencer **Sophia Culpo** has a degree in nutrition, too! "I believe our bodies are incredible vessels that need to be properly taken care of. Our skin is no different—in fact, it's our biggest organ! And it's not just the skin on our faces that matters. Taking care of your body is a way of thanking the home that we live in every day." She thinks that what you put in your body is just as effective as any skincare. Sophia likes to focus on getting skincare needs from nutrient-rich whole foods, like fruits, vegetables, healthy fats, and supplementing her diet with Vital Proteins Collagen Peptides.

She also swears by the Facial Radiance intensive peel by First Aid Beauty. It's a 3-minute mask that uses a combination of lactic and salicylic acids and mushroom enzymes to exfoliate and remove dead skin cells. Her biggest splurge is the Déesse LED mask by Shani Darden. "It's expensive, but it does amazing things for my skin. There are six treatment modes for a range of skincare concerns such as acne, fine lines, wrinkles, scarring, elasticity, etc. I try to use the mask nightly for about 10–15 minutes. My favorite setting is the Blue Light Mode, which has antibacterial properties to kill acne-causing bacteria. I also love the Blue & Green Mode to even out pigmentation and reduce scarring."

Body-positivity influencer and designer of Girl with Curves **Tanesha Awasthi** swears by Neutrogena Alcohol-Free Toner. She's been using it since it first came out and tells everyone she knows about it because it's inexpensive, great for all skin types, and gets the job done without all the froufrou and extra ingredients that aren't necessary when it comes to a toner.

Lauren Orlando of *The Sister Diary* podcast says, "After visiting the dermatologist last year, I started using the CeraVe Hydrating Facial Cleanser. It's super affordable, less than $20, and I've found it to be super effective! A pricier skincare product that I'm absolutely obsessed with right now is the Sunday Riley C.E.O. Glow Vitamin C + Turmeric Face Oil."

11

Chapter

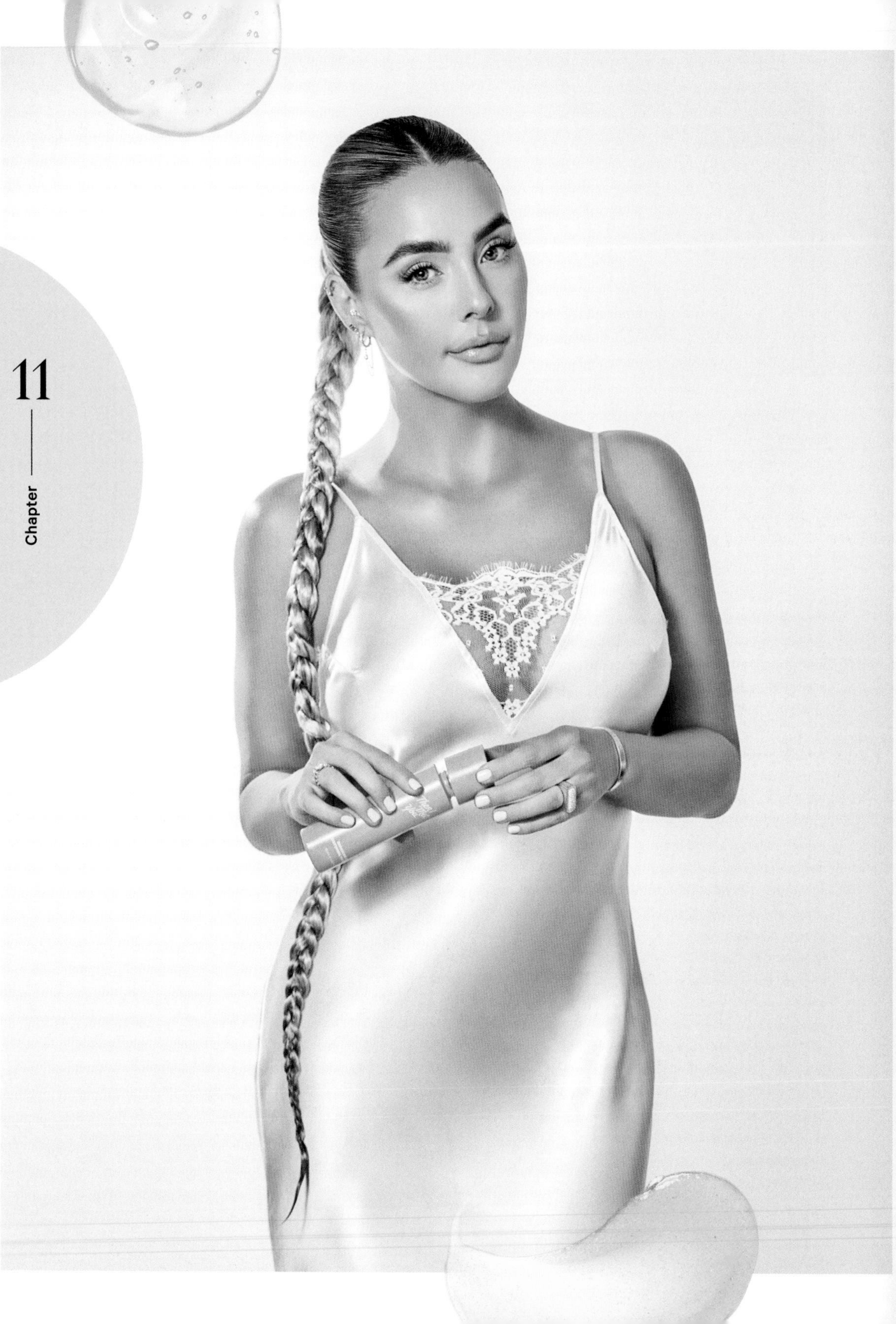

HIGH & LOW: LET'S TALK PRODUCTS

Sometimes you're ballin' and sometimes you're on a budget—we've all been there. This is one of my favorite series & posts to do on *The Skinny Confidential* blog, inspired by the time I was so broke that I couldn't afford any of the products I wanted—so I had to get really creative and find solid dupes.

IT'S TIME TO TALK HACKS, MKAY?

HIGH

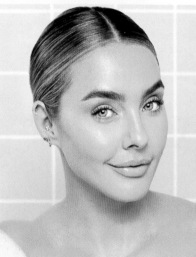

PRODUCT NAME: Dr. Dennis Gross Vitamin C + Collagen Brighten & Firm Vitamin C Serum

PRICE: $78

WHY IT WORKS: This specific serum contains vitamin C technology & a complex that neutralizes free radical damage & firms the skin while also getting rid of hyperpigmentation & dark spots. The overall goal of this is to focus on brown spots, fine lines & wrinkles. You're also going to see brighter, clearer skin.

PRODUCT NAME: Elemis Pro-Collagen Cleansing Balm

PRICE: $64

WHY IT WORKS: I love how this balm makes my skin feel. It doesn't feel stripped after you use it. It basically melts your makeup away & smells like a spa. It has collagen & makes your skin feel nourished & plump. This is a perfect product to use as a first cleanse.

PRODUCT NAME: *The Skinny Confidential* Ice Roller

WHY IT WORKS: We went over this in chapter 3, but for a refresh: a chic, solid, effective ice roller that holds cold for hours & hours (in fact, it even stays cold when it's not in the freezer) with a user-friendly (and pink) ridged silicone grip.

PRODUCT NAME: Joovv Therapy Infrared Light

PRICE: $295–$6,000

WHY IT WORKS: Red light therapy is the wellness phenomenon that I'm here for. My husband & I are both big fans of the Joovv lights. He has the huge one & I love the mini.

The benefits of red light therapy are kind of endless, but here are some: boosts collagen, rejuvenates skin from the inside out, helps with burns & healing, helps with scars & wrinkles, and has shown improvement in people with hyperpigmentation, vitiligo, eczema & psoriasis.

PRODUCT NAME: Tata Harper Hydrating Hyaluronic Acid Floral Essence

PRICE: $72

WHY IT WORKS: This bottle is big, hefty & filled to the tippy-top. It lasts forever, smells delicious & isn't too overwhelming. It rejuvenates the skin & is lovely under or over moisturizer. This specific one has a hydrating essence that plumps the skin & is great for fine lines, wrinkles & hyperpigmentation.

GET THE F●CK OUT OF THE SUN

PRODUCT NAME: Botanical Beauty Vitamin C Face Oil

PRICE: $12.95

WHY IT WORKS: If I'm going for a cheaper vitamin C, I always go for a vitamin C oil. I prefer it over a cream if I'm trying to save money. This specific one also has raspberry seed oil, cranberry seed oil & grapeseed oil. It really provides a softness & suppleness to the skin while also plumping. It's non-greasy & non-oily, even though it's an oil. It has vitamins A & E, as well as omegas, which we love, plus it's vegan, cruelty-free, water-free & won't clog your pores.

HOT TIP *Witch hazel is fab if you have hemorrhoids, especially post-birth—it's your best friend. It's an astringent that's super soothing & is a great toner for your face, too. Just be sure to invest in two bottles so the one you use on hemorrhoids isn't touching your face.*

PRODUCT NAME: Red lightbulbs

PRICE: $10–$25

WHY IT WORKS: These work for all the same reasons the Joovv lights work—red light therapy for all! Seriously, it lowers cortisol & increases melatonin production. We put red lightbulbs in our bedroom & it just really sets the mood for sleep & relaxation. Another affordable tip is to turn your iPhone onto red light mode.

PRODUCT NAME: DIY Lavender Lemon Face Mist

PRICE: $5–$15

DIRECTIONS: Purchase a 4-ounce dark glass or BPA-free plastic spray bottle & fill it with a bit less than ½ cup of distilled water, 2 teaspoons of witch hazel, 2 drops of lemon essential oil & 5 drops of lavender essential oil. Give it a shake & spritz away.

WHY IT WORKS: I like to use something like this at night because lavender calms you down. Another reason this is great at night is that citrus oils can increase your chance of sunburn, which we never want.

Witch hazel: An amazing toner for the skin. It can help with irritations & large pores and help manage oiliness.

Lemon essential oil: A great source of vitamin C that can help lessen the appearance of freckles & dark spots. It has antiseptic properties that can help clear the skin.

Lavender essential oil: Super relaxing & can help heal acne breakouts because it's antibacterial.

If you're feeling crazy, jazz up your face mist with a couple drops of rose hip or jojoba oil or replace the distilled water with tea! Peppermint tea to refresh, chamomile tea to calm, or green tea to nourish. SPRITZ, SPRITZ, SKINNIES!

PRODUCT NAME: Organic, cold-pressed oil

PRICE: $10–$20

WHY IT WORKS: As I said in many other sections of this book—OILS, OILS, OILS!! They're the secret to youthful, beautiful skin. Every girl should have organic grapeseed oil on hand. It's moisturizing, contains vitamin E, doesn't clog pores, is great for sensitive skin, tightens pores & reduces the appearance of scars.

PRODUCT NAME: Ice

PRICE: $0—that's right. it's fucking FREE

WHY IT WORKS: As I said earlier in the book, dunking your face in a bowl of ice water might be my favorite tip in the world. It's like magic & totally free.

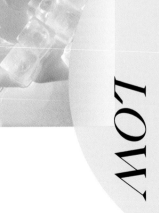

LOW

Katherine Schwarzenegger Pratt

/ @katherineschwarzenegger

BESTSELLING AUTHOR AND ANIMAL
WELFARE ACTIVIST

My favorite skin care product under $50 is definitely my go-to face wash, which is called Brave Soldier Clean Skin. It takes off all my makeup and leaves my skin clean but not stripped of my natural oils, which I love because my skin tends to run dry. My biggest skincare splurge is Dr. Barbara Sturm Hyaluronic Serum. I always heard about her hyaluronic acid, and never really understood what it was all about. I was given a sample of it, and I was totally amazed at the effect it had on my skin, so I splurged and ordered a full bottle. It gives my skin a feeling of being hydrated without all the excess oil and products that are left on my face from other products I've tried. I use it in the morning and at night and am obsessed right now.

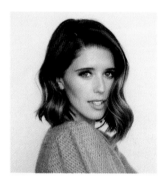

Vani Hari

/ @thefoodbabe

CO-FOUNDER OF TRUVANI AND
INFLUENCER BEHIND *THE FOOD BABE*

Organic sesame oil is the one ingredient that I love. I put it on before I shower or take a bath, for smooth soft skin. I always feel like I've been through an expensive spa treatment after. It's shocking to most people that you can use oils before bathing to seal in your skin moisture. It's my secret trick to avoid dry, scaly skin. I also smear it all over my belly (especially during pregnancy) before going to bed and use it as makeup remover. My biggest splurge is probably expensive natural lipstick in bright red . . . I love a bright lip! Clove + Hallow makes a killer color called Flaming Coral that I get so many compliments on.

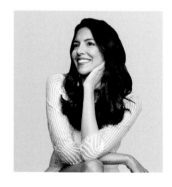

GET THE F♥CK OUT OF THE SUN

Jenna Rennert

/ @itsjennarennert

BEAUTY, FASHION, AND WELLNESS
EXPERT AND FORMER BEAUTY
EDITOR AT *VOGUE*

I was the beauty editor at *VOGUE* for
seven years—it was my job to find the
coolest and the most hardworking
skin care, hair & makeup products and
share them with the world. So when
you ask what's the most effective, let's
just say I know a thing or two about
beauty products.

The most effective skincare product I've tried is an acne treatment
that's $6 and available at the drug-
store. I know, too good to be true,
but trust me here. It's from Clean &
Clear—the brand is Persa-Gel. It's 10%
benzoyl peroxide, which reaches deep
into a zit (overnight! daytime! whenever!) to heal it from the inside out.
It dries up the breakout super fast. In
other words, it's epic.

In the splurge category, I could go
on . . . and on . . . and on. But for the
sake of finishing this book, I'll give you
two. La Mer Crème de la Mer, aka the
holy grail of all moisturizers. This stuff
is crazy hydrating, can heal a rash or
sunburn (don't go in the sun!). I once
said in an interview that my most
obnoxious beauty editor habit was
slathering this expensive face cream on
my body (especially during the winter
on dry spots) because it really is that
good. I later heard from a celebrity hairstylist friend that the Kardashian clan
did this same thing to help prevent
stretch marks during pregnancy. What
did I tell you? Holy. Grail.

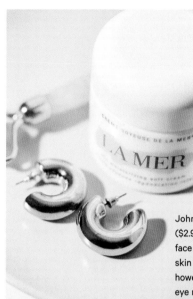

The second splurge item is basically an expensive bottle of magic
water. I use SK-II Facial Treatment
Essence every single morning when I
wake up. It's not a toner, not a serum
but an ESSENCE made of Pitera—
the story begins at a Japanese sake
brewery where workers had wrinkled
faces but very young, smooth-looking
hands after handling the fermented
sake formula for years. I can't speak to
the science, but this stuff gives you a
serious glow.

Farrah Brittany Aldjufrie

/ @farrahbritt

REAL ESTATE AGENT WHO
YOU MAY HAVE SEEN ON
*THE REAL HOUSEWIVES
OF BEVERLY HILLS*

Johnson's Head-to-Toe Baby Wash
($2.99)—I have been using this as a
face wash for years. It's gentle on the
skin (because it's meant for babies!);
however, it also dissolves ALL of your
eye makeup, so it's great if you've run
out of makeup-remover wipes. I cannot
stand leftover mascara/makeup residue. I buy this in bulk because it's so
inexpensive—I have a huge one in
my shower and a smaller one on my
counter. It's also great because it can
double as a body wash or shaving gel!
And it's cute, yellow, and nostalgic :)

SkinMedica TNS Essential Serum
($281)—This is a two-part serum that's
filled with growth factors, peptides,
proteins, and antioxidants. It's one of
the bestselling and highest-rated antiaging serums out there. I do feel that it
plumps my skin and helps with everything from tightening to fine lines to
texture!

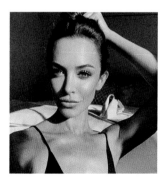

Erica Stolman

/ @fashionlush

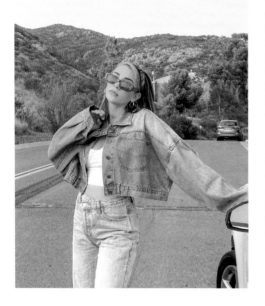

OK—so the absolute best skincare products I've tried under $50 is anything/everything from Versed! They sell the line at Target & it's honestly amazing. Clean products, simple ingredients & of course—great branding. My fave products from there are The Fix Emergency Eye Mask, Silk Slip lip oil, Found the Light vitamin C brightening powder, both their cleanser balm & cleansing gel & literally any of their serums. So yeah, like I said—everything from Versed is amazing.

As far as skincare splurges go—U Beauty Resurfacing Compound is my holy grail. I am not one to spend big on skincare, but this is one product I will buy over & over again. I don't know what kinda magic is in this bottle, but pretty much a week after I ran out of my first bottle, my skin showed it almost immediately. Within two days of getting my second bottle in the mail, my skin was clear & glowing again. The ingredients are clean, skincare gurus everywhere rave about it, and it literally gives you new skin.

GET THE F♥CK OUT OF THE SUN

Mandy Ansari

/ @mandy

MARKETING EXECUTIVE, LIFESTYLE INFLUENCER, AND MENTAL HEALTH ADVOCATE

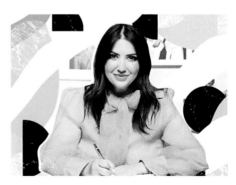

Rosewater has been used for centuries in Middle Eastern cultures (I'm Persian), and I'm never without it. With hydrating and soothing abilities, as well as natural antiseptic, anti-inflammatory, and antibacterial powers, it's one of those ultimate beauty powerhouses (often used by high-end beauty brands as a foundational ingredient for their bestselling products.) At under $10 a bottle, you'll up your whole routine with rosewater—whether you use it as a toner to hydrate & combat acne, under a sheet mask to boost its efficacy, on your dry scalp, or to balance your pH . . . you'll swear by it, too, once you give it a try. My splurge I will never abandon is the Dr. Dennis Gross Alpha Beta Extra Strength Daily Peel.

Jenna Kutcher

/ @jennakutcher

BUSINESS COACH, ENTREPRENEUR, AND PODCASTER OF *THE GOAL DIGGER PODCAST*

Primally Pure Cleansing Oil ($20!). I used harsh cleansers for years and chemical-laden products to clean my skin, not believing that naturally derived products could *really* work for my skin. Gave the clean stuff major side-eye since I thought that was for people with "naturally good skin." When I switched to using an oil cleanser, it almost immediately transformed the way my skin felt, so I ate my words real quick. It injected a TON of confidence to clean up my skincare act and bring nontoxic products into my life (and body!).

Major shout-out to the PMD personal microdermabrasion tool. I remember when I first bought it years ago and really mulled over its price tag, but I can testify that it's worth its weight in gold. I *still* get stoked to use it once a week, especially in seasons when I can't get regular facials (which, let's be honest, is like every season).

Gigi Goldman

/ @gigi.goldman

Kiana Cabell

/ @kianacabell

KOPARI BEAUTY CO-FOUNDERS

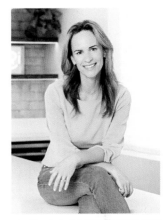

FYI: Kopari has always been a ride or die for me. I love their lip balm & I've been obsessed with them since they launched. The lip balm is so delicious that my husband likes to kiss it off my lips. They're amazing because they've figured out how to create the best experience with coconut oil. My other obsession is the coconut rose toner. It tightens and balances your skin. Kopari's products are super clean & they just get it. I love all their stuff, PLUS, they're not tested on animals and are non-GMO, free of parabens, sulfates, phthalates, & gluten. Now, you're going to hear from the founders.

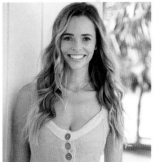

We both agree that it would have to be our Organic Coconut Melt. It's an amazing multipurpose product that hydrates like no other. I use it to remove makeup, cleanse my face, hydrate my bod, and moisturize my hair. Every member of Gigi's family (including the boys) uses it as well. It's $28, lasts a long time, and is the mother of all multitaskers.

For our splurge product on the other hand, we also agree that it's SkinCeuticals C E Ferulic Serum. It's one product that, while expensive, is worth the spend because we've noticed significant results from using it regularly. It's packed with antioxidants, vitamins C & E, and has really helped to brighten our skin and diminish our dark spots.

Heather McDonald

/ @heathermcdonald

ACTRESS, COMEDIAN, AND AUTHOR

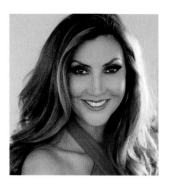

My favorite product under $50 is Olay Total Effects Refreshing Citrus Scrub Cleanser. I always say go cheaper on cleanser and eye makeup remover. Spend a little more on the actual skin cream you put on before your makeup and before bed that seeps through. My biggest splurge is the Chanel Sublimage La Crème 50g. I tend to have dry skin, especially right out of the shower. It just immediately moisturizes it and keeps me dewy all day long. It gives a great glow through your makeup, and I never feel dry when I have that on. Because it is so pricey, every time I buy it, which lasts for several months, the person at the counter is so happy they made a big sale that I insist on them giving me small samples (which are very generously sized) to keep with me when I travel and do stand-up comedy on the road.

This is the hottest skincare tip I learned from my friend Jule. The most amazing hack ever.

A baby washcloth is going to be gentler, softer & just better overall for the fragile skin on your face. You can find cute ones on Amazon that are pre-rolled with a festive bow or find them at any baby store or drugstore. They look so good on display in your bathroom & they're ready to go for when you want to take your makeup off.

BENEFITS OF USING A BABY WASHCLOTH ON YOUR FACE:

- 💜 Easy to use & wash.
- 💜 Won't pull the skin down.
- 💜 Antibacterial & hypoallergenic.
- 💜 Free from chemicals & dyes.
- 💜 Super soft because they're meant for a newborn's bum.

I thought this hack was genius, because washing your face is hopefully something you do every single night. You know I'm a huge fan of cleansing balm because it's so buttery—so when I take off my makeup, I throw some of the balm on my face, do a little facial massage, leave it on for 10 minutes & then gently take it off by patting upward with this baby washcloth.

Now, you can go get yourself some baby washcloths specifically for your face & keep them away from your significant other. OH, and colors matter! For my baby washcloths I went with pink because it's said to show a woman's beauty in the best way possible. It lifts your spirit & I'm going with it!

SKIN SPECIFICS AT ANY AGE (AKA BOOKMARK THIS PAGE):

EARLY TEENS–EARLY 20S:

CLEANSER: Use a cleanser that removes eye makeup. I'm a fan of cleansing balm or oil to remove makeup, and those are nice products for teenagers to start out with.

MILD ACID: Get a mild acid if you're suffering from acne. When I was this age, I started using a salicylic acid. Do not use a glycolic acid, though—that's the one that gave me hyperpigmentation on my face. I'm not a skincare expert, but I saw what happened to my own face.

MOISTURIZER: A light, plumping one with SPF—duh. Try to find something that works with an SPF of 40–50. SPF keeps you looking young and is oh-so important.

VITAMIN C: Also add in a vitamin C serum or cream for bonus points if you want to be extra proactive.

20S–MID-30S:

CLEANSER: A good cleanser that removes makeup.

ACID/TONER: Lactic or salicylic acid plumps the skin and keeps it dewy.

VITAMIN C SERUM: This is a must according to Dr. Dennis Gross.

EYE PRODUCT: Personally, I love an eye balm with caffeine because it tightens the eyes without giving you milia.

RETINOL: A retinol product a few times a week does the trick.

OILS, ALWAYS: Oils are the key to youth. You should always have some oils in your bathroom or on your vanity.

MOISTURIZER: Try to get a plumping moisturizer for your specific skin type with SPF (again, DUH). I like to have at least SPF 50.

EARLY 40S:

EXFOLIATING CLEANSER AND CLEANSING BALM: Alternate using these each day.

GLYCOLIC ACID: Introduce a glycolic or lactic AHA acid. Obviously, do your research to see what's best for your skin type.

FACIAL MIST: So many experts say to look for a mist with hyaluronic acid.

VITAMIN C: This is a very important skincare ingredient. I'm telling you, be sure it's in your skincare routine by now.

A DELICIOUS OIL: Again, it's the key to youth. I like grapeseed, rose hip, argan, or jojoba.

EYE GEL OR BALM: As I said above, I love a balm with caffeine in it.

RETINOID: According to the experts, you really want this in your routine at this age.

BOMBASS MOISTURIZER: Yes, you guessed it—with SPF.

MID-40S–100 (FOR SURE I WANT TO BE DOING SKINCARE WHEN I'M 100):

CREAM CLEANSER: A thicker cream cleanser that targets wrinkles and removes makeup.

EXFOLIATING CLEANSER: Use this every day.

ACIDS: Lactic, salicylic, or glycolic will do.

FACIAL MIST: Again, with hyaluronic acid.

EYE PRODUCT: The lighter the better here. Don't go for something too heavy.

VITAMIN A: Aka a retinoid.

OILS, OILS, OILS: Oil it up head to toe, especially at this age.

VITAMIN C: A serum or a cream, but it needs to be there.

MOISTURIZER: With SPF, of course.

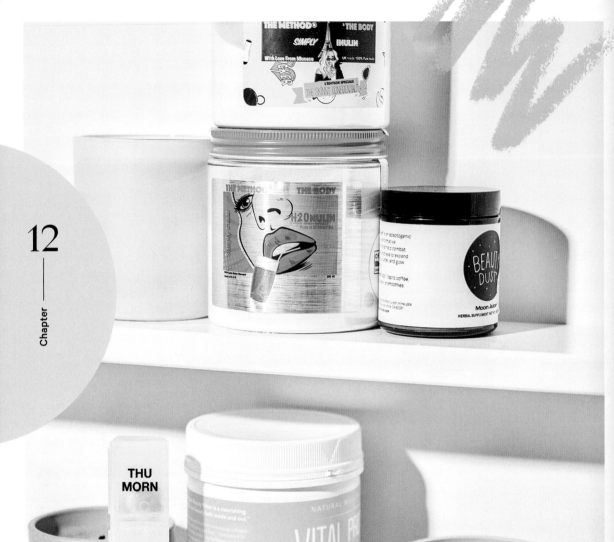

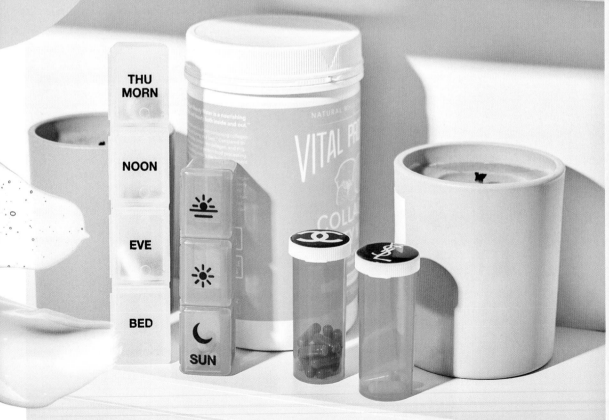

GLOW
FROM
THE
INSIDE
OUT

We've talked about everything under the sun, but I still have goodies in store for you! THAT'S RIGHT, we're going to talk all about foods, drinks, vitamins & minerals to eat for tight, youthful, pretty, plump skin at any age.

Think hydration hacks, your new favorite spa water & a collagen plumping smoothie. We even talk booze. Yes, the best booze options for your skin. Seriously like pink kombucha vodkas with a sprig of rosemary, K?

As everyone on the planet would agree, when you eat better you feel better, and when you feel better you look better.

Uma Ghosh / @umagd

CERTIFIED HEALTH COACH AND SCULPTURAL
FACELIFT THERAPIST

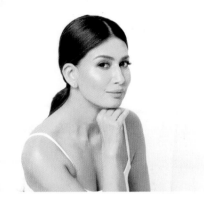

We all know beauty is more than skin deep, and our goal is to glow inside and out. And for that, we definitely need an integrative holistic approach to beauty and skin.

Holistic skincare is not simply another term for organic skincare. And it's not some New Age-y, esoteric trend only fit for people who believe natural things are the only way to go. It's actually a healthy and balanced lifestyle that has nothing to do with buying exclusive products.

A holistic health approach simply means looking at and treating something as a whole, and not just parts of it. In the case of our skincare, putting an expensive moisturizer on our face is not enough. It treats only one part of the skin—the outer layer—while the overall health of our skin depends on our mind, body & soul. Our skin depends on many factors, from the ingredients we use, our lifestyle choices (diet, exercise), the environmental stressors we meet, to our emotional & mental well-being.

A few years back, when I was a super busy TV and media entrepreneur, I used to work 18 hours a day, managing my home, attending events, socializing, traveling extensively, filming and managing my various TV shows, and managing other aspects. I was sleep-deprived, had little time to take care of myself, was stressed; I paid no attention to what I ate, so started the bloating, the melasma, dark circles, and chapped lips, cracks & wrinkles in my early 30s. Every time I looked in the mirror, I could not comprehend how my clear, clean, glowing skin had flipped to this.

To treat myself somehow, I fell into an endless cycle, trying out different chemical treatments, peelings, and skincare creams, relying on one doctor after another for my melasma. I suffered

for 10 years with all the expensive treatments and products, but nothing worked.

I eventually realized our environment and inner imbalances (physical, emotional, mental) can have serious consequences for our health; thus we need to take everything into account if we would like to restore that balance.

That's how my journey into holistic healthcare started.

THE HOLISTIC APPROACH TO SKIN

When we discover that we are not handling the stress our bodies are under, it's not as simple as regulating the initial root cause that will solve the issue. You have to start by reducing your stress significantly to find an overall balance for your mind, body & spirit.

Creating a ritual for yourself is ideal here. I want to help you come up with some techniques that keep you grounded without completely interrupting your life. You can start just like I did, by simple breathing exercises and then move to 5 minutes of meditation, and now, after many years of being consistent, I see amazing results.

Here are some simple examples of self-care to try:

1 Take a breath! And meditate.
Meditation is the most powerful stress-relieving tool we have. And the beautiful part about it is that once you have some training in a style you love, not only will you look more rested, your body will perform at the top of its game.

These are the benefits of breathing and meditation:

♥ Slows down the aging process.
♥ Improves self-confidence & mood.
♥ Helps you make healthier choices.

A few pranayamas for healthy skin. The first one is Kapalbhati. Kapalbhati gives you a forehead that shines from the outside, and it also strengthens your concentration power & increases your intellect. When you do Kapalbhati pranayama, toxins in your body are eliminated through exhalation and all the systems of your body are detoxified.

HOW TO DO IT:

1 Sit comfortably in Sukhasana, or the Easy Pose, and place your palms on your knees.

2 Direct your focus and awareness to the belly region and inhale deeply. While inhaling, pull your stomach in, getting your navel as close to the spine as you can.

3 Now exhale by relaxing completely, followed by an automatic inhalation. During exhalation, there will be a hissing sound. At that point, feel that all the toxins and negative energies from your body are getting eliminated.

4 Repeat at least 20 times.

ANULOMA VILOMA

This pranayama is very helpful in respiratory diseases like asthma. This breathing exercise is the best way to manage tridoshas in the body. Doshas are nothing but impurities in our bodies. When the tridoshas are not balanced in the body, we suffer from diseases.

HOW TO DO IT:

1 Sit comfortably in the Easy Pose. Now close your eyes and begin taking full deep breaths in and out through the nose.

2 Bring your left hand to a Vishnu mudra; curl the ring, index, and middle fingers into the palm, and leave the thumb and small finger free. Now press the left nostril with your thumb and breathe in through the right nostril only to the count of four.

3 Release your thumb and slowly exhale by emptying the lungs.

4 Now press the right nostril by using your small finger, and inhale on filling your lungs.

5 Repeat the steps, alternating the breath from the right to the left, making it smooth and effortless.

Aim to do at least eight rounds.

BAHYA PRANAYAMA

Bahya pranayama helps to prevent constipation, acidity & gastric issues and cures hernia completely. It also helps with the reproductive system and diabetes.

HOW TO DO IT:

1 Sit in the Easy Pose and close your eyes while keeping your spinal cord and head erect.

2 Breathe in deeply (inhale) and then exhale completely.

3 After exhaling, hold your breath and try to pull your stomach upward as much as you can. Pull up the muscles in the area below the navel.

4 Now move your head in the downward position in a way that your chin touches your chest. Hold this position for 5 to 10 seconds and assume that all the negativity from your body and soul has been eliminated. Now, relax and get back to the starting position.

5 Repeat this process five to 10 times.

IMPORTANT: If you are suffering from neck and back pain, do not move your head down. Just look straight and follow the same process.

2 Mindfulness Meditation

Mindfulness meditation is a mental training practice that involves focusing your mind on your experiences, emotions, thoughts, and sensations in the present moment. By choosing to turn your attention away from the everyday chatter of the mind and on to what your body is doing, you give the mind just enough to focus on so that it can quiet down.

Mindfulness meditation can involve breathing practice, mental imagery, awareness of body & mind, and muscle & body relaxation.

HOW TO DO IT:

Learning mindfulness meditation is straightforward; however, a teacher or program can help you as you start (particularly if you're doing it for health purposes). Some people do it for 10 minutes, but even a few minutes every day can make a difference. This basic technique will get you started:

1 Find a quiet and comfortable place. Sit in a chair or on the floor with your head, neck & back straight but not stiff.

2 Try to put aside all thoughts of the past & the future and stay in the present.

3 Become aware of your breath, focusing on the sensation of air moving in & out of your body as you breathe. Feel your belly rise & fall and the air enter your nostrils and leave your mouth. Pay attention to the way each breath changes and is different.

4 Watch every thought come and go, whether it be a worry, fear, anxiety, or hope. When thoughts come up in your mind, don't ignore or suppress them, but simply note them, remain calm, and use your breathing as an anchor.

5 If you find yourself getting carried away in your thoughts, observe where your mind went off to, without judging, and simply return to your breathing. Remember not to be hard on yourself if this happens.

6 As time comes to a close, sit for a minute or two, becoming aware of where you are. Gradually get up.

3 Positive Thinking

Your skin speaks volumes about your mental well-being. The perception of age isn't just physical. So, for example, even if you have some wrinkles, if your demeanor is positive, people will most likely think you are younger. People with healthier outlooks tend to take better care of themselves in terms of diet and exercise, which is good for the skin. Positivity also helps to deal with stress, which helps reduce the signs of aging.

- Being nonjudgmental toward ourselves and others.
- Detachment from outcome.
- Being in the moment (mindfulness).
- Writing in a journal.
- Practicing gratitude.
- Self-love.

4 Healthy Diet

Did you know a healthy diet can lead to healthier-looking skin?

How we eat is probably just as important when it comes to skincare as what we put onto our skin. The condition of our skin reflects what we put in our body, and a healthy diet is an "inside-out" approach to healthy skin. The healthier and more balanced our diet is, the more it will show on our skin outside.

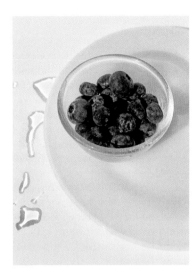

FOODS WE SHOULD EAT

Fiber

Fiber-rich foods include beans, lentil, chia seeds, flaxseed meal, whole wheat pasta.

Vitamins

Eat a lot of raw vegetables and fruit—that's the state with the highest quantity of vitamins.

Antioxidants

Antioxidant-rich food includes dark green vegetables, tomato, berries, beans, apples, pecans, grapes, nuts.

Healthy Fats

Healthy fats include avocado, walnut, flaxseed, olive oil, nut butter. Omega-3 fatty acids include fish, flaxseed, walnuts.

MORNINGS ARE KEY

I try to have a very strict morning routine with a big cup of hot water with lemon, a slice of ginger root, a sprig of mint & sometimes a dash of cayenne. I find when I start my day off with that, it sets the tone for everything else.

You should know my morning routine is completely meant to keep my cortisol down. That means a lot of bossa nova jazz music, tangerine oils going in my ceramic oil diffuser, lots of grapefruit essence candles & typically I'll sip my hot water concoction while I do something called the Morning Pages, which is a practice where you write your thoughts down on three (precisely three) pages every morning. Think of it like a mind dump for anything you're thinking. It can really help clear the mind so that you can get on with your day.

Knowing I'm getting my cortisol down while also doing something good for my skin in the morning (HOT WATER WITH LEMON!) just sets me up for a good day. Cameron Diaz says the first thing she does in the morning is drink water. This may sound like basic, expected advice, but she says to think of your body like a plant. It needs to be watered to grow. When it comes to skincare, I incorporate it into my morning and nighttime routine because it's super refreshing and rejuvenating for the skin. At this point, my skin craves it every morning.

Importance of Self-Care

Self-care and skincare go hand in hand. When you're taking care of your skin, you look better and feel better. If you're not taking care of yourself, you're an asshole to everyone around you. Self-care makes you feel sane and makes you a better human. Like right now: I'm getting my makeup done by Glamsquad (shout-out to Jeannine). I'm working and practicing self-care at the same time. I like to do what I call "passive multitasking"—I'll go get a facial and return emails at the same time, or I'll get a laser treatment and post to Instagram. I try to batch important tasks for work with my self-care routine. Of course, there are times where I'll shut off. For instance, if I go to a Korean bathhouse, I can't bring my phone in.

Kimberly Snyder

/ @_kimberlysnyder,
@sollynabyks

FOUNDER OF SOLLUNA AND BEST-SELLING AUTHOR

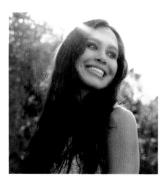

Meditation is a habit that I've been developing for years that makes a huge difference in my skin. We often think of meditation as a more spiritual practice, and don't usually connect the dots between meditation and skin health. Stress manifests in the skin, in the form of inflammation and wrinkles, and meditation has become my tried-and-true practice for reducing daily stress.

There is a lot of research on the topic to provide this connection. For example, a 2013 study found that mindfulness meditation can reduce chronic inflammation, which can lead to rapid aging and wrinkles. Additionally, stress and anxiety can promote wrinkle development due to high levels of cortisol, which breaks down our skin's collagen. Meditation offers stress-relieving benefits by bringing our mind to the present and lowering cortisol levels.

When we are more present in our bodies through meditation, we also tend to make better food choices the rest of the day, become more confident and less swayed into self-doubt & comparisons—all of which helps us to feel and look better in our skin.

Plus, meditation helps us connect back to ourselves and the inner light within us, which in and of itself helps create an amazing magnetic glow! Beauty sleep is real—I need at least 8 hours. The more I sleep, the better my skin looks. I attribute this to hormone regulation and just pure REST.

SKIN BENEFITS OF EXERCISE

This is so annoying, but actually very important: You should really be taking off your makeup before you exercise. Leaving your makeup on while you sweat will create those small white bumps (I get them under my eyes) called milia. I know firsthand that this happens because I used to do a lot of hot yoga with my makeup on. It was so noticeable that it was making my pores get clogged.

If you're like me and only wear makeup about two days a week (YES! Contrary to popular belief, I don't wear makeup that much), try to make those your workout days. It's nice to give your skin little makeup breaks throughout the week. If you're going to exercise with skincare on, make sure it's a bouncy, lightweight moisturizer or an oil like grapeseed, rose hip, or jojoba. Oil that shit up while you work out, then have a sauna or steam room sesh. CHECK on the glow after a workout—nothing prettier than a woman who just exercised. ORGASM CHEEKS! Pretty, fresh, alive!

Something to note: I like to avoid running. Why? This may be controversial, but I feel like it sags my skin! My face, my knees, my stomach, all pounding on the pavement, sags the skin. I swear! So instead, I walk everywhere. I walk while I'm on conference calls, to grab coffee, and when I go to the farmer's market.

I even went as far as getting a treadmill desk in my office—major efficiency points! Now I can walk on an incline and work on my phone.

And as far as workouts are concerned, I love low-resistance-level workouts. I feel like they don't spike my cortisol, which keeps my stress and belly fat down.

Hormones: Everyone should get their hormones tested—even if you're healthy. It tells you so much about your body. I know what's happening OUTSIDE, but what about *inside*? Why wouldn't I want to get my hormones checked if I had a lot of acne, major redness, or any kind of skin rash? When I get stressed out I notice tiny pimples on my lower cheek area and between my eyebrows. I had my hormones checked and found out I had extremely high cortisol, which is connected to stress. Look for a hormone specialist & ask for a full blood test panel. It will tell you if your thyroid is out of whack, what your testosterone levels are, and even give you insulin details.

Leyla Milani-Khoshbin

/ @leylamilani

CO-FOUNDER AND CEO OF
HAIRTAMIN AND LEYLA MILANI HAIR

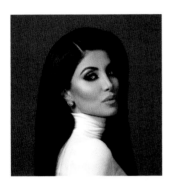

Get your hormones checked early. My GOD, has this been life-changing for me. From how I look to how much energy I have to finally conquering my adult acne, it all comes down to what's going on internally—especially for women who go through pregnancies. After my second pregnancy is when I just did not feel like myself. I was always tired, cranky, moody, had constant neck/shoulder pain—you name it. It wasn't until I started reading about hormone changes and found an incredible functional medical doctor who really helped put me on the right path.

DIET

Your skin picks up your healthy habits. The second I wake up I drink a mixture of water, lemon, and a little pinch of sea salt. Sometimes if I'm feeling bougie, I add fresh ginger clove slices. It works like a charm. Lemon keeps the body alkaline and the salt works for extra hydration. Then I meditate while letting the light in my room cascade over me. Meditation helps zen me out. And last, I move. Usually a walk to the coffee shop. But I always start the day with these three things: WATER, LIGHT, MOVEMENT.

Watermelons and cucumbers are skin foods. Unsalted raw nuts do really good things, too, because they're full of healthy fats, which promotes plump skin. I notice I look healthy when I'm nourishing my body with superfoods.

Green drinks all day, please! Kale, spinach, cucumber, ginger, pearl powder, a handful of berries, and some unsweetened coconut milk and I'm good to go.

Paola Alberdi

/ @paolaalberdi

LEADING FASHION AND LIFESTYLE
INFLUENCER OF *BLANK ITINERARY*

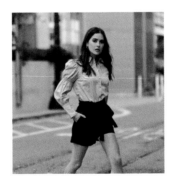

I think I have realized that no matter how many amazing and expensive products I use, if I don't have a healthy diet, my skin shows it. Yes, there are great products that have made a difference and help my skin, but the biggest daily habit that works for me is having a good diet. A diet with lots of vegetables and healthy fats and low in dairy and sugar has been shown to have great benefits for your skin. If you are spending a lot of money on trying all the products out there and are still frustrated, a good place to make some changes is your diet.

"We often focus much of our attention on treating skin from the outside in, but I've always been mindful of treating it from the inside out, and creating a treatment plan that addresses both. Live a healthy lifestyle. I do not mean to sound cliché, but it wouldn't be cliché if it weren't true. Drink water. Exercise. Use a humidifier to avoid the skin's exposure to dry air. Take cold showers. Use a moisturizer to seal the skin from negative environmental influences. My favorite and most trusted tip: de-stress. Whatever that means to you. For me? Daily meditation. Cortisol, what many people refer to as the "stress hormone," regulates many of the body's natural processes, such as metabolism, immune function, inflammation, and stress response. When our bodies produce excess cortisol, it negatively impacts the face & body skin health and causes dehydration, oil production, acne, weight gain, insomnia, etc. All of these negatively affect the skin and negatively affect life. It is proven that daily meditation and exercise can stabilize cortisol levels, thereby alleviating any factors damaging your skin you're in direct control of. Finding an outlet that allows you to stabilize your cortisol levels and center your mind & body will have a bigger ROI than absolutely anything you can buy. Your mind and body can be your best friends or your worst enemies—choose wisely."

/ **Dr. Jason Diamond** / @drjasondiamond
BOARD-CERTIFIED FACIAL PLASTIC SURGEON SPECIALIZING IN FACIAL SCULPTING, ANTIAGING, AND FACIAL REJUVENATION, AS WELL AS SKIN INTEGRITY AND HEALTH.

GET THE F●CK OUT OF THE SUN

EATING AND SUPPLEMENTS

What food you put on your skin or in your body can really make all the difference when it comes to the plumpness and dewiness in your skin. Here are some other things you can incorporate—but *it's important to note that you talk to your health care provider before starting any supplements.*

Probiotics:

HUGE fan of probiotics. Love a kombucha/champagne situation & also kimchi. But I also take probiotics every single day. Whether it's a pill or through food, or through coffee (heeeey inulin— more on that coming up), I need to get probiotics in.

OK . . . here's my experience/ knowledge on taking a daily probiotic.

Can we get real for a second? If I have to take antibiotics for some reason & if I DON'T take a probiotic (or eat yogurt/drink kombucha/chow down on kimchi), I get a yeast infection.

I also notice my skin isn't as clear if I forget to take them. A clean gut is key for flawless skin.

My favorite form of a probiotic to take is an acidophilus &/or eat a fermented food/drink.

Multivitamins:

After speaking with tons of doctors, they all recommend a multivitamin. I like a clean, non-GMO vitamin with extra omega, vitamin D, and biotin.

Chlorophyll:

We talked about chlorophyll in chapter 9, but I want to mention it here, too. Chlorophyll is an energy/ immunity booster, hormonal balancer & FABULOUS detoxifier. It's FILLED with vitamins, minerals & essential fatty acids, too. One of my favorite benefits? It promotes digestive health, so if you have any gut issues—DRINK UP!

SPA WATER FOR GORGEOUS SKIN

Just take your favorite glass water pitcher and add the ingredients below.

Pink Potion:

Jalapeño, lemon, pomegranate seeds, pinch of turmeric powder

Citrusy Lime-Aid:

Lemon, lime, mint, and ginger

Morning Spa Water:

Meyer lemons, fresh mint, cloves, and ginger—I also love a dash of cayenne in it, too.

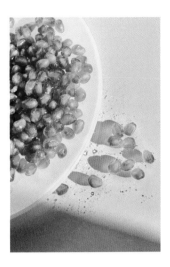

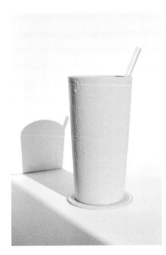

Katie Wells

/ @wellnessmama

WELLNESS INFLUENCER AND ENTREPRENEUR

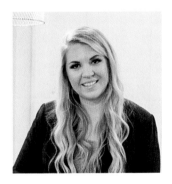

I originally got the advice to grow and regularly eat broccoli sprouts from my doctor as a way to help support my thyroid, but these nutrient-dense sprouts are also great for skin health. They're high in sulforaphane, which is anti-inflammatory and great for the liver. Supporting the liver is another good way to ensure skin health! My trick is to blend up the sprouts and drink as a smoothie.

FOODS FOR GLOWING SKIN:

INULIN

Inulin is a pure fiber powder derived from chicory root or artichoke root. My friend Ingrid told me about this gem. Inulin is a prebiotic—think of it like a healthy food for your probiotic to eat.

Inulin is so good in coffee or tea because it fills you up. Also, if you're into intermittent fasting, it won't mess up your fast! Seriously, if you don't have time for breakfast, throw a spoonful of inulin powder into your coffee tumbler & run out the door.

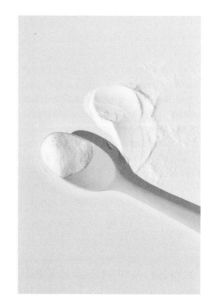

INGRID'S FRENCH HIGH-FIBER LE CHOCOLATE CHIP COOKIE Á LA FLEUR DE SEL

(COURTESY OF INGRID DE LA MARE-KENNY)

INGREDIENTS:

4 tbsp coconut butter, room temperature
½ cup tahini
½ cup fiber syrup or honey
½ cup Sukrin Gold or pure cane sugar
1 egg, room temperature
1 egg yolk
1 tsp vanilla extract
1 cup + 2 tbsp potato starch
6 tsp Simply Inulin
¾ tsp baking powder
⅔ packet instant yeast
1 tsp sea salt
2 cups bittersweet or semisweet
    chocolate chips
A couple pinches of flaky sea salt, such
    as Maldon or fleur de sel

DIRECTIONS:

In the bowl of a stand mixer, beat the coconut butter, tahini, Sukrin Gold sugar, honey (or fiber syrup) on medium speed for 2–3 minutes until fluffy.

Stop the mixer & scrape down the sides. Add the egg, egg yolk & vanilla and continue to mix for another minute, stopping to scrape down the sides of the bowl to be sure the eggs are incorporated.

In a small bowl, whisk together the potato starch, Simply Inulin, baking powder, instant yeast & sea salt.

With the mixer on low speed, add the dry ingredients until just combined. Then add the chocolate chips. Don't overmix. Cover the dough & refrigerate for an hour.

Preheat the oven to 325°F & line two baking sheets with parchment paper or silicone baking mats.

Form the cookies into rounds using an ice cream scoop or your hands. For small cookies, make each one 1½ inches round; for larger cookies, make them 2 inches round. Place them evenly spaced on the baking sheets & bake one sheet at a time in the middle rack of the oven.

Let them cool for 30–40 minutes & sprinkle them with flaky salt.

CUCUMBERS

You just can't go wrong with cucumbers, whether you eat them or put them on your skin. You know the classic image of someone at a spa with a towel around their head and cucumber slices on their eyes? That's because they're high in vitamin C, making them great for reducing lines and wrinkles. So slap those cucumbers on your eyes all day long.

They are also great for reducing swelling and water retention because they're a diuretic. Plus, if you have a burn, putting cucumbers on it will soothe and cool it.

PLUMPING CUCUMBER POTION

INGREDIENTS:
3 cucumbers
½ stalk of celery
Ginger clove
½ peeled lemon

DIRECTIONS:
Juice or blend (I prefer to juice).

WATERMELON

Watermelon is a diuretic, which means it's going to flush you out. Watermelon is full of water, 92 percent water, to be exact. It's also full of potassium, selenium, zinc, and helps promote collagen formation. Plus, watermelon is filled with amino acids and has blood-building chlorophyll, making it great for circulation.

SPICY WATERMELON JERKY

INGREDIENTS:
A big-ass organic watermelon
Cayenne powder
As much lime as you want!

DIRECTIONS:
Cut watermelon into 1-inch slices. Discard ends & remove rinds.

Cut slices down to about ¼ inch thick, then lightly sprinkle with cayenne powder.

Place the watermelon in a dehydrator, then squeeze a little lime on top. Dehydrate at 135°F for 18 (yes, 18) hours.

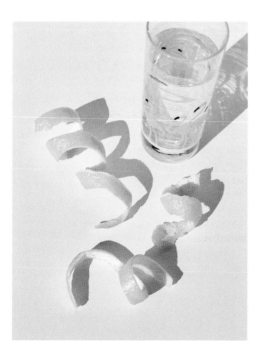

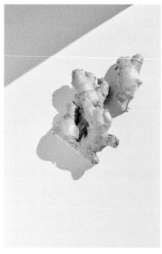

WALNUTS AND PECANS

Nuts are another food that are high in healthy fats and rich in omega-3 & omega-6—prime skin conditioners. You shouldn't go overboard with nuts, though, because they can cause inflammation; a little handful a day is great. Nuts also contain one of my favorite things for your skin, selenium. Selenium actually works with vitamin E to coat your cell membranes to create a protective layer. It neutralizes free radicals, soothes redness, and fights inflammation—which we always want.

THE NANZ'S HOLIDAY PECANS

INGREDIENTS:
1 egg white
or both!
1 tbsp water
1 cup sugar
¾ tsp salt
½ tsp ground cinnamon
½ tsp ground nutmeg
1 lb. pecan halves OR WALNUTS

DIRECTIONS:

Preheat the oven to 250°F & grease a baking sheet.

Beat together egg white & water until you get a frothy-like consistency. In a separate mixing bowl, mix sugar, salt, cinnamon & nutmeg.

Slowly add pecan halves to egg whites, stirring to cover the nuts evenly. Toss everything into the sugar mix until it's evenly coated.

Delicately spread the pecans on the ready-to-go baking sheet.

Bake at 250°F for 50 minutes to 1 hour (checking on them regularly). Stir every 15 minutes while they're in the oven. ENJOY!!

CINNAMON

I cannot have coffee without it. It curbs your sweet tooth & can help balance your blood sugar (coffee can cause your blood sugar to rise). I envision myself drinking cinnamon stick tea by the fire every day—obviously that doesn't happen. But whenever I get a chance to drink my drink with real cinnamon sticks, I take it—it's always better. Usually I just use organic Saigon cinnamon. It can also be added to French toast, pancakes & skinny waffles.

THE PREGGER'S PANTRY CINNAMON/CIDER BRUSSELS SPROUTS

MAKES 4 SERVINGS

INGREDIENTS:
1 tbsp extra virgin olive oil
2 cups brussels sprouts
1 Honeycrisp apple, diced
1 large pear, diced
½ cup spiced apple cider
1 tsp cinnamon

DIRECTIONS:

In a large pan over medium heat, heat oil. Cook brussels sprouts (cut side down), flipping once until browned for 10 to 12 minutes.

Add apple & pear; cook until soft for 5 minutes. Add cider and cinnamon; simmer, stirring, until all liquid cooks away.

GREEN TEA/MATCHA

Green tea is great for reducing redness. I like to put a spoon in ice water so it gets super cold, then wrap a wet green tea bag around it—a perfect travel hack. By putting it around your eyes, it will improve the elasticity of the skin around your eyes, plus tighten it, too. I love to get my green tea in by making matcha lattes. Also, green tea and matcha contain EGCG, a powerful antioxidant that helps with DNA repair.

THE SKINNY CONFIDENTIAL MAGICAL MATCHA LATTE

INGREDIENTS:
Almond milk or nut milk of choice
Inulin powder
Organic matcha powder
Cinnamon stick

DIRECTIONS:
Pour some almond milk and a scoop or two of inulin into your milk frother.

While that's heating up, take your cup & add a scoop of matcha & a cinnamon stick.

Pour the almond milk into your cup, stir & enjoy.

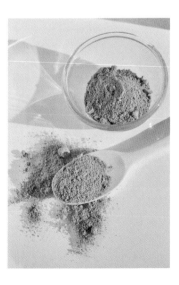

ALMOND BUTTER

I'm obsessed with eating almond butter because I truly feel like eating healthy fats reduces fine lines and wrinkles. When I was pregnant, I was really listening to my body. Something I noticed was that whenever I started my morning with a workout, having a scoop of almond butter made all the difference. In fact, if I went to Pilates without having a scoop of almond butter I felt faint. This tells me that it's amazing fuel for your body & your body really does crave healthy fats. So many models I talk to snack on almonds to make their hair silky & smooth. You should know there are amounts of vitamin E for healthy skin, hair & nails.

KRISTIN CAVALLARI'S ALMOND BUTTER SUGAR COOKIES
MAKES 24 COOKIES

INGREDIENTS:
1 stick unsalted, grass-fed butter, softened
1 cup raw coconut sugar
½ cup raw almond butter
1 large egg
1½ cups oat flour
¾ tsp baking soda
½ tsp pink Himalayan salt

DIRECTIONS:
Preheat the oven to 350°F & line two baking sheets with parchment paper.

Using a mixer, cream together butter, sugar & almond butter until fluffy. Add the egg & mix to combine.

In a separate bowl, mix flour, baking soda & salt with a spoon. Add the dry ingredients to the wet ingredients & mix well.

Spoon tablespoon-size balls onto the prepared baking sheets, keeping a little space between each ball.

Bake for 10 minutes, or until golden brown.

The cookies are thin—keep a close eye on them so they don't burn.

ARTICHOKES

There's nothing better than a delicious artichoke salad with lemon, olive oil, a little sea salt, and some black pepper. Don't overlook artichokes, because they're full of fiber. But the main benefit I like about artichokes is that they make you shit. That's right, they make you go to the bathroom. So, when you get all those toxins out of you, it's also eliminating toxins from your skin. You should know artichokes are not only full of fiber, they're also low in fat, high in vitamins, and loaded with magnesium, which, again, makes you go to the bathroom. Artichoke extract is even known to be a little skincare secret. So, if you ever see a serum, toner, or essence with artichoke extract, pour that shit on your face.

Also rich in vitamin C & therefore good for collagen production.

Anyway, since I got you drooling over artichokes, here's a salad recipe from Il Pastaio, the best Italian restaurant in LA :

LOS ANGELES' HOTTEST ARTICHOKE SALAD

(INSPIRED BY IL PASTAIO)

INGREDIENTS:

Baby artichoke hearts
Arugula
Shaved parmesan cheese
Italian olive oil
Lemon juice
Sea salt

DIRECTIONS:

Toss everything together & VOILÁ.

PAPAYA

I took papaya enzymes when I was pregnant & it helped ease my heartburn a lot. Papaya contains vitamin A & the papain enzyme. A papaya enzyme facial mask is always a good idea, too. In fact, Dermalogica Daily Microfoliant uses papain as the exfoliating agent. Eat the seeds of the papaya, because they're super high in antioxidants, which is so good for the skin. Not only that, they're a good dose of fiber, too!

BRAD EVARTS AKA DAD'S TUNA SALAD AND PAPAYA RECIPE

INGREDIENTS:

1 ripe-to-touch strawberry papaya
6 oz white albacore tuna
3 tbsp avocado oil mayonnaise
2 tbsp mustard
1 lemon
pinch of salt and pepper

DIRECTIONS:

Wash papaya by cutting it in half, and add the seeds of papaya to a large mixing bowl.

Add all other ingredients to the bowl and whisk together.

Towel-dry papaya, then scoop the tuna mixture into each half of the papaya.

Top with a squeeze of lemon.

HOT TIP

Add healthy fats to your diet. Whenever I don't get enough healthy fat, I notice that my skin is fucked. I really try to implement a lot of avocado oil, olive oil & coconut oil, or just plain avocados, into my diet. I like to keep almonds in my purse & you can catch me putting black sesame seeds, chia seeds & hemp seeds on my fruit every morning. All these things are going to help keep your skin plump & youthful. If you want even more fatty acids in your diet, pop an omega-3 pill.

BONE BROTH

When I was in college, I'd buy some frozen bone broth at the grocery store & defrost it. Then I'd heat it up in the microwave (yes, I know, but sometimes ya gotta do what ya gotta do) or on a stovetop in a teakettle. After that, I'd add lemon (duh), chili flakes, apple cider vinegar & chopped carrot or herbs. SOOOOooo, ta-da: fresh chicken BONE BROTH, college-y soup. I was on a major budget & had to be creative to get the most amount of nutrients aka bang for my buck.

Bone broth contains hyaluronic acid. This is an ingredient a lot of top-notch dermatologists use in their products. It's also used in fillers—so what we want to do is drink that hyaluronic acid. It promotes clear skin by reducing acne, rosacea, eczema & psoriasis. It also really helps with cell repair, which in turn helps with dark circles under the eyes. It's even known to prevent stretch marks during weight gain or pregnancy, since there's collagen in it. SOME people even report that bone broth gets rid of their cellulite because of the collagen.

CURRY GIRLS KITCHEN'S CHICKEN BONE BROTH

(& USE ALL PARTS OF THE CHICKEN'S BONES WITH SKIN, BUT NO WHITE MEAT!)

INGREDIENTS:
6 organic backs
6 organic legs
12 organic drumettes or wings
12–14 organic feet
4–6 organic thighs
3 large onions, rough-chopped
4 celery ribs with some leaves from the
    inner stock
6 large carrots, scrubbed clean
1–2 leeks, both white and green parts
Entire head of garlic clove smashed,
    unpeeled is fine, too!
10 peppercorns
1–2 bay leaves
1 tbsp Celtic sea salt
¼ cup apple cider vinegar
12–14 cups of water
Fresh parsley and dill

DIRECTIONS:
Place washed chicken parts, all but thighs, in a stockpot. Next, layer all vegetables over chicken parts. Place thighs over vegetables. Add spices and seasonings, but not the fresh parsley and dill. Cover with water. Do not fill water to top; really, just cover the ingredients with water. Once you've completed stacking the vegetables, bones, and water, don't touch or stir for the hours it cooks. In the last hour of cooking, add the dill & parsley.

Bring stock to a boil. Partially cover and let simmer for 12–20 hours. I like to "put up" my stock in the afternoon and let it simmer all night. Ohh, how the house smells so yummy!

In the morning, separate all the bones, meat & veggies. Save the onions, leeks, garlic & carrots to later puree and add back into 4 cups of stock for a warming veggie soup. Refrigerate and/or freeze any leftovers for later soup makings. Use the chicken meat to add to soup or make enchiladas, fajitas, or a yummy chicken salad or pasta dish. Lots of ideas to use your chicken!

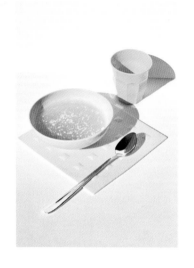

BONE BROTH,
page 225

CITRUSY LIME-ADE,
page 219

GET THE F♥CK OUT OF THE SUN

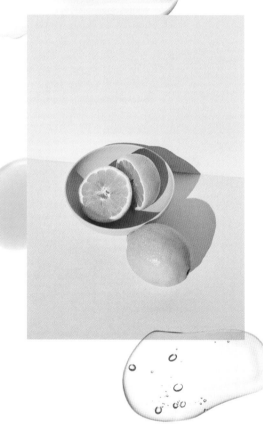

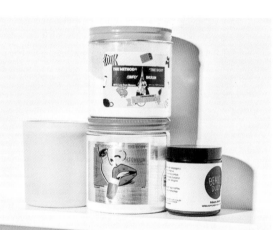

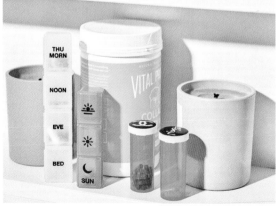

SUPPLEMENTS & MULTIVITAMINS,
page 219

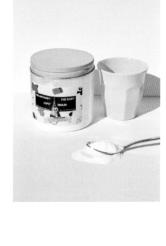

INULIN CHOCOLATE CHIP COOKIES,
page 220

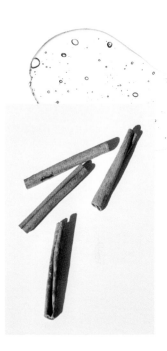

GREEN TEA/MATCHA LATTE,
page 223

GLOW FROM THE INSIDE OUT

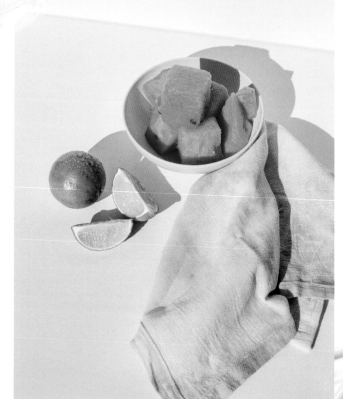

SPICY WATERMELON JERKY
PAGE 221

QUICK SKIN POTIONS TO ADD TO YOUR DIET

AMINO ACIDS: These are going to give a smoother, firmer look to your skin. They really are the building blocks of your hair & skin.

APPLE CIDER VINEGAR: This can be used as an astringent on your skin and is also known to detoxify & burn fat when you drink it.

ARGAN OIL: Many French women swear by argan oil, and it's also popular in Morocco. I like to use it to remove my makeup or in a salad dressing.

BEE POLLEN: Bee pollen has tons of vitamins, minerals & enzymes that benefit the skin. I love to dip a spoon in coconut oil & top with a tablespoon of bee pollen. Zing! Energy & skincare in a spoon.

BEETS: Extract from a beet has tons of vitamins and minerals and is known to plump the skin. I like to put beets in a blender with spinach & lemon & drink it down.

BROMELAIN: This is an enzyme from pineapple fruit that is known to help with oily or acne-prone skin. I took this a lot after jaw surgery because it helps with swelling.

CALENDULA: This was recommended to me by many skin gurus. It's a botanical that softens & plumps the skin and minimizes puffiness.

CAYENNE: Cayenne is really good for circulation, so it can help get the blood flow going in your face. Another plus is that it can plump up your lips.

CHAMOMILE: I use chamomile tea bags on my baby's eyes when they're puffy & swollen. It decreases inflammation & redness.

COCONUT OIL: This is an insane moisturizer and really holds in hydration on the skin. You can also use it as a lube. In fact, there's a great coconut oil lube called Woo. It's 100% natural & organic, pH-balanced, has only four ingredients, tastes like a vanilla cupcake (YUM) & I haven't had a UTI in the years I've been using it. Anyway, just don't put coconut oil on your face because it can clog your pores.

COLLAGEN: This is a hot protein that's very popular to nourish the structure of the skin. I love adding a little collagen to my smoothie, but you can also get collagen from bone broth, meats & fish, berries & citrus fruits.

FLAX SEEDS: These are such a good source of fiber & healthy fats. I like to add these to my smoothies or sprinkle over oatmeal or fruit.

HONEY: I always opt for honey in tea & fruit but tend not to go overboard with it because I don't want a ton of sugar. Organic, raw Manuka honey is my favorite. Some of the benefits are: heals burns when applied directly to skin, soothes a sore throat & can be used to treat acne (hormonal acne, specifically). It really helps keep the skin free of bacteria.

LEMONGRASS: Lemongrass tea is another one I'm obsessed with because it's super rich in vitamin C.

LEMON PEEL: There's this blender lemonade I love to make that uses 1 WHOLE LEMON. But the thing is, you actually use the whole lemon. (Quick recipe for ya: 2 cups of water, handful of ice, 1 whole lemon, a few tablespoons of coconut sugar, throw in some ginger & vodka if you're feeling crazy). Anyway, lemon peel is full of vitamin C & actually contains more vitamins & minerals than the inside. This will help your skin look healthier & prevent wrinkles. You could also zest a bit of lemon peel into all your recipes.

MAGNESIUM: Magnesium tea is calming, so it's really one of my favorite drinks to wind down with at night. Magnesium keeps things moving, wink-wink, which means it's going to improve the overall look of your skin. Magnesium lowers cortisol levels, which in turn balances hormones—that's so good if you're acne prone.

OLIVE OIL: A fabulous fatty acid. Use this in the best salad dressing in the world: 2 tbsp olive oil, 6 dashes red wine vinegar, ½ lemon squeezed, 1 tbsp spicy mustard, few dashes of Italian or French seasoning, 1 pressed garlic clove, pinch of salt. Shake it up or whisk, then enjoy over a salad.

GET THE F♥CK OUT OF THE SUN

PEARL POWDER: This magical amino acid has been used for thousands of years in China. Not just to wear, though—to eat! I sprinkle it in my smoothies every day. Pearl powder is exactly what you think it is: PEARL powder. If you want to do a quick hyperpigmentation mask to treat melasma, mix ½ teaspoon of pearl powder with a tiny bit of water and use a paintbrush to paint it on your face. You want it to have a pasty consistency.

RAW GARLIC: I pop raw garlic cloves like candy. Don't give a shit if my breath stinks because the benefits are too good. Garlic contains something called allicin that helps kill bacteria in the body. This is a really good for acne-prone skin. Garlic is also a powerful anti-inflammatory & helps blood circulation. When blood circulation is on point, we receive and absorb nutrients more efficiently.

RESVERATROL: This is full of many benefits like reducing redness, calming the skin & neutralizing free radicals because of its antioxidants. Oh & you wanna know how I get mine in? Wine. YES! It comes from the skin of grapes used to make wine. Sure, you can get resveratrol without drinking, but that cuts the fun in half.

ROYAL JELLY: This jelly is antiaging, packed with vitamins & heals from the inside out. It's what bees feed to their queen bee. Cool, right? The recommended way to take it is 1–2 teaspoons under the tongue, twice a day, preferably between meals (on an empty-ish stomach & with a bit of water).

SARDINES: Soap opera actress Susan Lucci's favorite snack? Sardines. She eats them for their omega-3 fatty acids, essential for smooth skin.

SEA SALT: This is so great for exfoliation but also good to ingest a bit because it can keep you hydrated & balance electrolytes. It's high in minerals & is known to detoxify the skin, increase circulation & give the skin a good dose of nutrients. I specifically love French, flaky fleur de sel salt. It has the best texture & you'll notice that it's different (better!) right away.

SELENIUM: Grab some eggs, sunflower seeds, spinach, shiitake mushrooms, or oysters, because they're full of selenium. This is going to combat damaging free radicals while strengthening your immune system.

SESAME SEEDS: These are full of antioxidants and anti-inflammatory properties. I like to eat black sesame seeds every day on all my fruit. They're full of essential fatty acids and lubricate the skin for that plump look. I also love a bit of sesame oil in a dressing or an Asian-inspired dish.

SHEA BUTTER: This is so popular among women for youthful skin, but you can also eat it—add it to any meal for a bit of flavor. However, you should also know that Cleopatra used this in her skincare routine, soooooooo we probably should, too, right? If you are going to eat it, go for only about 2 grams.

SPIRULINA: I eat spirulina every single day, Hawaiian spirulina to be exact. It's a natural appetite supressant & is so helpful for detoxifying your skin & body. It can help people who are prone to acne by controlling candida (yeast) overgrowth in the body, and it is packed with antioxidants.

VITAMIN E: When I was a little girl, I fell off my bike & fell hard. All I can remember is that I had a huge scab from my eye to my chin. My mom & dad left these tiny vitamin E capsules on my bedside table so that I could pop them open and apply them to my skin every night. Now it's years later & I don't have a scar. You can eat them or throw them on a salad, but you can also use them on a scar or scab. It's even more powerful if you combine them with vitamin C.

ZINC: Seeds, nuts, eggs, and shellfish all contain zinc. Eat your zinc because it's great for skin! I'm serious, it really helps with skin aging, which is what this book is all about—preventative care.

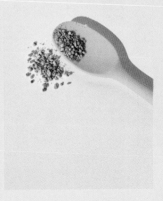

HOT PINK KOMBUCHA VODKA

INGREDIENTS:
1 oz. gluten-free vodka
3 oz. guava kombucha
Basil

DIRECTIONS:
Pour vodka over ice. Add kombucha on top (you can use any flavor—I love guava). Garnish with basil.

POMEGRANATE GRAPEFRUIT SPRITZ

INGREDIENTS:
Half-rim of coconut sugar
1½ oz. Blanco tequila
3 oz. pomegranate juice
1 oz. grapefruit, juiced
Pomegranate seeds
Mint leaves

DIRECTIONS:
Wet half of the rim of the glass with coconut sugar. Add ice to glass. Add tequila, pomegranate juice, grapefruit, and pomegranate seeds to shaker filled with ice—shake, shake, shake. Pour shaken medley into the cocktail glass. Garnish with mint leaves & few more pomegranate seeds. YUM.

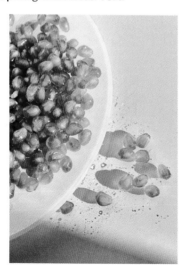

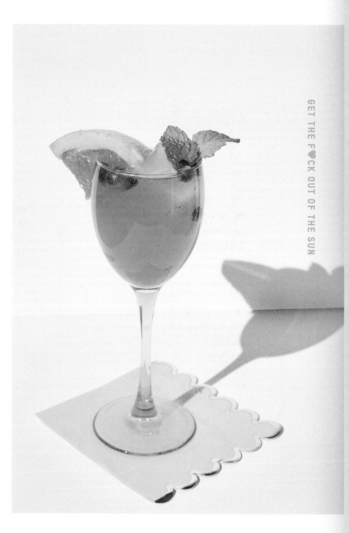

GET THE F♥CK OUT OF THE SUN

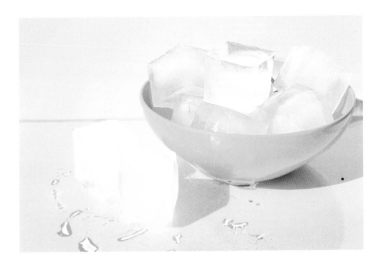

SKINNY WATERMELON MARGARITA

INGREDIENTS:

Half-rim of fleur de sel salt
Jalapeño, muddled (to taste—
    I LOVE A LOT!)
1½ oz. Blanco tequila
2 oz. watermelon, juiced
½ oz. lime, juiced
½ oz. lemon, juiced

DIRECTIONS:

Wet half of the rim of the glass with fleur de sel salt. Add jalapeño to taste into the bottom of the cocktail glass, muddle. Add ice to the glass. Juice watermelon. Add tequila, watermelon, lime & lemon to a shaker filled with ice—shake, shake, shake. Pour shaken medley into cocktail glass. Garnish with more jalapeño slices. CHEERS!

Dr. Harold Lancer ON DIET & SKIN:

We counsel patients on sleep, rest, and relaxation. We counsel them severely on nutrition, and so we actually have diets that influence less testosterone production, more estrogen production, or vice versa. Nutrition is hugely important for just about everything in dermatology. And so, some tips at home would be the following: We recommend as low a salt intake as possible. Preferably no added salt, because most food has some degree of salt in it. It dehydrates you and slows the metabolic process.

In general, dairy products slow digestion. When it comes to acne-prone skin or oil-producing skin, the less dairy the better. And it's not so much a matter of whether it's low-fat or no-fat, it's just a matter of dairy itself. It's not the biggest friend to the complexion. So salt, dairy, and then highly acidic things are inflammatory to the skin. They cause more of a water loss, more of a flushing to the skin. I tell patients, the more tasty something is, chances are your skin's not going to respond well.

Caffeine is a problem, too. It just makes the skin a little bit oilier, the pores larger, the skin a little bit more ruddy.

But I think the biggest offender is sugar. Sugar to the consumer just means birthday cake or donuts, and that's not really what it is. Fruit is a sugar, so you have to watch your fruits & vegetables. We recommend the low-glycemic fruits & low-glycemic vegetables.

Claire Grieve

/ @claire_grieve

CELEBRITY YOGA TEACHER, STRETCH THERAPIST, PLANT-CENTRIC HEALTH COACH, AND AUTHOR

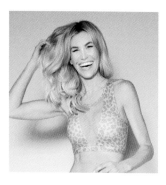

Attaining glowing skin from the inside out is really about being healthy in both your body and mind. All of my wellness programs include plant-centric foods, movement, mindfulness, and self-care. When all four of these things are at play in a healthful way, people truly radiate from the inside out. A nourishing diet is really important to gaining glowing skin. A good place to start is to focus on eating tons of vegetables and fruit—eat a lot of variety, or *eat the rainbow* to gain a robust variety of phytonutrients, vitamins, and minerals. This will support overall health that will radiate out of your skin. Vegetables and fruits also tend to be high in antioxidants, which help protect your body from free radicals that can cause signs of aging. Eating healthy fats, like avocado;

organic, cold-pressed, extra-virgin olive oil; and salmon, if you consume fish, will help give your skin a smooth, plump, and hydrated look. Foods that contain probiotics, such as kimchi and sauerkraut, also support great skin from the inside, as a balanced gut microbiome plays a huge role in your skin health.

Hydration is also really important for creating glowing skin. Drinking lots of filtered water throughout the day will ensure that your organs are working properly and that your cells are nourished, which will lead to radiant skin. I recommend drinking around 3–4 liters of water a day, depending on your weight, activity level, and diet. You can also boost your water intake by eating hydrating vegetables and fruits like cucumber, celery, watermelon, and lettuce. Exercise is also really important for healthy skin.

Moving your body helps to keep your systems moving and circulates blood and oxygen throughout your body and to your skin. Studies have actually shown that exercise can reverse the signs of aging in your skin! The last tip that I find people in our culture tend to struggle with the most is *rest and rejuvenation*. Getting ample sleep, 8–9 hours a night, is essential for good skin. This is the time that your cells repair themselves, and it should not be overlooked. Beauty sleep is a real thing! Meditation and restorative yoga are also great activities for glowing skin. Taking time to be mindful and to rest and rejuvenate helps to reduce stress, and therefore cortisol, which can contribute to inflammation and breakouts. When you lower your stress levels, you boost your skin's radiant power.

On top of all of this inside work, it's important to *take great care of your skin on the outside* with good

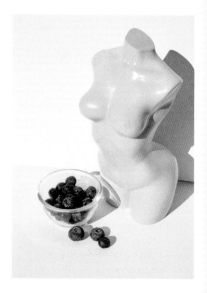

cleansing habits and products, too! One of my favorite practices is gua sha with organic oils. This massage technique helps to improve circulation to the skin, and also promotes lymphatic function and collagen production, which lead to beautiful glowing skin.

I drink a green goddess smoothie daily, and it truly helps me to have vibrant, glowing skin. There are so many amazing skin-health-boosting ingredients in this smoothie. Coconut water and zucchini are hydrating foods and support smooth, healthy skin. Pineapple, kiwi, chia seeds, and flax promote healthy digestion, which helps keep your skin looking fresh and blemish-free. Chia seeds and flax also supply the skin with healthy fats and omega-3s that will keep your skin looking luscious and smooth. The spinach and alkalizing greens will help alkalize your body, which is an important condition for smooth, vibrant skin. It is said that alkaline foods help to reduce skin inflammation, breakouts, and dryness.

GREEN GODDESS SMOOTHIE

INGREDIENTS:

¼ cup frozen pineapple
¼ cup frozen kiwi
½ cup of frozen wild
  blueberries
½ frozen peeled zucchini
1 cup organic spinach
1 tbsp almond butter
1 tbsp chia seeds
1 tbsp ground flax meal
1 tbsp of alkalizing greens
1 dash of Ceylon cinnamon
1 cup coconut water (choose
  a coconut water with no
  added sugar)
Ice to your desired level of
  thickness

DIRECTIONS:

Put all of your ingredients in a
high-power blender and blend
until smooth. Enjoy!

Jesse Golden

/ @jessegolden

HATHA YOGA TEACHER, HOLISTIC
HEALTH PRACTITIONER, AUTHOR

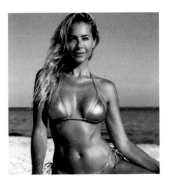

Nutrition and wellness have everything to do with our skin health. No matter how great of a product we put on our skin topically, if we are not also taking care of our nutrition and overall wellness, then we are only resolving half of the equation.

One of my favorite examples of how powerful nutrition is for our skin, is that you can literally eat your sunscreen, meaning that through a variety of food sources (antioxidants, microalgae) and supplements (astaxanthin), you can provide your body with UV protection internally. This helps avoid sunburn and even gives you a natural glow from the inside out. Not only that, but "sun spots" that often get blamed on sun exposure are sometimes a result of too much protein and sugar intake and can be reversed when we minimize those foods and incorporate an increased variety of fruits & veggies.

Another way nutrition affects our skin is via the microbiome of our digestive system.

Poor gut health is one of the primary issues those dealing with acne or any kind of skin or health issue have in common. Known as the gut/brain connection or, in this case, the gut/skin connection, it's the understanding that good health starts in the gut. Just to give you an idea, 70 percent of our body's immune system is in the gut. So if the gut is not healthy and there is a direct connection to our skin, then it will show up on the face in the form of acne or a rash. Once you get your gut microbial ecosystem healthy, your skin and health will flourish.

Some simple ways to repopulate healthy gut flora are through: probiotics (both supplements and fermented foods), prebiotics (minerals), eating a healthy non-inflammatory diet, reducing stress, and minimizing alcohol, antibiotics, and over-the-counter pain medications, which can all kill off the good bacteria and overgrow the bad bacteria.

The face is a direct representation of what is going on internally. TCM (traditional Chinese medicine) has mastered this through face mapping, depicting exactly which organ is affected on which area of the face. These are some of our bodies' first signals to us that something is imbalanced and needs attention. By making internal changes through diet and traditional treatment with Chinese herbs, we can begin to heal our bodies internally so that the face can reap the rewards externally.

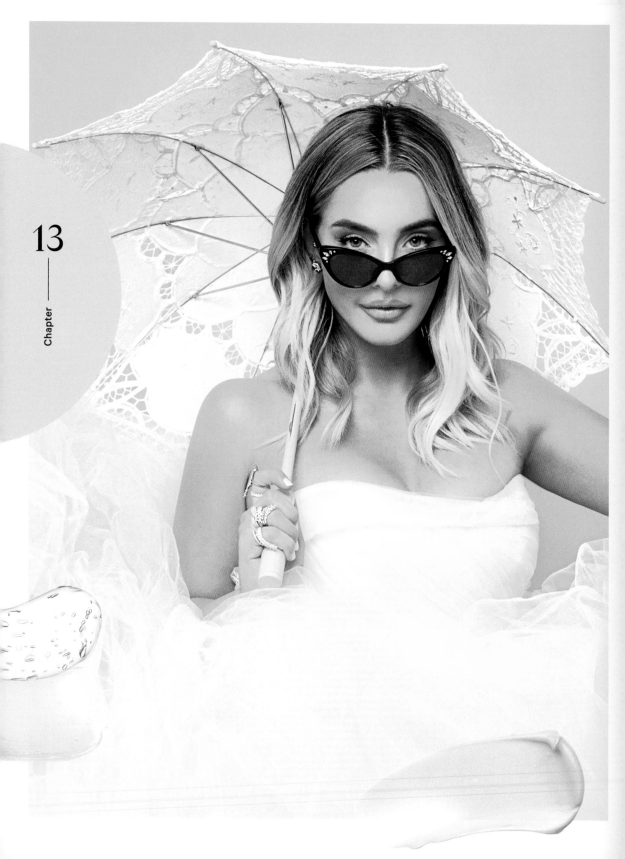

13

WHAT I WISH I KNEW

There are so many beautiful women who have spoken out saying that they wish they had known about preventative beauty. So, dedicating a chapter to people who look fucking fabulous who also happen to be 50+ is CRUCIAL. It's important to showcase both sides: the people who are practicing preventative beauty and the people who have been there, done that.

Of course, these beautiful, iconic women look amazing, but they have also really experimented. They will also tell you what they wish they knew: Some say they wish they spent more time in the shade, stopped using baby oil & were more diligent with their night cream. You know I also asked them their favorite products, too. AND THEY SPILL, MKAY!

You will get all the feels because you'll hear from people like Jillian Michaels, Jill Zarin, Patricia Altschul, Bobbi Brown, and Kate Somerville.

Annabelle DeSisto

/ @annabelledesisto

PODCASTER, COMEDIAN, CREATOR AND HOST OF THE *ADDERALL AND COMPLIMENTS* PODCAST

I swear on all my cats' lives when I say this: If I could get every minute back of my life that I spent hating myself for how I looked, I would get years & years of my life back. I would tell myself that the days you couldn't even get out of bed because you were crying while looking in the mirror, you were just as intelligent, beautiful & funny then as you are now. I would tell myself: Wash your face, don't wear cheap foundation, don't hold your T-Mobile Sidekick against your cheek, don't eat soy, don't listen to Jessica Simpson (you can listen to her music on your iPod Nano, just don't listen to her about a $65 acne cure), and, most important, the texture on the outside of your face doesn't dictate the value that you bring to this world. You have more going on in this world than just your pores.

FIRST THINGS FIRST. HERE, ACCORDING TO MY RESEARCH, ARE SOME BIG NO-NOS I PICKED UP:

Instead of using baby oil in the sun, opt for sunscreen.

Long gone are the days of lying out with baby oil, right? I hope so. Baby oil attracts the sun to you, which makes the UVA & UVB rays stronger, so basically they penetrate deeper into the skin. Unfortunately, it does the opposite of sunscreen—SO YOU WILL LEAVE WITH A FAT SUNBURN. And worse, skin damage.

Instead of the tanning bed, opt for a spray tan.

Tanning beds use unwavering, intense UVA & UVB rays. They are more dangerous than the real sun & should be avoided at all costs. Bye-bye, Playboy Bunny tan line. Get on board with spray tans. Here are some tips for ya:

- ♥ Shave, exfoliate & even dry brush before your tan.
- ♥ Get a manicure after & a pedicure before.
- ♥ Lay a towel down so the tanning solution doesn't stain the bottoms of your feet.
- ♥ Use a baby wipe to clean your palms & bottoms of your feet RIGHT after.
- ♥ Wear loose clothes, like a maxi dress & flip-flops to let your tan sink in.

Instead of over-exfoliating, opt for an oil cleanser.

Microbeads and particles in exfoliant can put little tears in your skin & cause damage. Using a cleansing balm, or literally "oil as cleanser," is a gentle, sure way to get off all of your makeup. You just take the oil or cleansing balm & massage it over your face in upward circles. Take a damp microfiber or baby washcloth & dab the product off your face. It takes all your makeup off in the gentlest way. Then, continue with your other cleanser & steps in your skincare routine.

Instead of smoking cigarettes, opt for a CBD pen.

I'm obsessed with my rose gold CBD pen. 1:00 A.M. used to be my bedtime. Like, wtf anxiety. Now I go to bed around 10-ish, which has been life-changing. Need my beauty sleep! A CBD pen is fun because you can lie in bed, hopefully on a silk pillowcase (LOL), take two puffs & BOOM—you're asleep.

CBD is known to help with arthritis, joint pain, stomach cramps, period cramps, swelling, aches, colds, anxiety, depression, eczema, psoriasis, rashes, YOU NAME IT. Also, it's known as a safe alternative to painkillers & some prescription drugs. Sometimes I like to put a few drops under my tongue & let it dissolve. EASY. It immediately makes me feel chill & relaxed. I am actually floored how well CBD oil works—I mean I try a lot of wellness shit, you know? And this, THIS works. It's relaxing without a high. It helps with anxiety, but not in a druggy way. It combats inflammation & does it fast.

Since sleep is the key to the sleep, CBD is your friend. And while we're on the subject of CBD, you must meet my friend, CBD expert Anna Margaryan of @Pellequr in Beverly Hills. She'll give you all the deets:

♥ Cannabidiol (CBD) is a potent antioxidant and has anti-inflammatory and pain-relieving properties. These properties allow it to relax the skin, prevent drying, and help with wounds while shortening healing time.

♥ CBD may also improve the skin's defense mechanism and ability to regenerate, which would result in relieving and eliminating many skin problems.

♥ Prior to using CBD, or any product, on your skin, ensure that it is safe, lab-tested, certified, and falls in line with your personal values.

♥ CBD is an antioxidant with regenerative qualities to help offset damage from sun, pollution, and aging. You can use it when you are feeling pain, a skin flare-up, or skin irritations. It seems everyone's complexion can stand to benefit from an application of cannabidiol.

GET THE SKINNY

ON THESE ICONIC INFLUENTIAL WOMEN:

Jillian

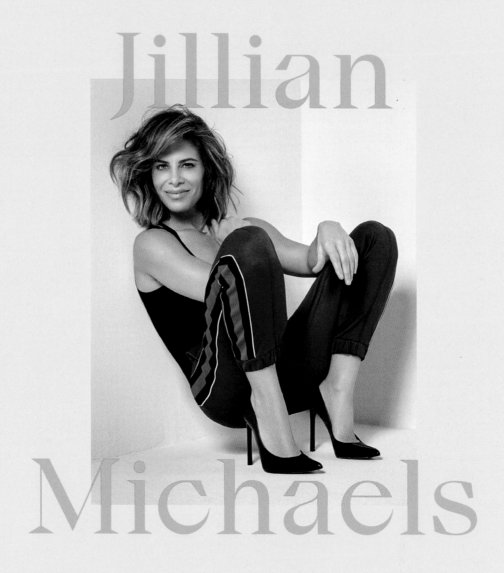

Michaels

/ @jillianmichaels

PERSONAL TRAINER, BUSINESSWOMAN,
AUTHOR, AND TELEVISION PERSONALITY

The cheapest thing that I would probably use would be any sort of omega oil. Sometimes I'll just literally put straight organic olive oil on my skin, and there's no chemicals, no garbage, no nothing. And honey or sugar scrubs—things that are exfoliating and moisturizing, and pretty much cost nothing and have zero chemicals.

Biggest splurge would be, and they are not green as far as I know . . . I'm ashamed to admit it, but they're so good: Dr. Harold Lancer products are just, I mean, they're expensive but his Glycolic 20% is really good. I use that one every day. Normally, I'm a hundred percent green, but his 20% glycolic, I think, is awesome.

Taking antioxidants—it's affordable and so worth it because, ultimately, we need to think about how to prevent oxidative stress, and in order to do that, you want to be consuming antioxidants. Clean, organic, food-based supplements with vitamins A, E & C are really important. I like Alaya Naturals because it's all clean, ethically sourced & organic. And it's important when you take supplements that the vitamins are synthesized and come from real food. Otherwise, it's a waste of money and incredibly ineffective.

It's super important. You want to eat the rainbow, like legitimate rainbow fruits and vegetables. So it could be spinach, kale, raspberries, blueberries, pineapple, mango—anything with the As, the Cs, the Es. Even fish oil, taken in your omega-3s, is really good because it's anti-inflammatory. Their main benefit is brain health and heart health, but they are also really good for the skin.

Collagen supplements with MSM glucosamine are just supplements—we have food. Get clean fruits and vegetables, meaning not things that are high in pesticide residue, preferably through thin-skinned organic fruits and vegetables. And if you don't have the money, you do thick skin. So, for example, instead of raspberries, you have an orange because it absorbs and requires fewer pesticides. Or watermelon. It's high in lycopene, vitamin C, potassium, but it has a really thick skin so it doesn't absorb or require a tremendous amount of pesticides. Pumpkin, sweet potato—all these things have beta-carotene and vitamin A, and all those things will require fewer pesticides.

Now, if you can do organic, then yes, spinach, kale, raspberries, and blueberries. All that stuff is also great. It's basically the rainbow, you want to eat all the colors, and if it's thin-skinned or leafy greens, you want it to be organic. If you can't afford organic, thick skin is the way to go.

Usually morning and night I put on an omega or some sort of oil—I mix it up. It could be calendula oil or olive oil or coconut oil, and I usually put that on in the morning and at night. Then I take a warm washcloth and just kind of remove any makeup, dead skin, or whatever. I usually do a really light exfoliation, again with that warm washcloth, sometimes a sugar scrub. I don't get crazy with it, just a little bit to remove any dead skin. Then I usually put on a glycolic acid and a natural antioxidant blend of vitamin C products to give it a little more brightness. Then a little more natural oil moisturizer or whatever, it could be argan oil. I just mix it up and then use sunblock.

I think it's all about balance. As long as you don't hang your happiness or your worth or your value on your looks, at the end of the day, you're fine. I had a terrible nose and I wanted to fix it; it changed my life for the better. If it's something that bothers you and you want to fix it, by all means. I really don't know the health side effects of Botox or fillers because I haven't researched it. I've totally done Botox before and had fillers under my eyes when I was too skinny, but I wouldn't think of that as protecting your skin. It might help with the appearance of making you look less tired, but that's if you want to augment your lips—that's a choice, but it isn't fighting aging. But I think, if something bothers you, fucking fix it, by all means. ♥

Jill Zarin

/ @mrsjillzarin

PHILANTHROPIST, BUSINESSWOMAN,
AUTHOR, AND TV PERSONALITY
FROM *THE REAL HOUSEWIVES OF
NEW YORK CITY*

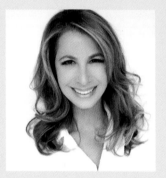

*WHAT HAVE YOU FOUND TO BE THE MOST EFFECTIVE SKINCARE
PRODUCT UNDER $50, AND WHAT'S YOUR BIGGEST SPLURGE?*

Pat Wexler has a daily moisturizer around $30 with SPF 20 that has been my
go-to product. I like to change my moisturizer too and just started using Luann
de Lesseps's new one, Sonage, and love it!

I have to admit that I get a spray tan on a regular basis. It is very safe. Although
it may not actually be true, I find it to be a natural SPF. I don't get tan or burn if I
have it on and I'm in the sun. This is just my opinion, but I've heard it from other
people, too!

*WHAT IS THE MOST
PRACTICAL, RELATABLE
ADVICE YOU'VE RECEIVED FOR
PREVENTATIVE SKINCARE?*

Sunscreen. Sunscreen is something I
will not go a day without. The sun is
what makes you age the fastest, so
when it comes to my face, I try to avoid
it at all costs. If I see a brown spot on
my skin, I know I need more protection.
I love Supergoop! or Drunk Elephant
for my face and COOLA for my body!
Freckles are a warning you are getting
too much sun. I play tennis every day
and only recently started wearing long
sleeves. I just can't afford to get too
much sun anymore, even if it is only
for 2 hours. I found an amazing line of
tennis clothes with the thinnest SPF
50 fabric. You can even jump in the
pool wearing it, which I love doing after
a long day of tennis. It is called Bobbe
Active. It makes you feel sexy and look
sexy! I am obsessed.

When I'm at the beach, I make sure
to stay in the shade under an umbrella
and wear sunglasses and a hat. As a
spray-tan lover, I'm happy being in the
shade on the beach and feel there's no
shame in a fake tan!

"As a spray-tan lover, I'm happy being in the shade on the beach and feel there's no shame in a fake tan!"

*WHAT WOULD YOU SAY TO
YOUR YOUNGER SELF ABOUT
SKINCARE IF YOU COULD?*

Do not pick your skin! If you leave that
pimple alone, it'll go away much faster
than if you attack it. I would also say
that when you start using a new product, make sure you give it enough time
to work and improve your skin. Change
does not happen after one use! Start
Botox early enough that deep lines
don't set in. Don't be a martyr—there
is no shame in doing what it takes to
look good. ♥

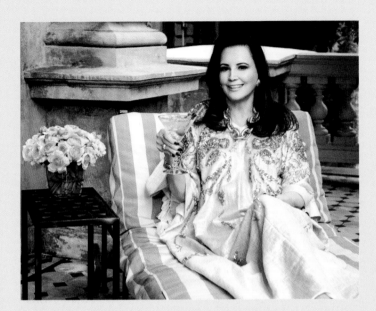

Patricia Altschul

/ @pataltschul

BELOVED MATRIARCH OF THE BRAVO HIT REALITY SERIES *SOUTHERN CHARM* AND MEGA-ENTREPRENEUR

"I have adopted the philosophy of less is more."

WHAT IS A HABIT YOU'VE DEVELOPED OVER THE YEARS THAT MAKES A DIFFERENCE IN YOUR SKIN?

A habit I've developed over the years that makes a difference is to double wash my face in the evenings. I start with Tasha Camellia Cleansing Oil, and after rinsing, follow with Dr. Dennis Gross All-in-One Cleanser with Toner. Every 2 days, I use Dr. Dennis Gross Alpha Beta Ultra Gentle Daily Peel or Huda Wishful Yo Glow Enzyme Scrub.

WHAT WOULD YOU SAY TO YOUR YOUNGER SELF ABOUT SKINCARE IF YOU COULD?

In my younger years, I made the mistake of applying too many products at once, which caused inflammation and breakouts. I don't believe in layering seven products on one's face at night; instead, I have adopted the philosophy of less is more.

WHAT IS AN UNUSUAL OR SOMEWHAT WEIRD PRACTICE YOU DO TO KEEP YOUR SKIN YOUTHFUL?

I brush my skin before I get into the bath or shower, which is unusual, since I don't know many people who do it. The other is that I use a tongue scraper to get rid of bacteria before brushing and flossing. The skin brush that I use is made by Yerba Prima and the tongue scraper is copper and was purchased on Amazon.

WHAT STEPS DO YOU TAKE DURING YOUR DAILY SKIN ROUTINE?

I cleanse my face once in the morning and apply Rhofade, which is a prescription for rosacea. The makeup I use is a combination of Armani and Chanel that has a SPF of 25. I apply the makeup lightly with a damp Beautyblender and set it with Huda Beauty Sugar Cookie powder. For brows I use all of the products from Anastasia Beverly Hills. I experiment with other brands; however, my lipstick has always been YSL number 22 followed by a gloss, usually a frosty pink. ♥

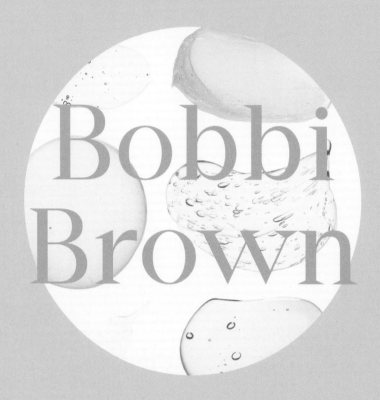

Bobbi Brown

WORLD-RENOWNED MAKEUP ARTIST,
BESTSELLING AUTHOR, SOUGHT-AFTER
SPEAKER, AND ENTREPRENEUR

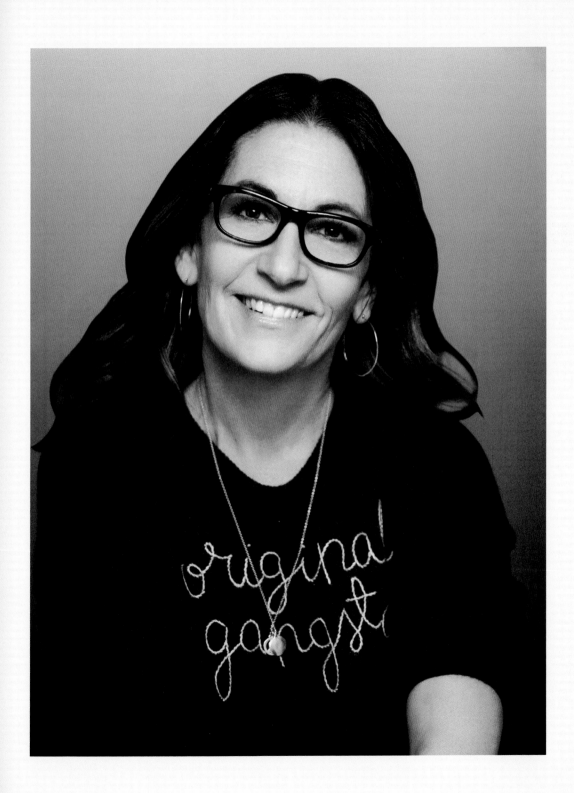

WHAT HAVE YOU FOUND TO BE THE MOST EFFECTIVE SKINCARE PRODUCT UNDER $50, AND WHAT'S YOUR BIGGEST SPLURGE?

Actually, my number-one go-to skin-care product is far under $50 and can be bought at any health-food store. It's a bottle of Apricot Kernel Oil, which is less than $10. Sometimes I add a few drops of essential oil—either neroli, orange, or lavender to make a miracle oil blend to restore my skin.

My biggest splurge is my favorite moisturizer, Augustinus Bader. To me, this cream is worth the price tag—it's changed my skin. It's somehow managed to even and tighten it.

WHAT IS THE MOST PRACTICAL, RELATABLE ADVICE YOU'VE RECEIVED FOR PREVENTATIVE SKINCARE?

To have good nutrition, to not smoke, to wear sunscreen, and to reduce everyday stress as much as possible. I believe these things, done in tandem, help preserve youthful, glowing skin.

WHAT IS THE WORST ADVICE YOU'VE EVER HEARD WHEN IT COMES TO TAKING CARE OF YOUR SKIN?

As I age, I still don't understand Botox as a means of preventing lines, or why anyone would choose that route instead of embracing the natural aging process. I think aging is of course what genetics gave you, but also lifestyle—I notice a serious difference in my face when my skin is taken care of through proper diet, hydration, sleep, reduced stress, and the use of good products.

"Your skin isn't the same every day, so my routine varies depending on my current needs."

WHAT IS A HABIT YOU'VE DEVELOPED OVER THE YEARS THAT MAKES A DIFFERENCE IN YOUR SKIN?

Drinking at least eight glasses of water a day—a couple of glasses with lemon. Water is a game-changer for your body, brain & beauty. Your skin looks plumper when you're hydrated. Water also flushes out toxins, which seriously improves the appearance of your skin. Adding lemon helps to cleanse and alkalize, and it adds an immunity-boosting dose of vitamin C. Drink lemon water before breakfast to get the maximum benefits.

WHAT STEPS DO YOU TAKE DURING YOUR DAILY SKIN ROUTINE?

Your skin isn't the same every day, so my routine varies depending on my current needs. In general, I start my day by washing my face with a regular cleanser. Then I layer different hydrating products, giving each a minute to sink in. In the morning, I use SPF, tap eye cream under my eyes, and put on moisturizer before my makeup. At night, after cleansing, I use a cream or oil, depending on how dry I am.

WHAT WOULD YOU SAY TO YOUR YOUNGER SELF ABOUT SKINCARE IF YOU COULD?

I didn't wear sunscreen when I was young, and I definitely didn't understand its importance for preventative skincare. I'd tell myself to add an SPF to my morning routine to protect my skin and prevent premature skin aging.

WHAT IS AN UNUSUAL OR SOMEWHAT WEIRD PRACTICE YOU DO TO KEEP YOUR SKIN YOUTHFUL?

The best thing I've found is lasers, which are unfortunately expensive and painful. Lasers reveal fresh, tighter, and more-even skin without changing the structure of your face, which to me is the most important.

WHAT ARE YOUR THOUGHTS ON PLASTIC SURGERY, BOTOX, FILLERS, LASERS, AND OTHER COSMETIC MEDICAL PROCEDURES?

My rule of thumb is to stick with procedures that make me look fresher and lifted—but, most important, still like me. Cosmetic medical procedures can alter your face to such an extreme that you no longer look like yourself, and there's no going back if you don't like it. That said, I tried Botox a couple of times, and I'm not a fan. I've used lasers to zap away sun spots and aid collagen production; after a lot of money and a little bit of pain—the treatment works wonders. ♥

Lisa Vanderpump

/ @lisavanderpump

STAR OF THE BRAVO HIT REALITY
SERIES *REAL HOUSEWIVES OF
BEVERLY HILLS* AND *VANDERPUMP
RULES*

HOW DO NUTRITION AND WELLNESS AFFECT YOUR SKIN?

I do think you are what you eat. I don't really eat junk food. Now, do I eat chocolate? Yes. But for the most part, I eat lots of vegetables and lots of fruit and a little bit of chicken and fish. And I do eat carbs as well, like pasta and bread. I also think a good workout every morning is good for you. I work out an hour day walking on the treadmill uphill.

WHY DO YOU TAKE CARE OF YOUR SKIN?

For me it's the essence of beauty. It's your foundation, how you look and how you feel about yourself.

WHAT'S AN UNUSUAL, SOMEWHAT WEIRD PRACTICE TO KEEP YOUR SKIN YOUTHFUL?

I do nothing. I have a light laser once a year. Brilliant, no downtime. [Dr. Simon Ourian] gives me some products, and that's it. I do Botox and things like that because that prevents wrinkles. I do think that when you have a little bit less expression in your face that it does save your face from making wrinkles. It's not just about what you look like now, it's preventative. ♥

WHAT HAVE YOU FOUND TO BE THE MOST EFFECTIVE SKINCARE PRODUCT UNDER $50, AND WHAT'S YOUR BIGGEST SPLURGE?

They're all under $50! I've used a lot of Neutrogena face wipes over the years. The important thing is to make sure you get all your makeup off and making sure your face is absolutely scrubbed clean before you go to bed. It doesn't matter how hard it is, that's the key to good skin. And a really good exfoliating cream. But I'm not fussy about skincare. Just keep the skin clean, out of the sun, and moisturized. I will say that I burned my hand quite badly about a month ago and it just wouldn't heal. So I put some Crème de la Mer on there, and within two days it was much better. I do think there's magic powers in it, but it costs a bloody fortune.

"...I'm not fussy about skincare. Just keep the skin clean, out of the sun, and moisturized."

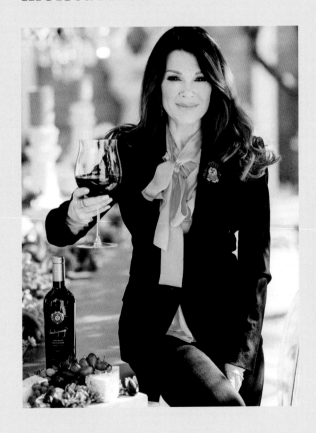

Kate
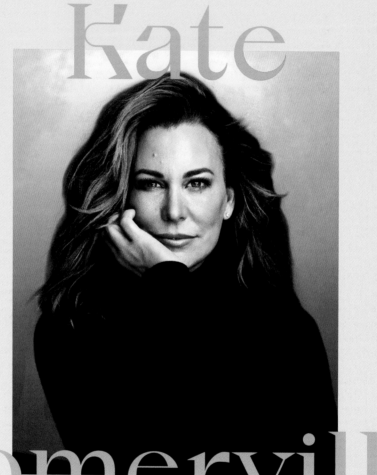
Somerville

/ @katesomervilleskincare

FOUNDER AND CREATOR OF
KATE SOMERVILLE SKINCARE AND KATE
SOMERVILLE SKIN HEALTH EXPERTS

WHAT'S THE BIGGEST MISTAKE YOU SEE PEOPLE MAKING WITH THEIR SKIN?

Wearing too much makeup and not exfoliating. Exfoliating is so important! I always recommend our ExfoliKate Intensive Exfoliating Treatment. This will gently dissolve and slough off dead skin cells, which cause a dull appearance to your skin and make wrinkles look more pronounced.

I've also seen people overstimulating or sensitizing their skin with too many products. I am all for using different actives or advanced ingredients and incorporating them into your routine properly, but unfortunately, sometimes people overdo it! This compromises your skin barrier, which can lead to other issues, including dryness, redness & acne. Should you find yourself in this situation, I recommend seeking out products with soothing peptides, ceramides—and just take it easy for a while.

HOT TIP

KATE SOMERVILLE: *As we age, we lose chemistry. So you want to put that chemistry back into the skin, and one of the top ingredients is hyaluronic acid, and we have it in mist spray form. So I spray that on and then I do a moisturizer that matches my skin type. For me, I'm almost 50, so I use things that have a lot of peptides, maybe retinols, vitamin C, but if you're younger and you're just starting to see the signs of aging, maybe a good moisturizer with lots of antioxidants.*

WHAT'S THE BEST TIP THAT PEOPLE CAN DO WHEN IT COMES TO FREE, AT-HOME SKINCARE?

Steam! It's absolutely the best rejuvenator, cleanser, and hydrator ever. Even steam from a hot shower or bath is great for opening your pores. I love putting ice on my eyes for de-puffing. Also, green tea bags are great for tightening skin. Just soak them and put them under your eyes, and then take cold spoons and massage after.

"I am all for using different actives or advanced ingredients and incorporating them into your routine properly, but unfortunately, sometimes people overdo it!"

IF YOU HAD TO PICK ONE HOLY GRAIL PRODUCT, THE BEST PRODUCT EVER, WHAT WOULD IT BE AND WHY?

Our Peptide K8 Power Cream. It has eight different peptides in it that have kept my skin young for 15 years! It reduces redness, yet it's one of the top antiaging moisturizers on the market. It's just a miracle cream for me!

WHAT'S A SMALL HABIT THAT PEOPLE CAN DO EVERY DAY THAT MAKES A BIG DIFFERENCE IN THEIR SKIN?

Moisturize, absolutely. You want to lock in all the hydration you can in the skin. Think about your skin as a piece of leather—if you let it dry and move it, it cracks. If you keep it hydrated and move it, it stays pliable and smooth. Look for products with hyaluronic acid. That will keep the skin plump and hydrated.

WHAT ARE YOUR THOUGHTS ON BOTOX, FILLERS & PLASTIC SURGERY?

Love it! I've been getting Botox since I was 23 years old—it has kept my skin without deep lines. Fillers are great to correct imbalances, keep the skin full, and keep plastic surgery at bay. Obviously too much is not good, either! I come from the plastic surgery world as well, so I've seen it help a lot of people—but I also think you can overdo it with anything.

At the clinic, we get to see something that has been nagging a client be instantly fixed—it's like instant gratification. If you have acne scars, we can fill them and make them flat. If you've lost volume in your cheeks, we can fix it within a minute. It's so gratifying to see how the clients feel more confident after visiting our Kate Somerville nurses. ♥

Gabrielle

Reece

/ @gabbyreece

PROFESSIONAL VOLLEYBALL LEGEND,
INSPIRATIONAL LEADER, AUTHOR, CREATOR
OF HIGHX, CO-FOUNDER OF XPT, AND
EXECUTIVE MEMBER OF LAIRD SUPERFOOD

WHAT HAVE YOU FOUND TO BE THE MOST EFFECTIVE SKINCARE PRODUCT UNDER $50, AND WHAT'S YOUR BIGGEST SPLURGE?

I will come at all of this from my outdoors and internal health point of view. I love the Epicuren Discovery X-Treme Cream Propolis Sunscreen SPF 45+. It doesn't make you break out, protects your skin with good ingredients, can handle a bit of sweat, and has a tiny bit of shine to give you that line-free look, but still works well with makeup. I am a big advocate of taking ingestibles to support external health—bone broth, fish oil, mineralized water—to internally help the external appearance. These not only are inexpensive but also will help us feel better as an entire organism. Nine birds with one stone. Also, last time I checked, sleep was free, even though it's precious.

WHAT IS THE MOST PRACTICAL, RELATABLE ADVICE YOU'VE RECEIVED FOR PREVENTATIVE SKINCARE?

To take care of your skin, but also not to "overdo" it. I don't know if you have ever experienced doing too much care to the skin (too many treatments, too many products, etc.), but it can almost irritate the skin vs. support the health and beauty of the skin. Also, Dr. Harold Lancer told me when I first met him at 24 not to start "messing with my face," because once you do one thing you will have to do another. He called it "chasing my face"—you do one treatment or change something and now you have to change something else, and so on and so on. Lastly, when my skin was not the way I wanted it or I was having strange breakouts, I learned to back away from it vs. to keep scrambling around to fix it. That obsessive approach can typically agitate everything; your skin and your spirit.

> **"Eating whole, real foods and even taking certain supplements support glowing skin."**

HOW DOES YOUR NUTRITION AND WELLNESS PLAN AFFECT YOUR SKIN?

I believe this is where the rubber hits the road. I appreciate skincare and beauty treatments, but I genuinely believe that skin is supported from the inside out. Sweat from exercise is good for your skin. Eating whole, real foods and even taking certain supplements support glowing skin. High-quality fish oils, chlorophyll, astaxanthin, and things like this are helpful to boost skin health.

WHAT STEPS DO YOU TAKE DURING YOUR DAILY SKIN ROUTINE?

I try to keep it simple. If the evening before I did a thorough regimen, then I will avoid washing my face in the morning. I believe overwashing and overcleaning your face (unless you live in a place with dirty air) can really strip away the needed oils for healthy skin. Possibly put on a sunblock if I'm headed out in the morning, but if I'm exercising, I just let it be.

I try to clean my face after big exercise or a long day as soon as possible. I like an African allafia soap or a Japanese charcoal bar. Nothing with too many stringent ingredients. Then I moisturize with radical moisturizer and throw some castor oil on my eyebrows and a hydrating lip balm on my lips.

WHAT IS AN UNUSUAL OR SOMEWHAT WEIRD PRACTICE YOU DO TO KEEP YOUR SKIN YOUTHFUL?

Nothing crazy, but I do a lot of sauna, and I think that helps support the health of my skin. Oh, that, and I did get roped into snail goo for your skin. That lasted about three times. ♥

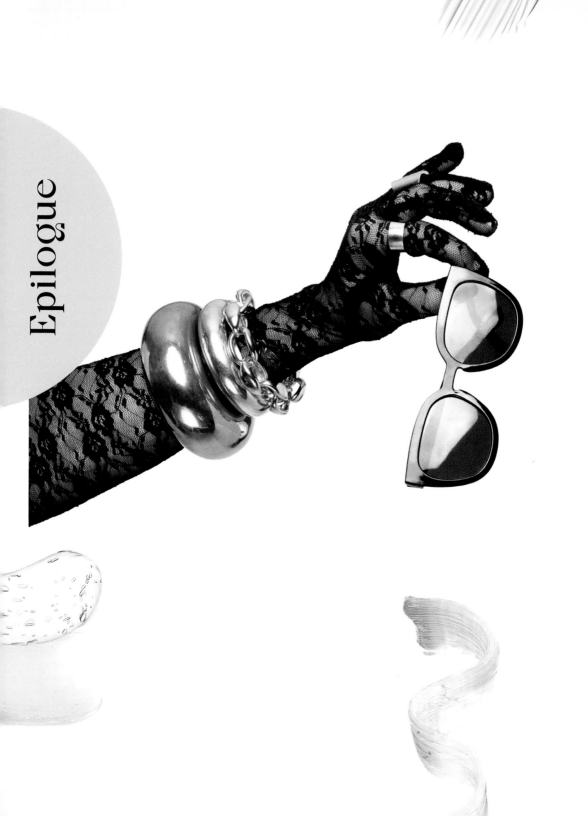

Epilogue

BURY
ME IN
THE
SHADE

All good things come to end—and that includes this happy hour–esque, self-care convo. So until next time, right? In all seriousness, please make this YOUR ultimate skincare bible. A resource you can refer back to. One you open when you have a pesky period pimple, wine face, or a wrinkle on your tit.

I hope you picked up little bits and pieces that work for you, whether that's putting a humidifier by your bed, adding a hyaluronic serum to your routine, or using an ice roller after a brutal hangover—surely you've picked up something to enhance your skin. Maybe even pass this book down to your kid? Share a Botox secret with a friend at a boozy brunch? Or shit, just take a pretty flatlay for your Instagram (you know I designed the cover for your feed).

When I was 16-ish years old, I did what basically everyone (probably you) did: I SUNTANNED. One day, I started to see this VERY obvious sun mustache on my upper lip. Then tiny brown spots on my forehead. A whole party of them, really. And after further investigation, I discovered I was "blessed" with hyperpigmentation.

At 17, there I was, at a real fork in the road. I could continue to lie in the sun and bake in the tanning beds like everyone else, or I could be preventative.

Preventative is a word that changed my life.

Every single day since I was 17, I formed small habits to actively invest in my skin, which are all things you read about in this book—tinting car windows, SPF daily, SO many hats, a skincare routine, driving gloves, you've heard it all by now. Being proactive as opposed to reactive. And eventually creating *The Skinny Confidential* out of small changes that make all the difference.

And that's my wish for you. To read this and feel an insane need to want to PREVENT the problem before it starts with those small changes.

Anyway, since the beginning of my blogging career, I've always said to chip away every day—go from A to B, rather than A to Z. When it comes to skincare, the same is true. Taking an extra 10 minutes every morning and night for YOU can make you a happier person. Skincare is not all about bougie pamper parties, and self-care is not selfish; in fact, they're both the opposite: They're essential to becoming the best version of yourself.

And before we finish off our glasses of dry champagne, it's not simply just about looks—it's about feeling good, investing in yourself, and shining from the inside out with CONFIDENCE.

As I found myself night after night, morning after morning, in front of the computer writing, I realized that the underlying theme throughout this book is my desire to help you glow from the inside out. For you to feel confident in your skin and feel proactive with your approach. And why not spend time on your mind, body, soul, relationships, and SKIN? ULTIMATELY, it's very much a 360° approach, right?

If this book can influence ONE person to spend an extra 10 minutes a day on self-care, or even convince someone to start being preventative by wearing hats and using sunscreen, I'll die happy.

BUT LIKE PLEASE,

BURY ME IN THE SHADE.

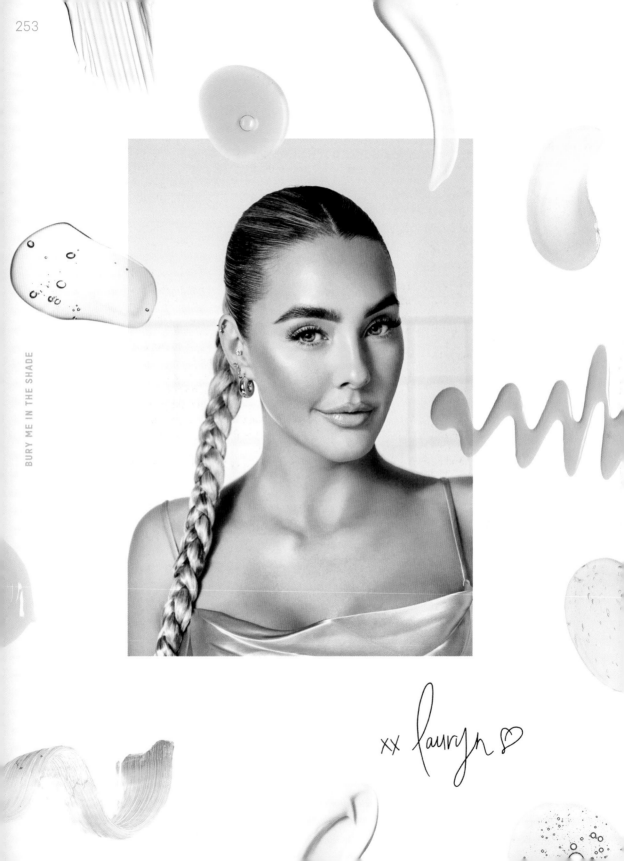

BURY ME IN THE SHADE

xx lauryn ♡

ACKNOWLEDGMENTS

O h fuck, I have to get my shit together to thank all of the incredible people who have helped me along the way (THERE ARE A LOT).

OK, so this book would have NEVER happened without YOU, the community. Truly, the platform would not exist without all of you. This book was created because of your excitement and passion around skincare. That's right—your tips, tricks, and questions. I hope that you continue to use this as your go-to skincare resource. Thank you all for your support, always.

To my dad (DADDY!), Brad, who always encouraged exploration without judgement and told me to be my own boss. You've never thought any of my dreams were too crazy, and you've always supported me along the way. I am an entrepreneur because of YOU. I look up to you—you are funny, charismatic, and the best father. Let's just say I can see why your restaurant is always packed.

I'd like to very much acknowledge my stepmom, Julie Evarts, who has been a role model when it comes to creativity, hosting, and making the home a sanctuary. My dad is lucky to have you. You have embraced our family with such grace. I adore you.

Speaking of siblings, my sisters, Faye and Mimi, and my brother, Myles—you're all as real as they get. I'm so happy to have you all as lifelong friends. Faye—you make me laugh like no other; Mimi—you've been by my side with *The Skinny Confidential* since the beginning and you have such creative taste; Myles—you're always in on the joke. I love you. Thanks for making family dinners COLORFUL.

Obviously, I wouldn't be here without my mom, Wendy, who was constantly on my ass about sunscreen and truly made me fall in love with skincare. I'll never forget when you told me to put sunscreen on my arms and legs when I was, like, 6. The reason I read and write daily is because of you—you taught me my two greatest loves. Thank you and I wish you were here.

I also wish my grandma, Mary Evarts, "The Nanz," was here, too. Every day I practice getting outside of myself because of you—I miss you. When I am sad, I look outside at the shrubs and think of you and smile.

My godparents, Michael and Jennifer Bell, who oh-so-graciously allowed me to live in their home for 5 years while I was a broke bartender launching *The Skinny Confidential*. You fed me, provided wine (so much wine!), laughs, and a safe space to write the blog and raise my chihuahua, Pixy. So much love for both of you.

Thank you to my in-laws, Gary and Lisa Bosstick, who encouraged me, even when I pulled out my huge Canon camera, to take pictures of the food at every single fancy restaurant. You must have thought I was crazy, but your support was and is invaluable. You both are always there for me when times are tough.

My brother- and sisters-in-law, Jordan, Tara, Nico, and Leah. SO, SO, SO happy we're now related—aren't you? LOL. You guys make everything more fun—and Nico, it's real fucking nice to have a lawyer in the family. I know everyone agrees.

My cutest nephew, Daxton (there's no one more handsome than you), and my darling niece, Luna (Zaza's first friend).

To the Abrams publishing team—Danielle Youngsmith, Diane Shaw, Glenn Ramirez, Katie Gaffney, Natasha Martin, Jessica Weiner, Mamie Van Langen—thank you for keeping me on a strict timeline and fully "getting" it. It's rare to find a publishing team who is so open. Rebecca Kaplan, my editor—the

ACKNOWLEDGMENTS

second I got on the phone with you, I knew I had to work with you. You're exactly what this industry needs. You are on the pulse. Janis Donnaud, my lit agent—you are smart, savvy, and know how to get a book deal done.

My manager, Alix Frank, who keeps my ass organized like no other. Alix, I cannot thank you enough for the contributions you have made to growing *The Skinny Confidential*. I always say you're a bulldog even though you look like a delicate butterfly. Love you.

Hilary Kenmare: THIS BOOK WOULD HAVE NOT HAPPENED WITHOUT YOU. You are so fucking valuable to our team and truly the most efficient person on the planet. I think I would be on Mars without you? Your kids are so lucky to have you as a mother—intelligent, well spoken, funny, you do it all really. Thank you for the countless hours you have spent working on this book with me. I talk to you more than my husband—LOL. But really, WE NEED TO DO A VIRTUAL HAPPY HOUR TO BLACK OUT AND CELEBRATE.

I also want to shout out my sexy, sassy, smart friends: Westin Mitchell (you've helped so much on the business creativity; you're a killer. You are truly my best friend, I adore you); Erica Stolman (I've known you since I was 12, you're like a sister to me; there's no one that gets me more than you); Gillian, Mauricio, Wolfie, and my goddaughter, Coco Couturier (there's nothing better than a homemade pizza and champagne day at your pool. I love all four of you more than life); Kim Kelly (one of my favorite friends and the best workout partner in all the land); Ingrid De La Mare-Kenny (my beautiful, dynamic friend and someone who always seems to be so in-tune with me—mind, body, and spirit—I appreciate your energy so much); Faith, Niel & Aspen Robertson (Aperol and Tajin for life with 560 conversations going on at the same time); Betsy Parker (for being one of my first friends in LA and kicking my ass in Pilates); Carly Zuffinetti (best mom ever and the kindest soul); Anna Margaryan (you are funny as shit and helped me so much during my postpartum anxiety and depression—you're a real one); and Dante & Rocco Petrillo, Erik/Cheryl/Brandon/Chad Vogt, Alex Ciccolo, Steve Houck, Danny Kurtzman, Chris Beaton, Lucy Jones, Jackie Becerra—I love each of you very much.

I have to shout out my team: Ansley Patterson, Mimi Evarts, George Talavera, Arielle Levy, Kelsey Long, Shawn Knudsen, Mackenzie Robinson, Samantha Heapps, and Taylor O'Connor (aka The Barenaked Cucumber). Honestly, the people around me are killers. I'm so lucky.

To all the major experts, doctors, celebrities, and influencers who took their precious time to contribute to this book: your valuable tips made this book. Thank you. I am forever grateful.

Last, but certainly not least, to my husband, Michael, who wears blue light glasses so I can work on the computer in the dark, and who has been a skin guinea pig for me for years. He encourages my entrepreneurial side and even took the time to share his skincare routine in this book. Michael, you are consistent and stable and have believed in me since we were 12 years old. You have never once told me not to go after a goal. You think crazy ideas are good ideas, but help me refine them so I don't go overboard. You not only let me take chances, you stop everything you are doing and take them with me. You really are the best husband, teammate, co-host, father, chihuahua dad (to Pixy and Boone—my sweet dogs), and partner I could ask for. You deserve a lot of sexual favors for all the time I have spent on the computer . . .

And to my sweet Zaza, my daughter . . . the brightest light in my life. Some hopes: I hope I can be as funny and smart and feisty as you one day. I hope you have this book on your vanity when you're older. And I hope you wear sunscreen and a good plumping serum. I've never loved anyone like I love you.

xx Lauryn

PHOTO CREDITS

FRONT COVER PHOTO:
Tan: Alexandra DiMarchi
Brows: Helena Tamargo
Hair: Hayley Heckmann
Makeup: Janelle Faretra
Styling: Jordan Marx
Nails: Queenie Nguyen

BACK COVER PHOTO:
Tan: Alexandra DiMarchi
Brows: Helena Tamargo
Hair: Hayley Heckmann
Makeup: Janelle Faretra
Styling: Jordan Marx
Nails: Queenie Nguyen

MAKEUP SWATCHES:
artcasta/Shutterstock.com,
Fotaro1965/Shutterstock.
com, Karen Rosalie, Kat Ka/
Shutterstock.com,
Kittibowornphatnon/
Depositphotos.com,
Kittibowornphatnon/
Shutterstock.com, Ninell/
Shutterstock.com, photolime/
Shutterstock.com,
timquo/Shutterstock.com,
YuliaLisitsa/Shutterstock.com

PHOTOS COURTESY OF:
Hrush Achemyan: 108 (far left)
Adrianna Adarme: 178 (second from left)
Paolo Alberdi: 217 (third from left)
Farrah Brittany Aldjufrie: 205 (third from left)
Patricia Altschul: 241 (second from left)
Justin Anderson: 156
Christine Andrew: 74 (far left)
Mandy Ansari: 206 (second from left)
Tanesha Awasthi: 199 (fifth from left)
Sivan Ayla: 27
Rocky Barnes: 147
Dr. Daniel Barrett: 164 (second from left)
Becca Batista and Kianna Cabell: 207 (Gigi Goldman picture)
Indy Blue: 111 (third from left)

Mimi Bouchard: 67 (second from left)
Kaitlyn Bristowe: 190 (second from left)
Max Bronner: 2–3, 30, 234, 250
Bobbi Brown: 243
Kenzie Burke: 114
Riawna Capri: 110 (far left)
Kristin Cavallari: 10
Jennifer Cawley: 248 (Gabrielle Reece swim picture)
Jade Chapman: 142 (far left)
Delaney Childs: 191 (fourth from left)
Amber Fillerup Clark: 86 (far left)
Sophia Culpo: 199 (fourth from left)
Sonya Dakar: 98
Dara Dorsman: 95 (top right)
Ingrid De La Mare-Kenney: 113 (second from left)
Dr. Lara Devgan: 132 (far left)
Dr. Jason Diamond: 164 (far left)
Dr. Kay Durairaj: 165 (sixth from left)
Lauryn Evarts: 53 (second from left)
Jesse Golden: 233 (third from left)
Claire Grieve: 232 (far left)
Dr. Dennis Gross: 8, 134 (far left), 164 (fifth from left)
Amelia Hamlin and Delilah Hamlin: 126
Vani Hari: 204 (second from left)
Melissa Wood Health and Michelle Rose: 62 (second from left)
Marianna Hewitt and Lauren Gores: 48
Carlene Higgins and Jill Dunn: 95 (third from left)
Uma Ghosh: 212
Dr. Andrew Jacono: 135 (second from left)
Mandy Mallen Kelley: 40
Chriselle Kim: 25
Elizabeth Kott: 62 (far left)
Candance Kumai and Jack Jeffries: 112 (far left)

The Ladygang and Claire Leahy: 138
Dr. Harold Lancer: 105 (second from left), 165 (seventh from left)
Sarah Nicole Landry: 198 (second from left)
Nikki Lee: 110 (second from left)
Sarah Lee and Christine Chang: 94 (far left)
Arielle Levy: 61, 66–67 (gua sha and shave your face), 76–77 (, 90–91, 105 (far left), 185, 186 (far left)
Arielle Lorre: 124 (second from left)
Georgia Louise: 133 (second from left), 164 (third from left)
Maggie MacDonald: 21 (second from left)
Dr. Anjali Mahto: 35
Katie Maloney: 78
Shea Marie: 143 (second from left)
Tiffany Masterson: 122 (far left)
Heather McDonald: 208
Hunter McGrady: 178 (third from left)
Teddi Mellencamp: 178 (far left)
Jillian Michaels: 238
Leyla Milani-Khoshbin: 217 (second from left)
Colleen Morgans: 148, 152
Danna Omari: 62 (third from left)
Madison Orlando: 198 (far left)
Joshua Ostrovsky: 160
Whitney Port: 92
Alexandra Potora: 74 (second from left)
Katherine Schwarzenegger Pratt: 204 (far left)
Jenna Rennert: 65
DeAnna Rivers: 179 (sixth from left)
Dom Roberts: 53 (far left)
Cindy Romero: 126
Karen Rosalie: 6, 10, 12–13, 14, 16, 21 (bottom left), 22, 33, 37, 43, 54, 69 (dry brushing), 78 (bottom

right), 87, 97, 116, 121, 123, 128, 131, 137, 162, 172, 173, 175, 180, 186 (top right), 192, 200, 202 (Lauryn close-up), 205 (product shot), 210, 226 (product shot), 253
Payton Sartain: 45
Jackie Schimmel: 87 (second from left)
Stassi Schroeder: 84
Emily Schuman: 145
Sarah Shen: 68–69 (ice roller, dermaplane, facial steamer, ice cubes, and product shot on far right), 83, 100, 183, 202, (ice roller), 203, 215, 219 (pink cup and pomegranate), 220, 221, 223, 226–227 (bowl, lemons, watermelon, cinnamon, and inulin), 229, 230, 231, 232 (top right)
Shoots & Giggles Photography and Margo Ducharme (Kimberly Snyder): 216 (far left)
Stephanie Simbari: 179 (seventh from left)
Molly Sims: 109 (third from left)
Kate Somerville: 165 (eighth from left), 246
Aimee Song: 124 (far left)
Patrick Starrr: 140, 141
Erica Stolman: 206 (far left)
Dr. Barbara Sturm: 164 (fourth from left)
Claudia Sulewski: 109 (second from left)
Kat Tanita: 79 (fifth from left)
That's So Sabotage Girls: 81
Christopher Tran: 5
Dr. Mona Vand: 198 (third from left)
Lisa Vanderpump: 245
Vashtie: 178 (fourth from left)
Clémence von Mueffling: 71
Katie Wells: 219 (third from left)
Kameron Westcott: 102
Ashley Wierenga (Topsie Vandenbosch picture): 190
Hyram Yarbro: 158
Jill Zarin: 240 (far left)

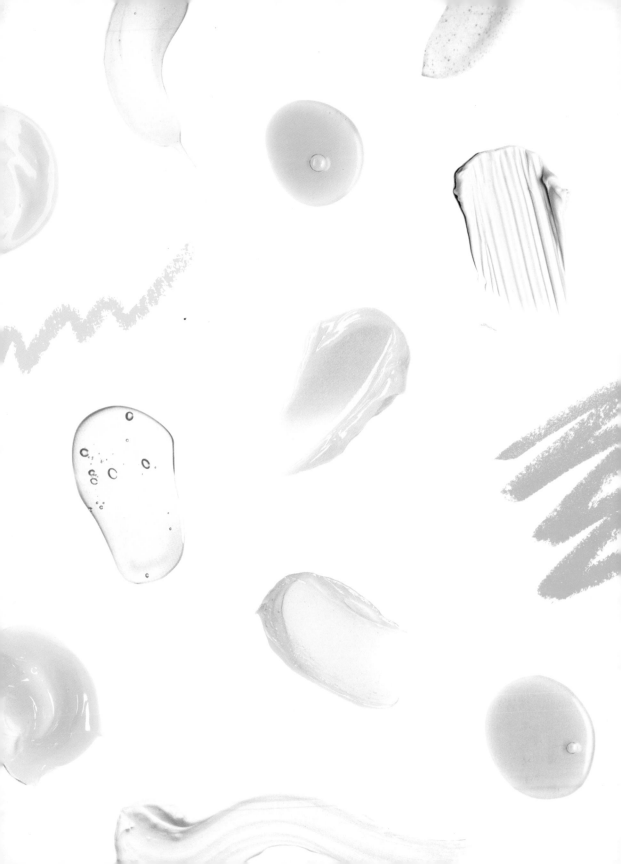